AF494755

Retinal Pigment Epithelium and Macular Diseases

Documenta Ophthalmologica Proceedings Series

VOLUME 62

Retinal Pigment Epithelium and Macular Diseases

Edited by

Gabriel Coscas
University Eye Clinic of Créteil, France

and

Felice Cardillo Piccolino
University Eye Clinic of Genoa, Italy

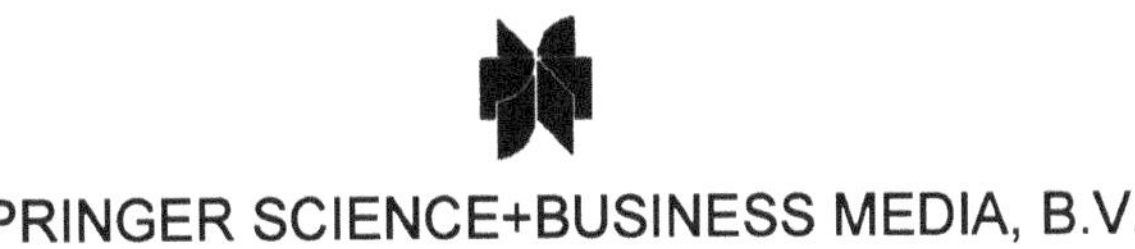

SPRINGER SCIENCE+BUSINESS MEDIA, B.V.

Library of Congress Cataloging-in-Publication Data is available.

DOI 10.1007/978-94-011-5137-5

Printed on acid-free paper

Dedication

"To my wife and my daughters and to all my group
in Créteil, with gratitude and love"
G.C.

"To my wife Luciana, for her loving support,
with gratitude and love"
F.C.P.

Acknowledgements

The editors express their sincere gratitude to Ms. Vanna Re, librarian of the University Eye Clinic of Genoa, for her valuable work in the preparation of this book.

Table of Contents

PART SIX: AGE-RELATED MACULOPATHY: DRUSEN

PART SEVEN: AGE-RELATED MACULOPATHY: CHOROIDAL NEOVASCULARIZATION

Preface

This volume of *Documenta Ophthalmologica* Proceedings Series collects the scientific papers presented at the 2nd International Symposium on Retinal Pigment Epithelium and the 4th Meeting of the European Macula Group held in Genoa, May 29–June 1, 1996. The Symposium on Retinal Pigment Epithelium was promoted by the University Eye Clinic of Genoa as the natural continuation of the first Symposium held with great success in Genoa in 1988. The previous Meetings of the European Macula Group were held in Coimbra (1988), Crete (1989) and Athens (1994). I was greatly pleased and honoured to host the fourth congress of this distinguished Society and I am grateful to Gabriel Coscas, José Cunha-Vaz and George Theodossiadis, founders of the Society, for selecting Genoa on this occasion.

The two meetings integrated well in an unicuum and brought together an exceptional number of outstanding retinal specialists coming from all over the world. All the aspects of the current research concerning retinal pigment epithelial and macular diseases were covered. Several interesting presentations regarded new techniques of retinal and choroidal imaging. A full session was dedicated to the latest advances in culture and transplantation of retinal pigment epithelial cells. Age-related macular degeneration was a major subject for discussion, including new approaches to treatment. This topic was highlighted by a mini-symposium on drusen, including a series of superb lectures on classification, clinicopathological studies, indocyanine green imaging, and laser treatment for prevention of choroidal neovascularization.

The sections of the proceedings reflect the sessions of the meeting. In this book the reader can find current knowledge as well as new trends and concepts on retinal pigment epithelial and macular diseases. Both clinical and experimental aspects are discussed, with excellent contributions by the leading experts in the field.

I wish to congratulate Gabriel Coscas and Felice Cardillo Piccolino for their successful work in editing this splendid book, which will be a lasting record of a memorable congress.

Mario Zingirian

1. A short history of the retinal pigment epithelium

T.J. WOLFENSBERGER

(Lausanne, Switzerland)

Introduction

During antiquity anatomical knowledge of the retina and its surrounding structures was limited[1]. Because of the macroscopic resemblance of the tissue to a fishnet, the name ἀμπφιβλεστροειδής – amphiblestroides (from ἀμφιβαλλειν – amphiballein = to throw around) alluding to a net that is thrown around a catch of fish – was coined by Herophilus around 320 BC. However, its principal role was not seen in acting as the visual receptor (a role reserved for the lens) but in carrying nourishment to the vitreous. This physiological concept satisfied most scholars and centuries went past with no real attempt to clarify the more fundamental role of the retinal tissues. The notion of a net-like structure was adopted by Celsus and then Galen, and it was finally the mediaeval scholar Gerard of Cremona who coined the Latin translation 'retina' in the 12th century. The term has remained in use for more then 800 years.

From the retina to the retinal pigment epithelium – the histology emerges

Anatomical knowledge stagnated for several centuries and it was not until the 17th century that Leeuwenhook broke new ground with the invention of the microscope. He vaguely described 'globular bodies' at the level of the outer retina in 1689[2], but it was the Dutch anatomist Frederic Ruysch who made the first real attempt to differentiate the layers of the posterior pole at the beginning of the 18th century. He described a distinct pigmented membrane (*tunica ruyschiana*) which comprised, according to him, the inner lamella of the choroid, most probably including the retinal pigment epithelium (RPE) although this was not explicitly stated[3]. This distinction was made because the choroid could be peeled of in two layers before gaining access to the retina. This multi-layer concept was confirmed a few years later by Johann Gottfried Zinn. In his seminal work *Descriptio anatomica oculi humani, iconibus illustrata auctore Johanne Gottfried Zinni*, published in 1755, he described the inner surface of the choroid with a thin layer of black pigment on it whose thickness decreases in old age[4]. In all these descriptions mention is made of pigment, although the source of it is assigned to the choroid exclusively. Even the great physiologist and natural scientist Albrecht von Haller (1708–1777)

G. Coscas and F. Cardillo Piccolino (eds.), Retinal Pigment Epithelium and Macular Diseases, pp. 1–4.
© 1998 Kluwer Academic Publishers.

observed this pigment, which he describes as a sort of inorganic mucus[5]. The first microscopical studies devoted at least in part to the RPE as a distinct entity date from 1790 when the Italian anatomist Carlo Mondini of Bologna described 'a real membrane formed of innumerable globules which make up an excessively delicate network'[6]. The next major anatomical discovery was brought about by an Irishman, Arthur Jacobs, who in 1819 described a membrane (*membrana Jacobi*), sometimes as dark as the choroid, which covered the retina externally[7]. This was later thought to represent the outer segments of photoreceptors tinged by adherent pigment. The first paper solely devoted to the RPE in its correct morphological sense was by the Englishman Thomas Wharton Jones, and appeared in the *Edinburgh Medical and Surgical Journal* in 1833[8]. He investigated the tissue of humans, cattle, horse and sheep and describes the epithelium as the 'pigmentum nigrum, a dark coloured matter that is found ... on the inner surface of the choroid where it has a very uniform character' (Fig. 1). His description of the RPE continues as follows: 'when ... the retina is removed, the inner surface of the choroid is found covered by a dark-coloured matter, which may be detached in small pieces. This matter is of a brown colour in the human eye, except over the tapetum in the ox where it is almost transparent. This is what is commonly called the tapetum nigrum.' He then adds a crucial statement 'But, according to my observations, it is a continuous and curiously organised membrane – *the seat of the pigment, but not the pigment itself*, which I shall therefore call the membrane of the pigment.' He then looked at the spread out and flattened tissue under magnification: 'if a portion of this membrane be examined by the aid of the microscope, it is seen to consist of very minute plates, of an hexagonal form, accurately joined together by their edges, in which plates are deposited numerous black particles, which are to be considered as properly constituting the pigment, but not essential to the hexagonal plates composing the membrane; because these may and do exist without the black particles.' He corroborated his hypothesis by examining albino tissue and discovered 'that the colouring matter is certainly absent, but ... I have found the membrane of the pigment to exist.' He added 'the hexagonal cells appear to be united together by means of mucous or cellular tissue, which is easily torn by a little traction, so that the fragments of the membrane always present a

Art. IX.—*Notice relative to the* Pigmentum Nigrum *of the Eye*. By Thomas Wharton Jones, Esq. Surgeon.

The *Pigmentum Nigrum* of the eye is that dark-coloured matter which is found on the posterior surface of the *iris*, on the ciliary processes, and on the inner surface of the choroid.

Fig. 1. The first paper entirely dedicated to the retinal pigment epithelium was published in 1833 by Thomas Warton Jones in the *Edinburgh Medical and Surgical Journal.*

serrated edge, the angles being those of hexagons.' A few years later Carl Ludwig Wilhelm Bruch (1819–1884) published his major contribution on the morphology of the RPE with his seminal work 'Untersuchungen zur Kenntniss des körnigen Pigments der Wirbelthiere'[9] in which he described the tapetum of mammals which had hitherto received little notice, as well as the 'structureless membrane' underlying the RPE, subsequently known by his name.

Lessons in embryology and physiology

At around the same time that this morphological concept gained acceptance (Fig. 2), new knowledge on the embryology of the retinal pigment epithelium became available. The major issue that was hotly disputed at that time was the fate of the outer layer of the optic vescile. It was generally agreed that the inner layer developed into the retina and many scholars believed that the stratum pigmentum of the retina developed from the choroid and was thus of mesodermal origin. It was not until 1861 that von Kölliker finally showed convincingly that the RPE was derived from the outer lamella of the optic vesicle and was thus retinal and not choroidal in origin[10]. Further investigations on the histology of the RPE followed through the second half of last century by Kühne, who also gave the first demonstration of a physiological role of the RPE in the regeneration of visual pigment which he called rhodopsin[11]. A fundamental increase in our understanding of RPE physiology did, however, not materialize until well into the second half of this century.

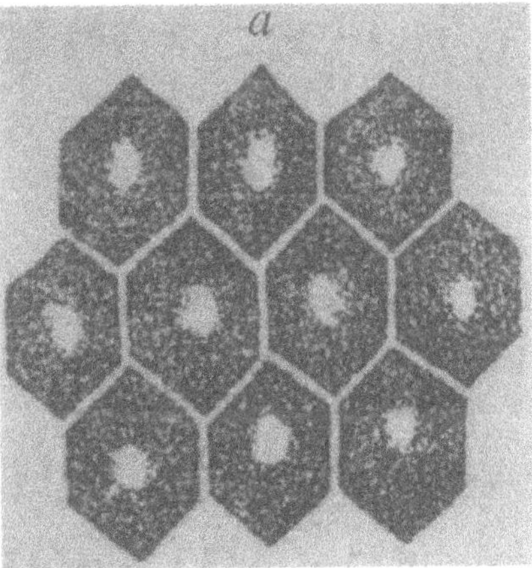

Fig. 2. One of the earliest original drawings of the RPE cells was done by Rudolf Albert von Kölliker in 1852 and published in his *Handbuch der Gewebelehre des Menschen.*

References

1. Magnus, H. Anatomie des Auges bei den Griechen und Römern. Leipzig: von Veit, 1878.
2. Leeuwenhook, A. First microscopic description of cones and rods. Phil Trans R Soc. 1689.
3. Ruysch, F. Thesaurus Anatomicus, vol. 2. Amsterdam: Wolters, 1702.
4. Zinn, J.G. Descriptio Anatomica Oculi Humani. Göttingen: 1755.
5. Haller, Av. Elementa Physiologiae Corporis Humani, vol. V. Lausanne: Grasset, 1763: 365–383.
6. Mondini, C. Commentationes Bononienses. 1790.
7. Jacobs, A. An account of a membrane of the eye, now first described. Phil Trans R Soc Lond. 1819: 300–307.
8. Wharton-Jones, T. Notice relative to the pigmentum nigrum of the eye. Edin Med Surg J. 1833; 40: 77–83.
9. Bruch, C.L.W. Untersuchungen zur Kenntniss des körnigen Pigments der Wirbelthiere. Zürich: 1844.
10. Kölliker, A. Entwicklungsgeschichte des Menschen. Leipzig: 1861.
11. Kühne, W. Zur Photochemie der Netzhaut. Untersuch Physiol Inst Univ Heidelberg. 1877; 1: 1–14.

Hôpital Ophtalmique Jules Gonin
University of Lausanne
15 Av. de France
1004 Lausanne
Switzerland

2. Blood–retinal barrier and new perspectives of management of retinal disease

J.G. CUNHA-VAZ

(Coimbra, Portugal)

The most important function of the blood–retinal barrier (BRB) is maintenance of the homeostasis of the retina environment by separating the retina from the systemic blood circulation. The organization of the BRB is such that the retina is protected from blood-borne compounds, since a strict homeostasis of the neuronal environment and an intact barrier are essential for optimal retina functioning. For treatment of diseases involving the retina, drugs must pass the BRB in a significant amount to have therapeutic effect. Drug entry into the retina, must take into account the plasma concentration profile of the drug, the volume of its distribution, the rate of metabolism of the drug, its plasma protein binding and the relative permeability of the BRB for that drug. All parameters affect the therapeutic efficacy of the drug and are also relevant for potential side effects.

In order to obtain therapeutic drug concentrations within the retina, several drug delivery strategies are under current investigation, opening new perspectives for more efficient management of retinal disease.

Morphology, function and regulation of the BRB

The BRB is formed by a complex cellular system of endothelial cells, retinal glial cells and retinal pigment epithelial cells. The retina has two sites of direct contact with the blood, at the level of the retinal vessels and at the chorioretinal interface, the inner and outer BRB, respectively.

In the inner BRB, the lumen of the retinal capillaries is covered by endothelial cells which are the first structure in the frontier separating the blood and the retinal tissue (Fig. 1). The retinal endothelial cells (REC) have various functional and morphological differences in comparison with endothelial cells derived from peripheral organs. The REC possess narrow intercellular tight junctional structures[1]. The tight junctions are composed of a complex of belt-like zonula occludens. These narrow tight junctions hinder paracellular transport of hydrophilic compounds and force movements across the endothelial

G. Coscas and F. Cardillo Piccolino (eds.), Retinal Pigment Epithelium and Macular Diseases, pp. 5–11.
© *1998 Kluwer Academic Publishers.*

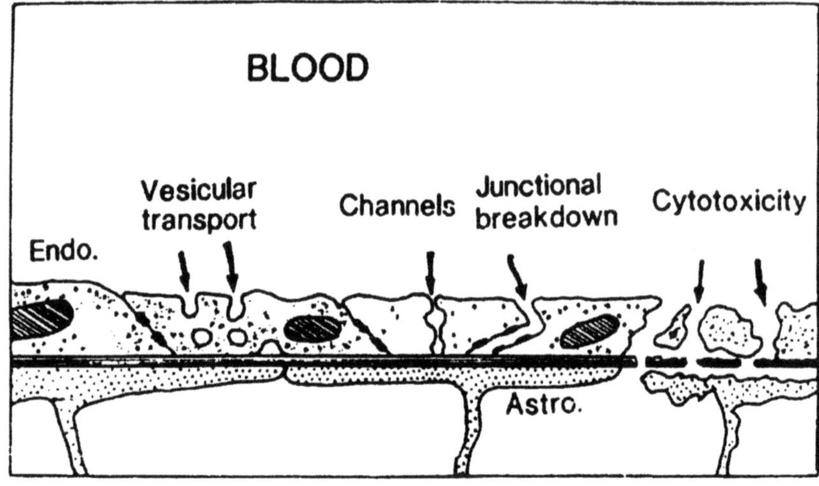

Fig. 1. Transport mechanisms across retinal endothelial cells.

cells themselves. Accessory roles appear to be played by the astrocytes which project their endfeet to the vessel walls, influencing the barrier function of these cells, and the pericytes.

In the outer BRB, the retinal pigment epithelium (RPE) is the first structure to be crossed or opposed by any substance originating from the blood and making its way into the retina. Adjacent epithelial cells are united by extensive zonulae occludentes, very similar to those described between the REC. These junctional structures, like the vascular ones, seal off the interepithelial spaces from experimental tracers. The RPE is formed by highly polarized cells which play a fundamental role in the regulation of the metabolic environment of the visual cells.

Metabolic barrier

Certain enzymes residing selectively in the REC and RPE constitute a metabolic barrier contributing to the protective function of the BRB. Fairly high activities of barrier-selective enzymes, including angiotensin converting enzyme, DOPA decarboxylase, γ-glutamyl transpeptidase (γ-GTP), pseudocholinesterase, monoaminoxidases and alkaline phosphatase, have been detected in these cells. Most of these enzymes are involved in the degradation of neurotransmitters released in the retina; in addition, compounds that have entered the BRB cells can be degraded into metabolites. Na^+, K^+-ATPase is localized predominantly in the abluminal membrane of the REC, and catalyses active transport of K^+ and Na^+ between blood and the retinal extracellular fluid.

Induction and maintenance of barrier function

Astrocytes and Müller cells surround the retinal vessels and may play an important role in the development and maintenance of the BRB. Astrocytic processes are not joined together and therefore allow substances that have crossed the endothelial barrier to diffuse into the retina. However, particularly during development and maturation, the presence of astrocytes is required to help differentiating a tight BRB. Chan-Ling and Stone[2], studying a model of experimental retinopathy of prematurity in cats showed that the retinal vessels lost their BRB characteristics in association with glial damage. They suggest that barrier properties are induced in the REC by the astrocytes and Müller cells.

The presence of the BRB has major implications for the passage of hydrophylic compounds into the retina. As a result, essential nutrients must be transported into the retina by means of selective carrier mechanisms. Several transport systems have been characterized, varying from passive transport to active and energy-requiring processes.

Passive transport

As early as 1958 Bleeker and Mas[3] had shown a good correlation between diffusion across the BRB and penetration into the vitreous and lipid solubility of compounds. Lipid-soluble substances penetrated according to their oil/water partition coefficient, the more fat-soluble substances penetrating more easily.

Personal studies in collaboration with David Maurice produced the first approximate value for the permeability coefficient of a substance at the level of the BRB. The results obtained showed that fluorescein, which has a molecular radius of approximately 5.5 Å, has a permeability coefficient at the BRB in the order of 0.14×10^{-5} cm sec^{-1} very different from the value of 3.9×10^{-5} cm sec^{-1} registered for vascular permeability in general[4], but comparable to the value of 0.16×10^{-5} cm sec^{-1} obtained by Crone[5] for the BRB for fructose (Table 1). It is particularly interesting to compare the value obtained for the permeability of the BRB to fluorescein, in a situation of

Table 1. Permeabilities of different cells and tissues.

			Permeability ($cm\ sec^{-1} \times 10^{-5}$)			
Substance	Molecular weight	Radius (Å)	BRB (*Ref.* 7)	BBB (*Ref.* 5)	Capillaries (*Ref.* 4)	Beggiatoa cells (*Ref.* 6)
Urea	60	2.6	–	–	9.7	1.6
Glucose	180	3.7	–	0.16	6	–
Sucrose	342	5.3	–	–	5.9	0.14
Fluorescein	376	5.5	0.14	–	–	–
Raffinose	504	6	–	–	5.9	–

simple diffusion, with the value found by Davson and Danielli[6] for the permeability of a cell, Beggiatoa, to sucrose (7–5.3 Å): they are similar. The passive transfer at the level of the BRB appears, therefore, to be extremely restricted, being similar to that considered for cellular permeability in general.

Active transport

Specific carrier systems mediating active transport of certain compounds into the retina have been identified. A selective glucose carrier system has been characterized which transports 2-deoxyglucose, mannose, galactose and glucose with a high capacity. In the brain vessels Glut-1 (55 kDa) is expressed asymetrically both at the abluminal and luminal membrane of the endothelial cell.

An active transport for organic anions has also been demonstrated at both the inner and outer BRBs[7]. Fluorescein has the characteristics of an organic anion. Using fluorophotometry techniques it was possible to characterize this active transport in a situation of 'uphill' gradient and using various inhibitors, competitive and metabolic. This transport showed a clear analogy with other transport systems for organic anions existing in the body, indicating that all ions with similar characteristics are actively transported by the BRB.

The function of this active transport process, at the level of the BRB, appears to be to block the penetration of organic anions from the blood into the retinal tissue and to pump them out whenever they are present. This pumping process may therefore be considered as an important part of the barrier mechanism specially for the removal of toxic agents from the retina.

Receptor mediated transcytosis and absorptive mediated endocytosis

Proteins can be transported through the barrier endothelial cells into the retina by means of receptor-mediated transcytosis. The initial step in this process is the specific interaction of a ligand with its receptor on the luminal side of the endothelial cell. The complex of receptor and ligand is endocytosed and endosomes cross the cell cytoplasm by means of diffusion. Receptor-mediated exocytosis at the abluminal side of the endothelial cell releases the peptide into the retinal interstitial space. One of the proteins that can cross the BRB in this manner is transferrin, for which the retinal endothelial cell possesses a relatively high density of receptors. Insulin-like growth factors (IGF) I and II and insulin can also be transported through the endothelium by means of transcytosis. Non-specific transcytotic passage of certain proteins such as glycosylated proteins has been called absorptive mediated endocytosis[8].

Modification or enhancement of transport of drugs into the retina

A transient increase in the permeability of the BRB can be achieved by modification of BRB properties (Fig. 1). Opening of the BRB, for instance, can be achieved by intracarotid infusion of a hyperosmotic solution such as mannitol or arabinose. Perfusion with such a solution for about 30 sec opens the BRB and BRB reversibly. Osmotically induced shrinkage of the retinal and brain capillary endothelial cells causes opening of the tight junctions. Other methods include perfusion with oleic acid or protamine. These, however, produce a non-specific opening of the BRB with associated opening of the blood–brain barrier and CNS side effects.

Hypertension also results in an acute induction of pinocytosis and a non-specific increase in the transport of injected compounds. Enhanced vesicular transport may also be caused by radiotherapy. The threshold energy for BRB dysfunction in the rabbit eye for white and blue light is $250\,\mathrm{J/cm^2}$ and $50\,\mathrm{J/cm^2}$, respectively[9]. Temporary light exposure may be proposed as an adjuvant to drug therapy to achieve penetration of the BRB.

Chemical modification of drugs to enhance BRB transport

Several chemical modifications leading to changes in drug transport have been described. The synthesis of analogues there are more lipophilic than the parent drug will increase their BRB permeability. Enhanced BRB transport is found for drugs with fewer hydrogen bonds than the parent compound.

Lipidization of drugs and the formation of prodrugs may require the existence of a so-called tissue sequestration system, since highly lipid soluble drugs will efflux rapidly from the nervous tissueback to the blood. Bodor et al.[10] have developed a strategy for the delivery of compounds into the CNS by sequential metabolism at the target site using enzymatic or chemical cleavage, based on the concept of prodrugs.

Another approach to enhancing drug transport across the BRB is the utilization of specific carrier systems which are present at the barrier level. Drugs may be modified so that their structures resemble endogenous ligands for a specific carrier system in the BRB, leading to uptake via the carrier. The use of L-DOPA together with decarboxylase inhibitors in Parkinson's disease represents a successful means of selectively enhancing drug uptake. The possibilities of using the endogenous transporters for the transport of (modified) compounds are limited, however, since most carrier systems are highly specific for endogenous ligands.

Liposome-encapsulated drugs

Drugs can be incorporated into liposomes with the intention of enhancing drug transport to the retina and brain. The disadvantage of using a liposome as a drug carrier, however, is its rapid uptake by the liver, lungs and spleen. One strategy to overcome this problem is the use of specific glycolipid ligands. Umezawa and Eto[11] reported that mannosylation of liposomes facilitated the entry of such liposomes into the brain.

The use of liposomes as drug carrier systems for the CNS in itself has been unsuccessful. However, selectivity of liposomes for the CNS can be significantly improved by the incorporation of a recognition marker such as mannose or sulphatide into the lipid layer, which may subsequently interact with specific surface molecules on the barrier cells.

Coupling of drugs to vectors

Another approach to obtain more selective BRB transport is coupling drugs to antibodies directed against specific epitopes present on the endothelial cell surface of the BRB. These antibodies, so-called vectors, may be used successfully to target drugs more specifically to the retinal tissue, as for the brain. Friden et al.[12] described a method of coupling radiolabeled methotrexate to the anti-transferrin receptor antibody, OX-26. Endothelial cells of the BRB possess a relatively high density of transferrin receptors and the ligand complex was transcytosed across the endothelial cells in the brain parenchyma.

Absorptive-mediated transcytosis can also be used for drug transport to the brain. Proteins undergoing transcytosis through the endothelium may therefore serve as drug delivery vector for the CNS. Smith and Boarchard[13] studied the mechanism of transport of albumin versus cationized and glycosylated albumin across monolayers of cultured cerebral endothelial cells. The transport rate of modified albumin was seven-fold higher than that of native albumin.

The use of antibodies directed against specific epitopes on the cerebral endothelial cells is an elegant technique to obtain more selective transport to the brain. Compounds with a molecular weight up to 40 kDa can be transported into the retina and brain using this strategy.

References

1. Shakib, M., Cunha-Vaz, J.G. Studies on the permeability of the blood-retinal barrier. IV. Junctional complexes of the retinal vessels and their role in the permeability of the blood-retinal barrier. Exp Eye Res. 1966; 5: 229–234.
2. Chang-Ling, T., Stone, J. Degeneration of astrocytes in feline retinopathy of prematurity causes failure of the blood-retinal barrier. Invest Ophthalmol Vis Sci. 1992; 33: 2148–2159.
3. Bleeker, G.M., Maas, E.H. Penetration of penethamate penicillin esther into the tissue of the eye. Arch Ophthalmol. 1958; 60: 1013–1020.
4. Vargas, F., Johnson, J.A. Permeability of rabbit heart capillaries to non-electrolytes. Am J Physiol. 1967; 213: 87–93.
5. Crone, C. The permeability of brain capillaries to non-electrolytes. Acta Physiol Scand. 1965; 64: 407–412.
6. Davson, H., Danielli, J.F. The Permeability of Natural Membranes. London: Cambridge University Press, 1952.
7. Cunha-Vaz, J.G., Maurice, D.M. The active transport of fluorescein by retinal vessels and the retina. J. Physiol. 1967; 191: 467–486.
8. Partridge, W.M. Blood-brain transport of nutrients. Introduction. Fed Proc. 1986; 45: 2047–2049.

9. Putting, B.J. The Effects of Light on the Blood-Retinal Barrier. Thesis, The Hague, 1993: p. 141.

10. Bodor, N., Prokai, L., Wu, W.M. et al. A strategy for delivering peptides into the central nervous system by sequential metabolism. Science. 1992; 257: 1698–1704.

11. Umezawa, F., Eto, Y. Liposome targeting to mouse brain: mannose as a recognition marker. Biochem Biophys Res Commun. 1988; 153: 1038–1044.

12. Friden, P.M., Walus, L.R., Musso, G.F., Taylor, M.A., Malfroy, B., Starzyk, R.M. Anti-transferrin receptor antibody and antibody-drug conjugates cross the blood-brain barrier. Proc Natl Acad Sci USA. 1991; 88: 4771–4775.

13. Smith, K.R., Boarchardt, R.T. Permeability and mechanism of albumin, cationized albumin, and glycosylated albumin transcellular transport across monolayers of cultured bovine brain capillary endothelial cells. Pharm Res. 1989; 6: 466–473.

Department of Ophthalmology and
Biomedical Institute for Research on
Light and Image
University of Coimbra
Portugal

3. Subretinal protein and serous detachment

M.F. MARMOR

(Stanford, USA)

Introduction

The term 'serous detachment' implies that subretinal fluid is proteinaceous. However, there has been little direct data on the movement of protein in or out of the subretinal space. This report summarizes recent experiments from our laboratory which investigated this issue and sought to clarify the role of protein in serous detachment in man[1-5]. These experiments also examine the effects of vitreous within the subretinal space, as may occur in rhegmatogenous detachment, and the source of protein when serous detachments form after focal ischaemia or toxic damage to the RPE and choroid.

Methods

These experiments all conformed to the Association for Research in Vision and Ophthalmology Resolution on the Use of Animals in Research. They were performed on pigmented Dutch rabbits weighing approximately 1.5 kg, sedated with acepromazine maleate (1 mg/kg, i.m.) and anaesthetized with ketamine hydrochloride (20 mg/kg, i.m.) and xylazine (2 mg/kg, i.m.). Experimental serous detachments were made as described previously[6] by injecting fluid into the subretinal space through a glass micropipette that passed through the limbus and across the vitreous space. The volume of fluid injected subretinally could be measured, as could fluid withdrawn for later chemical analysis. In different experiments, solutions were injected into the subretinal space, vitreous cavity or bloodstream. Injected materials included saline solution (Hanks' solution), autologous serum, bovine fluorescein isothiocyanate albumin (FITC albumin) or liquefied autologous vitreous. In some experiments, RPE damage was produced by intense light damage[7,8] or by the systemic administration of sodium iodate. Spontaneous detachments were induced by focal illumination of the retina after rose bengal administration, or intravitreal administration of the toxin *n*-ethylmaleimide. Albumin concentration in test fluids was measured by gel electrophoresis, comparing the stained bands to those produced by calibrated aliquots of pure rabbit albumin. FITC albumin concentrations were measured by fluorophotometry. Readers are referred to the original publications[1-5] for details of the methodology.

G. Coscas and F. Cardillo Piccolino (eds.), Retinal Pigment Epithelium and Macular Diseases, pp. 13–17.
© 1998 Kluwer Academic Publishers.

Results

Protein was injected into the subretinal space and its concentration measured in the vitreous, or it was injected into the vitreous and samples of subretinal fluid withdrawn for measurement[1,2]. The results of these experiments showed that albumin diffuses across the retina in either direction at a rate such that the concentration difference diminishes by 4–5% per hour (Fig. 1). In other words, saline within the subretinal space takes on protein from the vitreous, gaining about 5% of the vitreous concentration per hour; conversely, albumin within the subretinal space diffuses out into the vitreous so that the subretinal concentration is gradually diminished by about 5% per hour (correcting for changes in subretinal fluid volume).

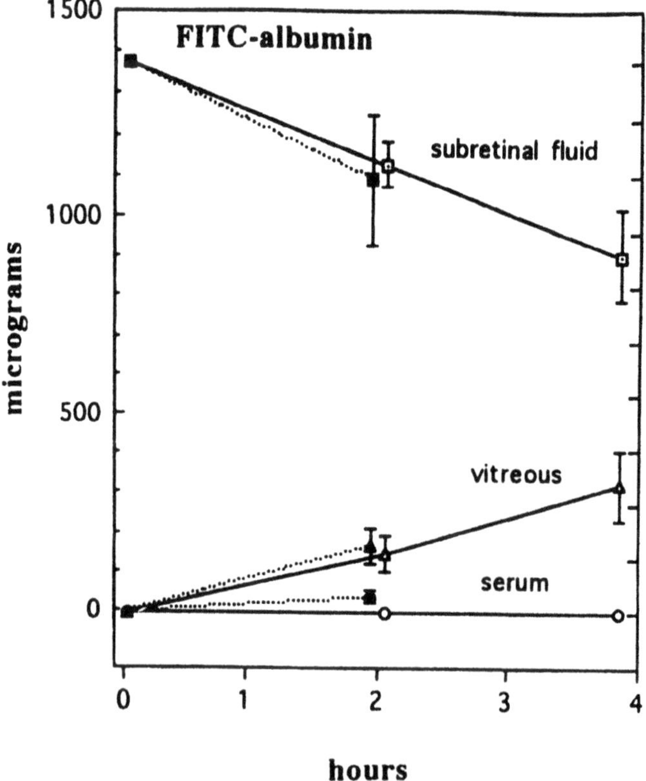

Fig. 1. Movement of albumin out of the subretinal space after subretinal injection of fluoresceinated (FITC) albumin. Solid lines represent normal RPE; dotted lines represent experiments with RPE damaged by intravenous sodium iodate injection. The total amount of albumin in the subretinal space diminished over time by diffusion into the vitreous, at a rate independent of RPE damage. FITC–albumin entered the bloodstream only after the RPE had been damaged. From Ref. 2.

These results are independent of the RPE, and depend only upon the concentration difference between subretinal space and vitreous. When the RPE is intact, there is virtually no movement of protein across the RPE in either direction. However, when the RPE was damaged with sodium iodate, protein entered the subretinal space from the choroidal extracellular fluid, or labelled protein could be observed to leave the subretinal space and enter the bloodstream. Interestingly, the rate of protein movement across iodate-damaged RPE was only about 25% of the diffusion rate across the retina.

Given that large protein molecules can move across the retina with reasonable facility, one might expect an even more facile movement of ions in water: solutions injected into the subretinal space equilibrated osmotically with the vitreous within a minute or less. This indicates that the vitreous and subretinal space are in osmotic equilibrium because of the ease of diffusion across the retina. A corollary of this observation is that protein in the subretinal space probably does not osmotically cause the filling or maintenance of serous detachments.

Although protein diffuses out of the subretinal space, when the concentration is higher than that of the vitreous, the protein concentration of subretinal fluid will also be influenced by ongoing fluid absorption across the RPE. We performed a series of experiments[3] in which liquefied vitreous, or a solution of albumin at vitreal concentration, was injected into the subretinal space to see how these processes might affect fluid that enters the subretinal space in rhegmatogenous detachment. Since there was little gradient for diffusion across the retina, the concentration of protein in the subretinal space rose as subretinal fluid was absorbed. This may be one mechanism by which protein is concentrated in subretinal fluid in rhegmatogenous detachments, since there is a continual entry of vitreal protein through the retinal hole as well as a continual absorption of water across the RPE. Of course, protein may also enter through the RPE if it becomes damaged as a part of the disease process.

The subretinal protein concentration will rise rapidly whenever the pigment epithelial barrier is damaged, by diffusion of protein from the very high concentrations in the choroidal extracellular space. This was demonstrated by injecting saline into the subretinal space, damaging the RPE with sodium iodate and measuring the protein content of the subretinal fluid. Experiments were also performed to determine the source of protein in detachments that formed spontaneously in models of disease. Two models were used. In the first, serous detachments were induced by photosensitizing rabbits with rose bengal and then producing choroidal thrombosis with exposure to light[4]. Serous detachments formed rapidly over the area of ischaemic injury, and subretinal fluid removed just 3 h after photosensitization had a concentration 68% of serum level. The subretinal protein concentration neared serum levels by 24 h (Fig. 2). Similar results were obtained from detachments that formed after intravitreal administration of *n*-ethylmaleimide[5]. The subretinal protein was roughly 70% of serum levels within 30 min (Fig. 2). Since these high

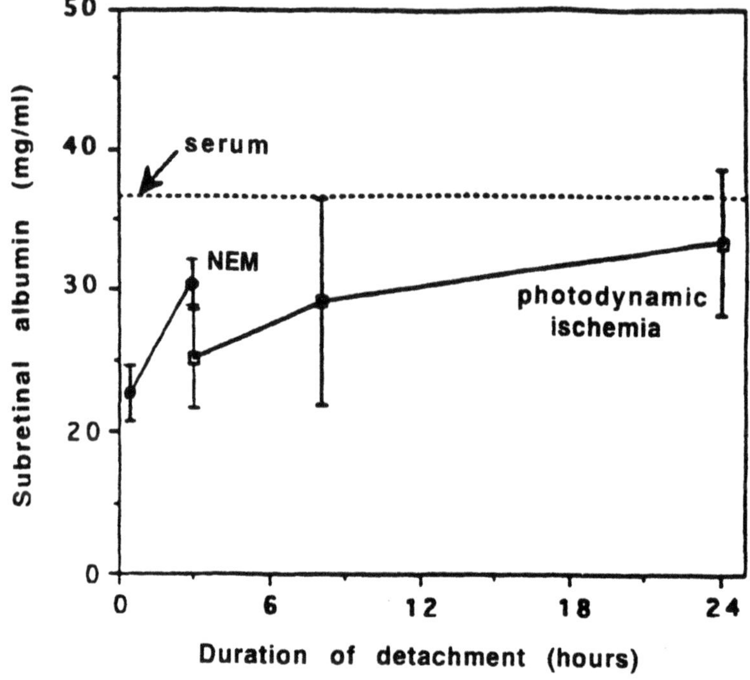

Fig. 2. Albumin concentration in the subretinal space in experimental detachments induced by intravitreal injection of *n*-ethylmaleimide (NEM) or by choroidal thrombosis as a result of intense light exposure in the presence of intravenous rose bengal (photodynamic ischaemia). The initial measurements showed a protein concentration 60–70% of serum levels, and the concentration rose over time. Modified from Refs 4 and 5.

concentrations could not possibly be achieved from the vitreous (normal vitreous protein is less than 1% of serum concentration), it appears that the source of protein in serous detachments is indeed the choroid. The fact that the initial subretinal fluid protein concentrations in our experiments was somewhat less than that of serum suggests that the fluid was a transudate across a partial barrier, rather than an exudate.

Discussion

These experiments show that the protein in serous detachments undoubtedly comes from the choroid, but they also show that protein will not remain in the subretinal space unless there is a continual influx. In the absence of new protein, the subretinal concentration would fall close to vitreal levels within a day or so, assuming that the fluid volume was stable. The rate at which the protein concentration falls would be slower if fluid was being absorbed simultaneously, although the overall concentration would still fall. A 'steady state' of subretinal protein can only be maintained if there is continued entry of protein as well as fluid entry in either a non-rhegmatogenous or rhegmatogenous detachment. This conclusion might be modified, however, to the extent that proteins become altered chemically or inspissated to lose diffusability. In rhegmatogenous detachments, protein entering the subretinal space from the vitreous can become concentrated over time as subretinal fluid is absorbed (although there is also a possibility of protein entry through the RPE if it should lose its barrier function at any point after detachment).

Subretinal fluid as well as protein is in a dynamic balance within any retinal detachment. Entry of fluid from the vitreous or through an RPE defect is offset by active transport across the RPE, and water diffuses across the retina in conjunction with osmotic adjustments. Since osmotic equilibrium is maintained continually between the subretinal space and vitreous, the mere presence of protein in the subretinal fluid is not sufficient to form or maintain serous detachments. Since the RPE has such an effective transport system, it has been postulated that in disorders such as central serous chorioretinopathy, where the area of leakage may be very small, fluid absorption may be compromised across a broad area of RPE (at least corresponding to the detachment)[9,10]. This absorption abnormality is probably most often a result of choroidal vascular pathology, which leads secondarily to relatively diminished water transport across the RPE.

References

1. Takeuchi, A., Kricorian, G., Yao, X.-Y., Kenny, J.W., Marmor, M.F. The rate and source of albumin entry into saline-filled experimental retinal detachments. Invest Ophthalmol Vis Sci. 1994; 35: 3792–3798.
2. Takeuchi, A., Kricorian, G., Marmor, M.F. Albumin movement out of the subretinal space after experimental retinal detachment. Invest Ophthalmol Vis Sci. 1995; 36: 1298–1305
3. Takeuchi, A., Kricorian, G., Wolfensberger, T.J., Marmor, M.F. When vitreous enters the subretinal space. Retina. 1996; 16: 426–430.
4. Takeuchi, A., Kricorian, G., Wolfensberger, T.J., Marmor, M.F. The source of fluid and protein in serous retinal detachments. Curr Eye Res. 1996; 15: 764–767.
5. Chon, C.H., Yao, X.-Y., Dalal, R., Takeuchi, A., Kim, R.Y., Marmor, M.F. An experimental model of retinal pigment epithelial and serous detachment. Retina. 1996; 16: 139–144.
6. Marmor, M.F., Abdul-Rahim, A.S., Cohen, D.S. The effect of metabolic inhibitors on retinal adhesion and subretinal fluid resorption. Invest Ophthalmol Vis Sci. 1980; 19: 893–903.
7. Wilson, C.A., Royster, A.J., Tiedeman, J.S., Hatchell, D.L. Exudative retinal detachment after photodynamic injury. Arch Ophthalmol. 1991; 109: 125–134.
8. Yao, X.-Y., Marmor, M.F. Induction of serous retinal detachment in rabbit eyes by pigment epithelial and choriocapillary injury. Arch Ophthalmol. 1992; 110: 541–546.
9. Marmor, M.F. New hypothesis on the pathogenesis and treatment of serous retinal detachment. Graefe's Arch Clin Exp Ophthalmol. 1998; 226: 548–552.
10. Marmor, M.F., Yao, X.-Y. Conditions necessary for the formation of serous detachment: Experimental evidence from the cat. Arch Ophthalmol. 1994; 112: 830–838.

Department of Ophthalmology
Stanford University Medical Center
Stanford, CA 94305-5308
USA

4. Ageing of the human retinal pigment epithelium

M. BOULTON and J. WASSELL

(Manchester, UK)

Introduction

The human retinal pigment epithelium (RPE) is a non-dividing system which throughout life undertakes a number of functions essential for the maintenance of photoreceptor cells. With increasing age, the RPE is seen to undergo structural changes, lose melanin (its light absorbing pigment), accumulate the age pigment lipofuscin, have reduced antioxidant capacity and progressively accumulate deposits on, and within, the underlying Bruch's membrane. These age-related changes in both the RPE and Bruch's membrane appear to be strongly associated with the pathogenesis of age-related macular degeneration (ARMD).

Age-related changes in cell density

RPE cell density has been reported to change with age; however, reports remain contradictory. In the peripheral retina, cell numbers have been found to increase, decrease, or not change with age[1, 5]. At the macula, Dorey et al.[4] and Watzke et al.[6] found RPE cell density to decrease with age. The resultant increase in cell area was associated with an increase in the height of RPE cells[4,7]. Furthermore, the age-related loss of the RPE was significantly slower in whites than in blacks[4]. By contrast, Gao and Hollyfield[5] found no age-related change in RPE cell density. The most comprehensive study to date by Panda-Jonas et al.[8] reported that RPE cell density decreases by about 0.3% per year with increasing age. Since the RPE is normally a non-dividing system, any insidious loss of RPE cells would result in an overall increase in the area of adjacent cells as they spread to fill in the gaps, affecting the photoreceptor/RPE cell ratio and hence RPE phagocytic load. Reports concerning age-related changes in the photoreceptor/RPE cell ratio are inconsistent. Dorey et al.[4] found the mean ratio of photoreceptors to RPE cells was higher in the macula than in either the paramacular or equatorial area, and that this ratio increased with increasing donor age. By contrast, a later study by Gao and Hollyfield[5] failed to reveal a difference in the photoreceptor/RPE cell ratio between the fovea and equator or an age-related increase in this ratio.

G. Coscas and F. Cardillo Piccolino (eds.), Retinal Pigment Epithelium and Macular Diseases, pp. 19–28.
© 1998 Kluwer Academic Publishers.

Age-related changes in pigment granule type and structure

Melanin

Melanin has a dual role within the retina, acting to absorb spurious light to increase visual acuity and as a protectant against oxidative damage[9]. The melanin content of human RPE cells shows a regional distribution, with levels decreasing from the equator to the posterior pole while showing a significant peak at the macula[7,10]. This peak may be attributed in part to the denser packing of melanin per unit area owing to the taller, narrower RPE cells in the macula compared with shorter, wider extra-macular cells[7]. The differential distribution of melanosomes is maintained throughout life but a significant decline in the total numbers of granules is observed in all regions after the age of 40[7,10,11]. When comparisons were made between three age groups (1–20, 21–60 and 61–100 years) the decline in melanosomes in the macular RPE between the early and late decades was about 35%. Taken as a percentage of cell volume, 8% of the cell is occupied by melanin in the first two decades of life, decreasing to 6% in the subsequent age group and to 3.5% in the oldest age group[7]. This loss correlates with the increase in the numbers of 'complex' melanin granules (see later).

Lipofuscin

Post-mitotic cells of various ageing tissues accumulate nondegradable lipid-protein aggregates within lysosomal residual bodies[12]. The generic name 'lipofuscin' has been given to this lipophilic material which appears to constitute heterogeneous groups of substances with characteristic physico-chemical properties, including a natural yellowish-green fluorescence when excited with ultraviolet light[13].

Lipofuscin is present within the human RPE as yellow-brown refractile granules which characteristically fluoresce under short wavelength light excitation[14]. Its progressive accumulation within the RPE has been reported to be bimodal[15] but more recent measures of RPE fluorescence *in vivo* indicate there is a continuous increase in RPE lipofuscin throughout life[16,17]. Topographically, maximal accumulation of lipofuscin granules occurs in the posterior pole, albeit with a decrease at the fovea[18]. This distribution of lipofuscin as a function of retinal location remains constant throughout life and correlates with the density distribution of rod photoreceptor cells across the retina[3,14,18]. The cytoplasmic volume of the RPE occupied by lipofuscin increases with age; by the age of 40 years some 8% of the cytoplasmic volume of macular RPE cells is occupied and by 80 years this figure has risen to 19%[7]. The cytoplasmic volume occupied by lipofuscin in the macula is greater than that in either the equatorial or peripheral RPE, i.e. approximately 19% as opposed to 13%.

Lipofuscin granules are thought to represent the life-long accumulation of lysosomal residual bodies containing the undegradable end-products of phagocytosis of photoreceptor outer segments[14,19–21] and, to a lesser extent, autophagy[14]. Whether some turnover of the constituent material of lipofuscin granules occurs throughout life is as yet unclear.

While it has been widely accepted that lipofuscinogenesis in the RPE occurs via lipid autoxidation and aldehyde/amine crosslinking reactions[9,22,23] it is likely that vitamin A is an equal, if not a more important, substrate. Several lines of evidence suggest that vitamin A metabolites may be more directly involved than lipid peroxidation products in the development of lipofuscin fluorescence within the RPE. Firstly, in both normal and RCS rats raised on diets free of all forms of vitamin A other than retinoic acid (which cannot be used in the visual cycle), the amount of lipofuscin accumulating in the RPE is dramatically reduced[20,24]. Additionally, a specific vitamin A-dependent fluorophore was isolated from lipofuscin-like material accumulating adjacent to the RPE in RCS rats[24]. This fluorophore was similar to the major orange emitting fluorophore of RPE lipofuscin. Second, Eldred and Katz[22] separated lipofuscin into ten fluorophores by thin layer chromatography. Two of these fluorophores co-migrated with retinol and retinol palmitate; a third, the major orange emitting fluorophore of lipofuscin, has been identified using fast atom bombardment mass spectrometry as an amphoteric quaternary amine that arises as a Schiff's base reaction product of retinaldehyde and ethanolamine[25]. Third, the development of lipofuscin-like fluorescence in the RPE of rats given intravitreal injections of iron or a lysosomal protease inhibitor was dependent on the availability of dietary vitamin A[26,27]. Vitamin A has also been directly localized to autofluorescent inclusions generated in the presence of the protease inhibitor[28]. Thus, both lipid autoxidation and vitamin A are likely to be major substrates in lipofuscin formation.

The morphology of pure lipofuscin granules is similar in all age groups, and evidence from a number of laboratories suggests that lipofuscin is a broad band absorber with a decrease in absorption from the shorter to longer wavelengths[22,29]. The fluorescent characteristics have long been studied and it is now generally accepted that lipofuscin has a number of fluorophores, including blue, yellow and orange emitters[10,30,31]. Furthermore, the proportion of the individual fluorphores in lipofuscin is age related[29,30]. The overall fluorescence intensity of the lipofuscin granules increased with increasing age; the emission and excitation peaks being about 40% higher in those over 60 y than in younger individuals.

There is considerable debate as to how lipofuscin affects cell function: some consider lipofuscin to be an inert substance which acts directly by congesting the cytoplasm (lipofuscin can occupy up to 30% of cell volume in certain tissues[12]), while others propose that lipofuscin is toxic and may act as a source of reactive oxygen species[3,9,32]. Lipofuscin granules located within retinal pigment epithelial cells have a significant potential for exerting deleterious reactions within component cells: lipofuscin can constitute up to 19% of cytoplasmic volume in later life[7] and pigment epithelial cells are constantly exposed to both light and high partial pressures of oxygen[33], both of which can contribute to a perfect environment for reactive oxygen species formation.

The first definitive demonstration of RPE lipofuscin as a free radical generator came from Boulton *et al.*[34], who showed that lipofuscin is a photoinducible generator of the superoxide anion and that this effect appeared to be wavelength dependent; superoxide anion generation was greatest in granules exposed to blue rather than red or full white light. The spectral dependence of superoxide anion generation by lipofuscin may explain the so called 'blue light hazard' to the retina. At wavelengths below 550 nm, extended irradiances produce actinic or photochemical lesions but are too low to produce thermal effects[35]. These photochemical lesions are prominent at the level of the retinal pigment epithelium and it has been noted that the action spectra for blue light damage is grossly similar to the broad band absorption spectra of both melanin[33] and lipofuscin[22,29]. Analysis of blue light photoreactivity in human RPE cells demonstrates a marked increase in the rate of oxygen photo-uptake as donor age increases, and this photo-uptake is largely due to lipofuscin[36]. Additionally, by incubating lipid membranes or enzymes with lipofuscin in an extracellular system, it has been shown that lipofuscin can induce oxidative damage to these membranes and inhibit enzyme function; these effects were mediated by the production of reactive oxygen species[37]. Further studies are required at the cellular level to confirm the extent to which lipofuscin is detrimental to retinal cell function.

Complex granules
With increasing age, melanin, lipofuscin and lysosomes can fuse to form complex structures (melanolipofuscin and melanolysosomes) within the RPE[14]. These complexes exhibit a regional distribution similar to that of lipofuscin, i.e. highest density in the macula and decreasing towards the periphery and fovea[7]. Expressed as a percentage of the area within the cell, the complex granules range from 3.3% in the first decade of life to 8–10% in the sixth. These complex granules may represent melanin in the process of repair, modification or degradation. The association of lysosomes with pigment granules (i.e. melanosomes, lipofuscin granules or pigment complexes) may explain the age-related change in the lysosomal enzyme content and activity of human RPE cells[38]. The overall activity of both acid phosphatase and cathepsin D, in all retinal regions, increases as a function of donor age. This association of lysosomes with increasing numbers of pigment granules may necessitate an increase in lysosome numbers in order to maintain the normal degradative cycle following outer segment ingestion by RPE cells.

Age-related changes in antioxidants

In order to prevent severe autoxidative damage to the retina the RPE is particularly rich in a variety of antioxidants such as vitamin E, superoxide dismutase (SOD), catalase, glutathione peroxidase and melanin[9,39]. There is limited information on the changes in antioxidant levels within the RPE with age. Friedrichson *et al.*[40] reported an age-related decrease in vitamin E levels in the macular RPE after 70 years of age, while levels in peripheral cells remained constant. This decrease corresponds to the time at which the incidence of ARMD starts to increase. Castorina *et al.*[41] have demonstrated an age-related correlation between lipid peroxidation and antioxidant enzyme activity in the rat retina. More specifically, Liles *et al.*[42] found that SOD activity in the RPE does not exhibit a significant correlation with ageing or ARMD, while catalase activity increases with both age and ARMD.

Bruch's membrane

Bruch's membrane is an acellular 'sieve-like' structure consisting of five sub-strata, two of which are basement membranes and two are collagenous, while the remaining layer is composed of elastin[43]. The progressive accumulation of debris, thickening, calcification and modification of collagen fibrils are all associated with the ageing of Bruch's membrane[44–46]. Lipid accumulation is a prominent feature in Bruch's membrane with age[47]. Such lipids consist largely of phospholipids, triglycerides, fatty acids and free cholesterol (there is little cholesterol ester), consistent with the lipids being of cellular origin[48,49].

In addition to alterations induced within Bruch's membrane, the diffuse accumulation of fine granular deposits on its innermost margin (i.e. above the RPE basement membrane) has also been observed[46]. These diffuse deposits between the RPE and its basement membrane have been termed basal linear deposits, diffuse drusen, or basal laminar deposits[46,50–52]. In association with these basement membrane changes, the basal border of the epithelial cells undergoes a reduction in the complexity of the basal invaginations suggesting a progressive decline of active transport with age.

Over the age of 40 years, focal aggregations of sub-pigment epithelial debris are observed and these excrescences on Bruch's membrane are called drusen[3]. These deposits can be found both internal and external to the RPE basement membrane[46]. Drusen are a common finding in the macular region and in the far periphery of older eyes[53]. Drusen exhibit a variety of clinical appearances but are generally described as hard or soft according to the nature of their margins and staining characteristics[46]. Hard drusen have distinct margins and a dense compact structure that stains intensely during fluorescein angiography, whereas soft drusen have blurred margins and stain relatively weakly. Histochemical studies suggest that the fluorescein-excluding drusen have a high content of neutral fats and lack protein, while conversely, fluorescein-staining deposits have high proportions of phospholipids and protein[3,54]. The former appear to be the type of drusen associated with disciform complications. The mechanism of drusen formation is unclear: some authors support the concept of the apoptosis of portions of RPE cell membranes and cytoplasm[55,56] while others advocate the extracellular aggregation of diffuse deposits derived from incompletely degraded components of photoreceptor cell phagocytosis[3]. Drusen show regional differences in that, although they occur in both the far peripheral retina and in the posterior pole, they only lead to sight-threatening sequelae in the central retina[57,58].

The progressive accumulation of debris, thickening, calcification and modification of collagen fibrils associated with ageing is thought to weaken Bruch's membrane, ultimately resulting in subretinal neovascularization[46,59]. In developed countries up to 90% of cases of legal blindness attributable to ARMD are a consequence of the neovascular or exudative form of the disorder[60]. The role of the RPE in modulating subretinal neovascularization is unclear but it has been demonstrated that the RPE exerts some control over the structure and function of the choriocapillaris[61,62] and that RPE cells proliferate around newly formed vessels, which if enveloped by RPE, halt the progression of the neovascularization[63]. However, the inability of the RPE completely to envelop subretinal new vessels may in part be due to the proliferative ability of RPE cells; the proliferative capability of RPE cells is less in older eyes than in younger eyes, opening the possibility that blood–retinal barrier repair is effected more slowly in the elderly[64,65].

The changes in inherent structure and the build-up of debris within Bruch's membrane may well result in the exponential decrease in the hydraulic conductivity of Bruch's membrane-choroid complex exhibits seen with increasing age, the most rapid decline occurring during the first four decades of life[67]. This age-related change is most pronounced in the macula, where there is an exponential decline of hydraulic conductivity with a half-life of 15 years, compared with 22 years for the peripheral fundus[68]. Such alterations impede the transport of nutrients to and from the retina and in the case of outflow may have a bearing on RPE detachments, i.e. water pumped from the retina towards the choroid may collect in the sub-RPE space if it cannot cross a lipid barrier in Bruch's membrane[69].

Consequences of RPE ageing

Although there is no direct evidence that the RPE is the primary site for any human retinal disease, age-related changes in the RPE and Bruch's membrane have been associated with a wide variety of retinal pathologies, in particular, age-related macular degeneration (ARMD). ARMD, which affects more than 35% of people over the age of 65 years and accounts for 50% of the blind registrations in this age group, is always associated with RPE atrophy, pigment dispersion and/or drusen[70,71].

The onset of ARMD has been linked with ageing changes associated with the RPE: progressive intracellular accumulation of lipofuscin, and the extracellular accumulation of lipids, basal linear deposits and drusen at the level of Bruch's membrane[32,59,72]. It has been postulated that the severity and nature of the age-related changes can define the type of ARMD excessive levels of lipofuscin being associated with atrophic ARMD and Bruch's membrane changes associated with exudative ARMD[59].

Conclusions

RPE ageing is considered to be a natural occurrence in all individuals; however, in some these changes are excessive and culminate in retinal degeneration. The risk factors responsible for RPE ageing are now being identified, as are the importance of the age-related modifications to retinal disease; lipofuscin accumulation and/or Bruch's membrane deposits are considered to be major contributors. In addition, the importance of reactive oxygen species and antioxidant levels are now becoming evident. Future research should increase our understanding of RPE ageing changes and hopefully allow intervention in the development of age-related eye diseases such as ARMD.

References

1. Tso, M., Friedman, E. The retinal pigment epithelium: III growth and development. Arch Ophthalmol. 1968; 80: 214–216.
2. Streeten, B.W. Development of the human retinal pigment epithelium and the posterior segment. Arch Ophthalmol. 1969; 81: 383–394.
3. Marshall, J. The ageing retina: physiology or pathology. Eye. 1987; 1: 282–295.
4. Dorey, C.K., Wu, G., Ebenstein, D., Garsd, A., Weiter, J.J. Cell loss in the ageing retina: relationship to lipofuscin accumulation and macular degeneration. Invest Ophthalmol Vis Sci. 1989; 30: 1691–1699.
5. Gao, H., Hollyfield, J.G. Aging of the human retina. Differential loss of neurons and retinal pigment epithelial cells. Invest Ophthalmol Vis Sci. 1992; 33: 1–17.
6. Watzke, R.C., Soldevilla, J.D., Trune, D.R. Morphometric analysis of human retinal pigment epithelium: correlation with age and location. Curr Eye Res. 1993; 12: 133–142.
7. Feeney-Burns, L., Hilderbrand, E.S., Eldridge, S. Aging human RPE: morphometric analysis of macular, equatorial and peripheral cells. Invest Ophthalmol Vis Sci. 1984; 25: 195–200.
8. Panda-Jonas, S., Jonas, J., Jakobczyk-Kmija, M. Retinal pigment epithelial cell count distribution, and correlations in normal human eyes. Am J Ophthalmol. 1996; 121: 181–189.
9. Handelman, G.J., Dratz, E.A. The role of antioxidants in the retina and retinal pigment epithelium and the nature of pro-oxidant induced damage. Adv Free Radical Biol Med. 1986; 2: 1–89.
10. Weiter, J.J., Delori, F.C., Wing, G.L., Fitch, K.A. Retinal pigment epithelial lipofuscin and melanin and choroidal melanin in human eyes. Invest Ophthalmol Vis Sci. 1986; 27: 145–152.
11. Schmidt, S.Y., Peisch, R.D. Melanin concentration in the normal human retinal pigment epithelium. Invest Ophthalmol Vis Sci. 1986; 27: 1063–1067.
12. Sohal, R.S. Age Pigments. Amsterdam. Elsevier/North-Holland Biomedical Press, 1981.
13. Brizee, K.R., Ordy, J.M. Cellular features, regional accumulation, and prospects of modification of age pigments in mammals. In: Sohal, R.S. (ed.), Age Pigments. Amsterdam. Elsevier/North-Holland Biomedical Press, 1981.
14. Feeney, L. Lipofuscin and melanin of human retinal pigment epithelium: fluorescence, enzyme cytochemical and ultrastructural studies. Invest Ophthalmol Vis Sci. 1978; 17: 583–600.

15. Weale, R.A. Do years or quanta age the retina? Photochem Photobiol. 1989; 50: 429–438.
16. Delori, F.C., Dorey, C.K., Staurenghi, G., Arend, O., Goger, D.G., Weiter, J.J. In vivo fluorescence of the ocular fundus exhibits retinal pigment epithelium lipofuscin characteristics. Invest Ophthalmol Vis Sci. 1995; 36: 718–729.
17. Hopkins, J., Von Ruckmann, A., Fitzke, F., Bird, A. Fundus autofluorescence in age-related macular disease. Invest Ophthalmol Vis Sci. 1996; 37 (suppl.): S114.
18. Wing, G.L., Blanchard, G.C., Weiter, J.L. The topography and age relationship of lipofuscin concentration in the retinal pigment epithelium. Invest Ophthalmol Vis Sci. 1978; 17: 601–607.
19. Feeney-Burns, L., Eldred, G.E. The fate of the phagosome: Conversion to 'age pigment' and impact in human retinal pigment epithelium. Trans Ophthalmol Soc UK. 1983; 103: 416–421.
20. Katz, M.L., Drea, C., Eldred, G., Hess, H., Robison, W.G. Influence of early photoreceptor degeneration on lipofuscin in the retinal pigment epithelium. Exp Eye Res. 1986; 43: 561–573.
21. Boulton, M.E., McKechnie, N.M., Breda, J., Bayly, M., Marshall, J. The formation of autofluorescent granules in cultured human RPE. Invest Ophthalmol Vis Sci. 1989; 30: 82–89.
22. Eldred, G.E., Katz, M.L. Fluorophores of the human retinal pigment epithelium: separation and spectral characteristics. Exp Eye Res. 1988; 47: 71–86.
23. Katz, M.L., Robison, W.G. Senescent alterations in the retina and retinal pigment epithelium: evidence for mechanisms based on nutritional studies. In: Armstrong, D.A. (ed), The Effects of Ageing and Environment on Vision. New York: Plenum Press, 1991: 195–209.
24. Katz, M.L., Eldred, G., Robison, W.G. Lipofuscin autofluorescence: evidence for vitamin A involvement in the retina. Mech Ageing Dev. 1987; 39: 81–90.
25. Eldred, G.E., Lasky, M.R. Retinal age pigments generated by self-assembling lysomotrophic detergents. Nature. 1993; 361: 724–726.
26. Katz, M.L., Nornberg, M. Influence of dietary vitamin A on the autofluorescence of leupeptin-derived inclusions in the retinal pigment epithelium. Exp Eye Res. 1992; 54: 239–246.
27. Katz, M.L., Christianson, J.S., Gao, C.L., Handelman, G.J. Iron-induced fluorescence in the retina: dependence on vitamin A. Invest Ophthalmol Vis Sci. 1994; 30: 37–43.
28. Katz, M.L., Gao, C.L. Vitamin A incorporation into lipofuscin-like inclusions in the retinal pigment epithelium. Mech Ageing Dev. 1995; 84: 29–38.
29. Boulton, M.E., Docchio, F., Dayhaw-Barker, P., Ramponi, R., Cubeddu, R. Age-related changes in the morphology, absorption and fluorescence of melanosomes and lipofuscin granules of the retinal pigment epithelium. Vis Res. 1990; 30: 1291–1303.
30. Eldred, G.E., Miller, G.V., Stark, W.S., Feeney-Burns, L. Lipofuscin: resolution of discrepant fluorescence data. Science. 1982; 216: 757–759.
31. Docchio, F., Boulton, M., Cubeddu, R., Ramponi, R., Dayhaw-Barker, P. Age-related changes in the fluorescence of melanin and lipofuscin granules of the retinal pigment epithelium: a time resolved fluorescence spectroscopy study. Photochem Photobiol. 1991; 54: 247–253.
32. Boulton, M.E. Ageing of the retinal pigment epithelium. In: Osborne, N., Chader, G.J. (eds.), Progress in Retinal Research. Pergamon Press, 1991: 125–151.
33. Marshall, J. Radiation and the ageing eye. Ophthal and Physiol Opt. 1985; 5: 241–263.
34. Boulton, M., Dontsov, A., Jarvis-Evans, J., Ostrovsky, M., Svistunencko, D. Lipofuscin is a photoinducible free radical generator. J Photochem Photobiol. B 1993; 19: 201–204.
35. Ham, W.T., Ruffolo, J.J., Mueller, H.A., Guerry, D. The nature of retina radiation damage as a function of wavelength, power level and exposure time. Vision Res. 1980; 20: 1105–1111.
36. Rozanowska, M., Jarvis-Evans, J., Korytowski, W., Boulton, M., Burke, J., Sarna, T. Blue light-induced reactivity of retinal age pigment. J Biol Chem. 1995; 270: 18825–18830.
37. Wassell, J., Moore, J., Boulton, M.E. The potential phototoxicity of retinal lipofuscin. Invest Ophthalmol Vis Sci. S375. 1996; 37 (suppl.).
38. Boulton, M., Moriarty, P., Jarvis-Evans, J., Marcyniuk, B. Regional variations and age-related changes of lysosomal enzymes in the human retinal pigment epithelium. Br J Ophthalmol. 1994; 78: 125–129.
39. Newsome, D.A., Miceli, M.V., Liles, M.R., Tate, D.J., Oliver, P.D. Antioxidants in the retinal pigment epithelium. Prog Retinal Eye Res. 1994; 13: 101–123.

40. Friedrichson, T., LeVan Kalbach, H., Buck, P., van Kuijk, J. Vitamin E in the macular and peripheral tissues of the human eye. Curr Eye Res. 1995; 14: 693–701.
41. Castorina, C., Campisi, A., Di Giacomo, C., Sorrenti, V., Russo, A., Vanella, A. Lipid peroxidation and antioxidant enzymatic systems in rat retina as a function of age. Neurochem Res. 1992; 17: 599–604.
42. Liles, M.R., Newsome, D.A., Oliver, D. Antioxidant enzymes in the aging human retinal pigment epithelium. Arch Ophthalmol. 1991; 109: 1285–1288.
43. Hogan, M.J., Alvarado, J.A., Weddell, J.E. Histology of the Human Eye. Philadelphia: Saunders, 1971.
44. Feeney-Burns, L., Burns, R.P., Gao, C.L. Age-related macular changes in humans over 90 years old. Am J Ophthalmol. 1990; 109: 265–278.
45. van der Schaft, T.L., de Bruijn, W.C., Mooy, C.M., de Jong, P.T. Basal laminar deposits in the ageing peripheral retina. Graefes Arch Clin Exp Ophthalmol. 1993; 231: 470–475.
46. Garner, A., Sarks, S., Sarks, J.P. Degenerative and related disorders of the retina and choroid. In: Garner, A., Klintworth, G.K. (eds), Pathobiology of Ocular Disease. Dekker: New York, 1994: 631–674.
47. Pauleikhoff, D., Harper, A., Marshall, J., Bird, A.C. Aging changes in Bruch's membrane: a histochemical and morphological study. Ophthalmology. 1990; 97: 171–178.
48. Sheraidah, G., Steinmetz, R., Maguire, J., Pauliekhoff, D., Marshall, J., Bird, A.C. Correlation between lipids extracted from Bruch's membrane and age. Ophthalmology. 1993; 100: 47–51.
49. Holz, F.G., Sheraidah, G., Pauliekhoff, D., Bird, A.C. Analysis of lipid deposits extracted from human macular and peripheral Bruch's membrane. Arch Ophthalmol. 1994; 112: 402–406.
50. Sarks, S.H. Ageing and degeneration in the macular region: A clinico-pathological study. Br J Ophthalmol. 1976; 60: 324–341.
51. Sarks, J.P., Sarks, S., Killingsworth, M.C. Evolution of geographic atrophy of the retinal pigment epithelium. Eye. 1988; 2: 552–577.
52. Loffler, K.U., Lee, W.R. Basal linear deposits in the human macula. Graefe's Arch Clin Exp Ophthalmol. 1986; 224: 502–506.
53. Eagle, R.C. Mechanisms of maculopathy. Ophthalmology. 1984; 91: 613–625.
54. Pauliekhoff, D., Zuels, S., Sheraidah, G.S., Marshall, J., Wessing, A., Bird, A.C. Correlation between biochemical composition and fluorescein binding of deposits in Bruch's membrane. Ophthalmology. 1992; 99: 1548–1553.
55. Burns, R.P., Feeney-Burns, L. Clinico-morphologic correlations of drusen of Bruch's membrane. Trans Am Ophthalmol. Soc. 1980; 78: 206–255.
56. Ishibashi, T., Sorgente, N., Patterson, R., Ryan, S.J. Pathogenesis of drusen in the primate. Invest Ophthalmol Vis Sci. 1986; 27: 184–193.
57. Foos, R., Trese, M. Chorioretinal junction: vascular characterisation of Bruch's membrane in peripheral fundus. Arch Ophthalmol. 1982; 100: 1492–1503.
58. Gass, J.D. Drusen disciform macular detachment and degeneration. Arch Ophthalmol. 1973; 90: 208–217.
59. Segato, T., Midena, E., Blarzino, M.C. Age-related macular degeneration. Ageing. 1993; 5: 165–176.
60. Hyman, L.G., Lilienfeld, A.M., Ferris, F.L., Fine, S.L. Senile macular degeneration: a case control study. Am J Epidemiol. 1983; 118: 213–227.
61. Korte, G.E., Gerszberg, T., Pua, F., Henkind, P. Choriocapillaris atrophy after experimental destruction of the retinal pigment epithelium in the rat. Acta Anat. 1986; 127: 171–175.
62. Sakamoto, T., Sakamoto, H., Murphy, T.L. et al. Vessel formation by choroidal endotheliala cells in vitro is modulated by retinal pigment epithelial cells. Arch Ophthalmol. 1995; 113: 512–520.
63. Miller, H., Miller, B., Ryan, S.J. The role of the retinal pigment epithelium in the involution of subretinal neovascularisation. Invest Ophthalmol Vis Sci. 1986; 27: 1644–1652.
64. Flood, M.T., Gouras, P., Kjeldbye, H. Growth characteristics and ultrastructure of human retinal pigment epithelium in vitro. Invest Ophthalmol Vis Sci 1980; 19: 1309–1320.
65. Boulton, M.E., Marshall, J., Mellerio, J. Human retinal pigment epithelial cells in culture: a

means of studying inherited retinal disease. In: Cotlier, E., Maumanee, I.H., Berman, E.R. (eds). Genetic Eye Diseases: Retinitis Pigmentosa and Other Inherited Eye Disorders. New York: Alan R Liss. 1982; 101–118.

66. Fisher, R.F. The influence of age on some ocular basement membranes. Eye, 1987; 1: 184–189.
67. Moore, D., Hussain, A., Marshall, J. Age-related variation in the hydraulic conductivity of Bruch's membrane. Invest Ophthalmol Vis Sci. 1995; 36: 1290–1297.
68. Starita, C., Hussain, A., Pagliarini, S., Marshall, J. Hydrodynamics of ageing Bruch's membrane: Implications for macular disease. Exp Eye Res. 1996; 62: 565–572.
69. Bird, A.C., Marshall, J. Retinal pigment epithelial detachments in the elderly. Trans Ophthalmol Soc UK. 1986; 105: 674–682.
70. MRC. Diseases of the eye. Working party report submitted to Neurobiology and Mental Health Board. London: Medical Research Council, 1983.
71. Egan, K.M., Seddon, J.M., Age-related macular degeneration: epidemiology. In: Albert, D.M., Jakobiec, F.A. (eds), Principles and Practice in Ophthalmology: Basic Sciences. Philadelphia: WB Saunders Co, 1994: 1266–1274.
72. Heidenkummer, H.P. Age-related macular degeneration: current aspects of pathogenesis and treatment. Eye Sci. 1991; 7: 6–20.

Department of Ophthalmology
Manchester Royal Eye Hospital
Oxford Road
Manchester M13 9WH, UK

5. Sub-RPE deposits might be related to defective ubiquitin-dependent proteolysis

K.U. LOEFFLER and N.J. MANGINI

(Frieburg, Germany and Chicago, USA)

Purpose

Sub-retinal pigment epithelium (RPE) deposits can be distinguished by their location, morphology and histochemical properties. Soft drusen and basal laminar deposit (BLD), especially, are considered of major importance in the pathogenesis of disciform age-related macular degeneration, and it has been speculated that certain components within these structures might be responsible for subretinal neovascularization. At present, however, not even the processes underlying the formation of drusen or BLD are known. Ubiquitin (Ub) is a member of the stress protein family that has been shown to be involved in the non-lysosomal degradation process of abnormal proteins, especially in neurodegenerative diseases. Using immunohistochemical methods, we investigate the human retina and RPE and in particular sub-RPE deposits for the presence and distribution of Ub and related enzymes.

Methods

We studied 30 human retinae from eyes enucleated for malignant melanoma or secondary glaucoma. Immunohistochemistry was performed on paraffin sections using antibodies (Abs) to ubiquitin (Ub), Ub conjugating enzyme (E2), Ub carboxyl-terminal hydrolase (PGP 9.5), and the photoreceptor proteins arrestin (Arr), rhodopsin (Rho), and phosphodiesterase (PDE). Immunoreactivity (IR) was tested using the ABC method, and results were visualized with DAB or AEC.

Results

In all specimens, Ub IR was seen throughout the retina, and Ub conjugating enzyme (E2) co-localized with Ub. Labelling with anti-PGP 9.5 revealed a specific pattern with predominant labelling of ganglion cells and nerve fibers, the inner plexiform layer and a distinct cell population at the outer aspect of the inner nuclear layer. Ub, as well as the related enzymes E2 and, albeit to

G. Coscas and F. Cardillo Piccolino (eds.), Retinal Pigment Epithelium and Macular Diseases, pp. 29–30.
© *1998 Kluwer Academic Publishers.*

a lesser extent, PGP 9.5 were also demonstrated in the RPE. Notably, sub-RPE deposits revealed a strong IR with anti-Ub but not with the related enzymes. Many drusen were intensely labelled, although there was some variation in staining pattern. Small sub-RPE deposits, probably corresponding to early BLD, were most consistently positive. Anti-Arr, anti-Rho, and anti-PDE staining was prominent in photoreceptors but also absent in drusen and BLD. No IR was observed at the choroidal aspect of Bruch's membrane with any of the Abs used in this study.

Conclusions

The presence of Ub and Ub-related enzymes in the RPE suggests that the Ub-dependent proteolytic pathway plays a role in the degradation and subsequent disposal of proteins from the RPE. The presence of Ub and/or Ub–protein conjugates, but not the related enzymes, in sub-RPE deposits could indicate that extrusion of otherwise indigestable material from RPE is somehow involved in the formation of drusen and BLD. Similar to the formation of extracellular deposits in some neurodegenerative diseases, one could speculate that certain proteins become ubiquitinylated within the RPE but that there is a defect in further degradation of the Ub-protein complex. Ub might be attached to somehow 'indigestable' proteins that are, therefore be extruded into the subRPE space. This could occur if the protein was too large to be processed by the proteosome complex. Alternatively, impaired degradation could be the result of a defect in the Ub processing system itself with subsequent extracellular accumulation of Ub–protein complexes. Our data do not distinguish these two possibilities. However, our data do support the concept that sub-RPE deposits are derived from RPE cells, and that these deposits are different from the age-related thickening of Bruch's membrane between the choriocapillaries. Using our technique, we could not demonstrate any of the investigated photoreceptor proteins in sub-RPE structures. This would indicate that they are not a major constituent of these deposits unless their configuration is altered in such a way that they are no longer accessible for the antibodies we used. Future studies will therefore concentrate on the further analysis of ubiquitinylated proteins within sub-RPE deposits.

Universitaets-Augenklinik
Sigmund-Freudstr. 25
D-53105 Bonn
Germany

6. Selective damage on retinal pigment epithelium causes photoreceptor cell death by apoptosis

H. MAEDA, N. OGATA, X. YI, M. TAKEUCHI, H. OHKUMA
and M. UYAMA

(Osaka, Japan)

Introduction

The retinal pigment epithelium (RPE) has a major role in maintaining the homeostasis and visual activity of the retina. Various pharmacological agents are known to affect the pigment epithelial cells primarily[1,2] or to affect the neurosensory retina and damage the RPE secondarily[3-5]. When the physiological functions of the pigment epithelium are altered the overlying retina is also affected, resulting in a decrease of visual function.

Ornithine is a non-protein amino acid which plays an important role in the urea cycle. Kuwabara *et al.*[6] and Ishikawa *et al.*[7] showed that an intravitreal injectyion of ornithine caused severe damage on the RPE and retina. However, these studies could not exclude the osmotic effects due to high-dose administration[8]. We showed that a small amount of ornithine selectively damaged the RPE with no initial effects on photoreceptors immediately after intravitreal injection[9-12]. It was of interest that the absence of RPE cells caused loss of the outer and inner segments, as well as the disappearance of the choriocapillaris and photoreceptor cells.

To determine whether the photoreceptor cell death in ornithine-induced retinopathy occurs by an apoptotic mechanism, we used TUNEL and electron microscopic analysis in rat eyes.

Materials and methods

We used 8-week-old Sprague–Dawley albino rats. The ornithine solution was prepared by dissolving L-ornithine hydrochloride (Sigma chemical Co., St. Louis) in physiological saline solution, pH 7.2, to a concentration of 0.25 mol/l (osmotic pressure 550 mOsm). We injected 0.01 ml of the solution into the vitreous cavity through the equator using a Hamilton microsyringe.

At 6 and 12 h and 1, 2, 4, 7, 14, 28 days after administration eyes were removed, fixed in 10% neutral buffered formalin fixation, embedded in paraffin, and subjected to histopathological examination. Apoptotic cells were detected using terminal deoxynucleotidyl transferase-mediated deoxyuridine

G. Coscas and F. Cardillo Piccolino (eds.), Retinal Pigment Epithelium and Macular Diseases, pp. 31–36.
© *1998 Kluwer Academic Publishers.*

triphosphate digoxigenin nick end labelling (TUNEL) assay, which stains the 3′-OH ends of fragmented DNA. We also used electron microscopy to detect the morphological changes of apoptosis.

Results

Six hours after ornithine administration, no positive signals were detected by TUNEL method: TUNEL-positive cells first appeared in the outer nuclear layer 12 h after treatment. Histopathologically, RPE cells were severely damaged and flattened. The outer segments of photoreceptors were also damaged; however, damage of the inner retina and choroid was not remarkable (Fig. 1). The number of TUNEL-positive cells increased with time exclusively in the outer nuclear layer. TUNEL-positive photoreceptor cells were most significant 2 days after treatment, while no morphological changes were observed in the outer nuclear layer, although the ganglion cell layer, inner nuclear layer,

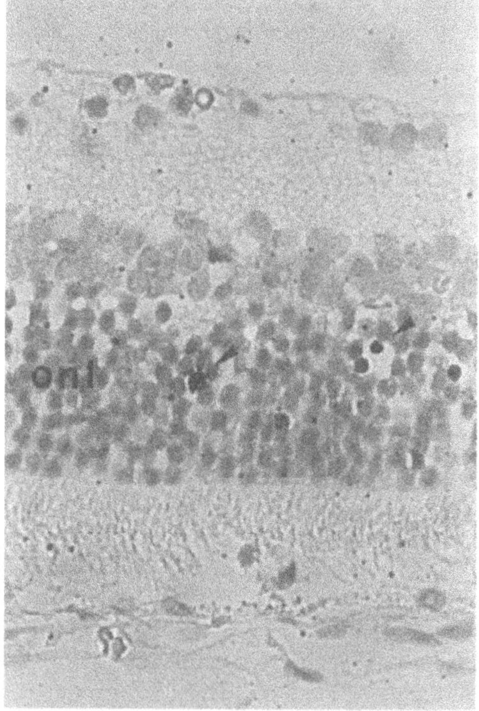

Fig. 1. In situ retinal labelling by the TUNEL method counterstained with methylgreen. Albino rat, 12 h after injection of ornithine solution. RPE cells were severely degenerated and became flat in appearance. TUNEL assay revealed a few positive cells (arrow heads) in the outer nuclear layer (onl) for the first time.

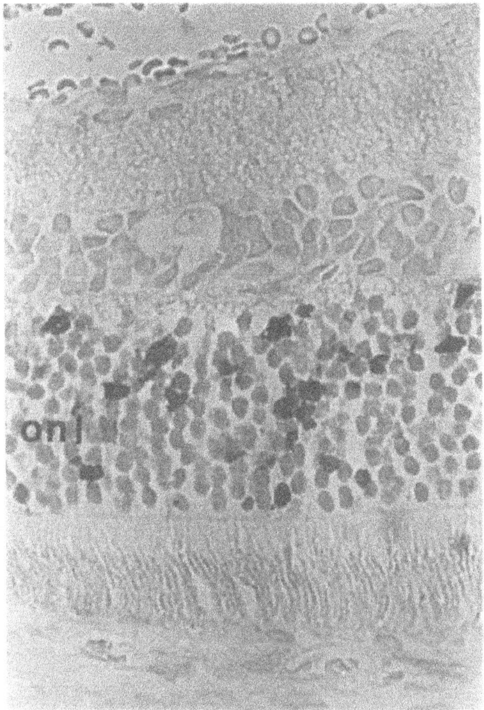

Fig. 2. In situ retinal labelling by the TUNEL method counterstained with methylgreen. Albino rat, 2 days after treatment. The retina maintained normal structure, although RPE cells were damaged and flattened. A large number of TUNEL positive cells were seen exclusively in the outer nuclear layer (onl), but the ganglion cell layer, inner nuclear layer, damaged RPE cells and choroid were negative for TUNEL assay.

damaged RPE cells and choroid were negative by TUNEL (Fig. 2). Electron microscopy revealed shrunken photoreceptor cells with pyknotic nucleis scattered in the outer nuclear layers.

Seven days after treatment, most of the damaged RPE cells had disappeared and the outer nuclear layer was disorganized. TUNEL-positive photoreceptor cells had markedly decreased in number. Fourteen days after treatment, the RPE cells and the outer and inner segments of photoreceptors had disappeared. The nuclei of photoreceptors were lying directly on Bruch's membrane and there were a few TUNEL-positive cells in the outer nuclear layer (Fig. 3). TUNEL-positive cells remained until 28 days after treatment when the photoreceptor cells had disappeared (Fig. 4).

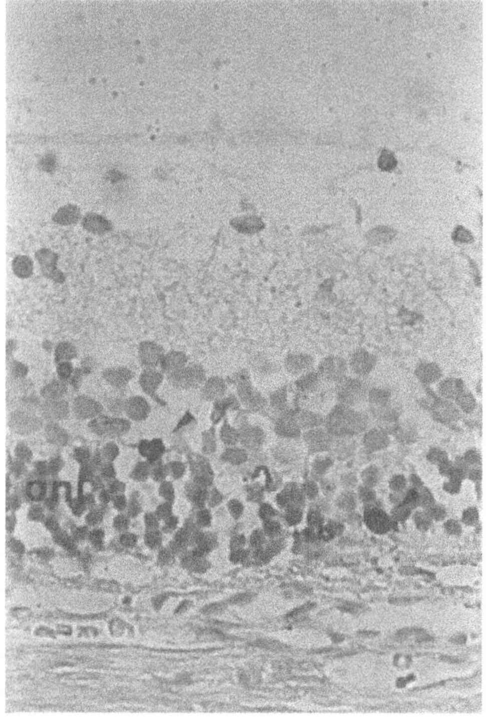

Fig. 3. In situ retinal labelling by the TUNEL method counterstained with methylgreen. Albino rat, 14 days after treatment. The RPE cells and the outer and inner segments of photoreceptors were disappeared. The nuclei of photoreceptors were touched directly on Bruch's membrane. There were a few TUNEL-positive cells (arrow heads) in the outer nuclear layer (onl).

Discussion

Apoptosis is a form of programmed cell death defined by characteristic morphological and biochemical changes. In the retina, apoptosis is observed in cell differentiation during the normal developmental process. Additionally, apoptosis is a primary mechanism of photoreceptor degeneration in retinal photic injury[13], experimental retinal detachment[14] and inherited retinal dystrophy[15,16] in mice and rats.

In general, it is difficult to distinguish *in situ* cells undergoing apoptosis by light microscopy. TUNEL is based on the specific binding of terminal deoxy-nucleotidyl transferase (TdT) to 3'-OH ends of fragmented DNA at the single cell level, and it stains early stage apoptosis in systems which precede gross morphological changes. In the present experiment, we observed apoptotic photoreceptor cells after intravitreal ornithine injection in rat eyes. Ornithine causes primary damage to the RPE; subsequently some of photoreceptor cells

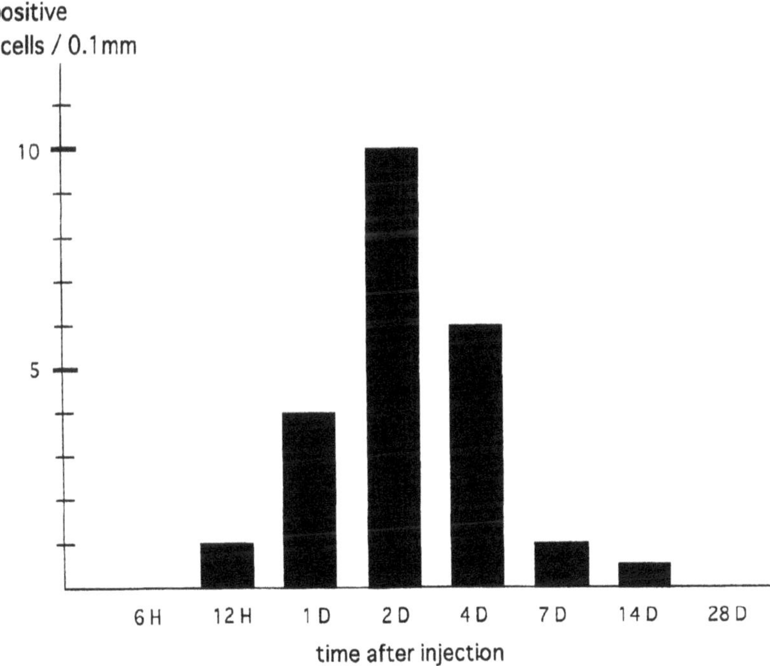

Fig. 4. Quantitative analysis of apoptotic cell death in the outer nuclear layer following ornithine injection. The first TUNEL positive photoreceptor cells were observed at 12 h after ornithine injection. The number of TUNEL positive cells increased through 2 days, then markedly decreased. TUNEL-positive cells remained until 28 days when photoreceptor cells had disappeared.

revealed evidence of apoptosis by TUNEL assay. TUNEL-positive cells were most significant at 2 days, before morphological changes were detected in the outer nuclear layers by light microscopy.

It is interesting that the damaged RPE showed no TUNEL-positive staining during all stages after ornithine injection. We suggest that this is because ornithine causes necrotic changes in the RPE.

As RPE cells play an important role to maintain the environment around photoreceptor cells, these findings suggest that dysfunction of RPE causes photoreceptor cell death which arises from apoptosis.

Acknowledgements

This study was supported in part by a Grant-in-Aid for Scientific Research from the Ministry of Education in Japan and the Science Research Promotion Fund of the Japan Private School Promotion Foundation. The authors thank Mr. K. Kobayashi for his technical assistance.

References

1. Lee, K.P., Valentine, R. Pathogenesis and reversibility of retinopathy induced by 1,4-bis (4-aminophenoxy)-2-phenylbenezene (2-phenyl-APB-144) in pigmented rats. Arch Toxicol. 1991; 65: 292–303.
2. Heywood, R., Gopinath, C. Morphological assessment of visual dysfunction. Toxicol Pathol. 1990; 18: 204–217.
3. Lasansky, A., DeRobertis, E. Submicroscopic changes in visual cells of rabbit induced by iodoacetate. J Biophys Biochem Cytol. 1959; 5: 245–261.
4. Gregory, M.H., Rutty, D.A., Wood, R.D. Differences in the retinotoxic action of chloroquine and phenothiazine derivatives. J Pathol. 1970; 102: 139–150.
5. Bellhorn, R.W., Bellhorn, M., Friedman, A.H., Henkind, P. Urethane-induced retinopathy in pigmented rats. Arch Ophthalmol. 1973; 12: 65–76.
6. Kuwabara, T, Ishikawa, Y., Kaiser-Kupfer, M.I. Experimental model of gyrate atrophy in animals. Ophthalmology. 1981; 88: 331–334.
7. Ishikawa, Y., Kuwabara, T., Kaiser-Kupfer, M.I. Toxic effects of ornithine and its related compound on the retina. Adv Exp Med Biol. 1982; 153: 371–378.
8. Marmor, M.F. Retinal detachment from hyperosmotic intravitreal injection. Invest Ophthalmol Vis Sci. 1979; 18: 1237–1244.
9. Uyama, M., Itagaki, T., Takahashi, K., Yamagishi, K., Ohkuma, H. Experimental ornithine-induced retinopathy. In: Zingirian, M. (ed). Retinal Pigment Epithelium. Amsterdam: Kugler & Ghedini, 1989: 45–52.
10. Takeuchi, M., Itagaki, T., Takahashi, K., Uyama, M.. Retinal degeneration after intravitreal injection of ornithine: 1: Early change after administration. Acta Soc Ophthalmol Jpn. 1990; 94: 1012–1023.
11. Takeuchi, M., Itagaki, T., Ohkuma, H., Takahashi, K., Uyama, M. Retinal degeneration after intravitreal injection of ornithine: 2: Late change after administration. Acta Soc Ophthalmol Jpn. 1992; 96: 161–168.
12. Takeuchi, M., Itagaki, T., Takahashi, K., Ohkuma, H., Uyama, M. Changes in the intermediate stage of retinal degeneration after intravitreal injection of ornithine. Acta Soc Ophthalmol Jpn. 1993; 97: 17–28.
13. Abler, A.S., Chang, C.J., Fu, J., Tso, M.O.M. Photic injury triggers apoptosis of photoreceptor cells. ARVO abstracts. Invest Ophthalmol Vis Sci. 1994; 35: 1517.
14. Cook, B,, Lewis, G.P. Apoptotic photoreceptor degeneration in experimental retinal detachment. Invest Ophthalmol Vis Sci. 1995; 36: 990–996.
15. Tso, M.O.M., Zhang, C., Abler, A.S. Apoptosis leads to photoreceptor degeneration in inherited retinal dystrophy of RCS rats. Invest Ophthalmol Vis Sci. 1994; 35: 2693–2699.
16. Chang, G.Q., Hao, Y., Wong, F. Apoptosis: final common pathway of photoreceptor death in rd, rds, and rhodopsin mutant mice. Neuron. 1993; 11: 595–605.

Department of Ophthalmology
Kansai Medical University
10–15 Fumizonocho
Moriguchi, Osaka 570, Japan

7. RPE lipofuscin in ageing and age-related macular degeneration

F.C. DELORI

(Boston, USA)

Introduction

Lipofuscin accumulates throughout life in the RPE as a result of oxidative damage to photoreceptor membranes. At old age, lipofuscin trapped in lysosomes is a major cellular constituent and can occupy as much as 25% of the free cytoplasmic space[1]. It has been postulated that excessive lysosomal accumulation of lipofuscin in RPE cells impedes metabolic activity of these cells and that lipofuscin contributes to the pathogenesis of age-related macular degeneration (AMD)[1-6]. These concepts are supported by the finding that elevated levels of lipofuscin in donor eyes are associated with decreased numbers of photoreceptors[7], and by the striking parallels in the age-relation and topography of lipofuscin in donor eyes and AMD[5]. Loss of visual function in inherited diseases such as Stargardt's disease[8] and Batten's disease[9] has also been associated with excessive accumulation of lipofuscin-like materials in the RPE.

Lipofuscin is a fluorescent pigment with a peak excitation in the UV and a broad range of excitation, from 300 to 500 nm[10-12]. The ability to excite lipofuscin with visible light made it feasible to elicit its fluorescence *in vivo*[13]. We have developed a fundus fluorophotometer for non-invasive measurement of the intrinsic fluorescence (autofluorescence) from discrete sites of the fundus[14]. The technique allows for the measurement of the absolute fluorescence intensity and for the determination of its spectral characteristics (which is essential for identifying the nature of the fluorophores). This report summarizes our findings in regard to non-invasive measurement of lipofuscin in normal subjects and in patients with AMD.

Methods

The fluorescence of the fundus is measured using a fluorophotometric method[14]. The fluorescence is excited using a xenon arc lamp and interference filters centered at 430, 470, 510 or 550 nm (halfwidth 20 nm). Excitation is focused in a 3° diameter retinal area for a duration of 180 ms (retinal radiant exposure 5–15 mJ/cm^2). The fluorescent and reflected light are collected from

G. Coscas and F. Cardillo Piccolino (eds.), Retinal Pigment Epithelium and Macular Diseases, pp. 37–45.
© *1998 Kluwer Academic Publishers.*

a 2° diameter sampling area (centered in the excitation field). Reflected light is eliminated by high pass detection filters, and the fluorescence, after dispersion by a monochromator, is spectrally analysed by a cooled optical multichannel analyser. The detection spectral range is 400–900 nm (spectral resolution 6 nm). Fundus reflectance spectrum are also recorded from the same retinal area by replacing the excitation filter with a neutral filter and omitting the barrier filter.

The subject's pupil is aligned under infrared illumination and the site of interest selected while viewing the fundus and using a fixation target. Each fluorescence spectrum measurement is followed by acquisition of a baseline spectrum to account for contributions of scattered lens fluorescence, stray fluorescence in the instrument, and dark/leakage current from the detector[14]. Acquisition of one spectrum takes 2 s and the entire protocol (two sites, fluorescence at four excitations, and reflectance) typically takes about 15 min.

All data are corrected for instrumental factors, excitation energies, and spectral sensitivity of the detection system. Fluorescence spectra are then individually corrected for the absorption of the ocular media (crystalline lens). This correction is based on an analysis of the reflectance spectrum acquired for each subject at 7° temporal to the fovea; the fundus is used as a reflector for a double pass measurement of lens optical density[15].

Results and Discussion

Intrinsic fundus fluorescence results principally from RPE lipofuscin

The spectral characteristics of *in vivo* excitation and emission spectra (Fig. 1) are in good agreement with spectra obtained for extracts of human RPE[10–12,16]. Although lipofuscin consists of at least 10 distinct fluorophores[11], only a few, the orange-red emitters, have excitation bands extending in the visible range. It is likely that the orange-red fluorophore VIII is the dominant lipofuscin fluorophore that is being sampled non-invasively.

The dominant fluorophore detected *in vivo* is located in the RPE (or its immediate proximity) based on the following evidence[16] first, lack of blood spectral signature on emission spectra shows that the fluorophore is located anterior to the choriocapillaris; second, foveal fluorescence arises posterior to the macular pigment since its spectral signature is superimposed on the foveal excitation spectra; third, fluorescence at about 15° from the fovea is affected by bleaching of rhodopsin: the fluorophore is located posterior to the photoreceptors; fourth, fluorescence from within a full-thickness macular hole has the same spectral characteristics as that measured at 7°T; the fluorophore is not located in the neurosensory retina; finally, fluorescence in patients with Stargardt's disease is highly elevated but the spectra have essentially normal in shape[17]. Increased accumulation of 'lipofuscin-like' material in the RPE is part of the pathology in Stargardt's disease[8].

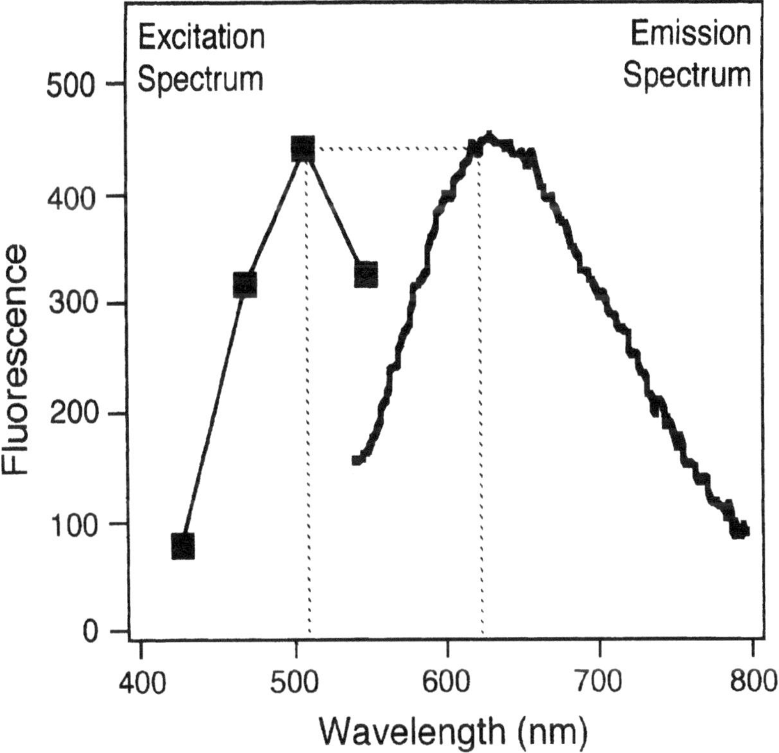

Fig. 1. Excitation spectrum (for emission at 620 nm) and emission spectrum (for excitation at 510 nm) recorded at 7° temporal to the fovea in a 54-year-old normal subject. Fluorescence is expressed in $(nJ.nm^{-1}.sr^{-1})/J$. The spectra were corrected for ocular media absorption.

Normal subjects

Fundus fluorescence is highest at the posterior pole, with a local minimum at the fovea, and it decreases towards the periphery[16]. This spatial distribution is consistent with that of lipofuscin distribution observed in donor eyes[3,18]. The foveal minimum is in part caused by absorption of the measuring light by macular pigment and RPE melanin (densest in the fovea). Using estimates of macular pigment density[19] and published RPE melanin densities[3,20], it can be estimated that fluorescence of lipofuscin at the fovea is about 20% lower than perifoveally.

Fundus fluorescence at the posterior pole increases significantly with age. In normal subjects, fundus fluorescence at 7°T (Fig. 2) and at the fovea increases significantly with age up to age 70 ($p < 0.0001$). This is consistent with observed increased lipofuscin in the RPE of aging donor eyes[18,21,22]. At age 70 the fluorescence is 3–7 times higher than at age 20. The emission

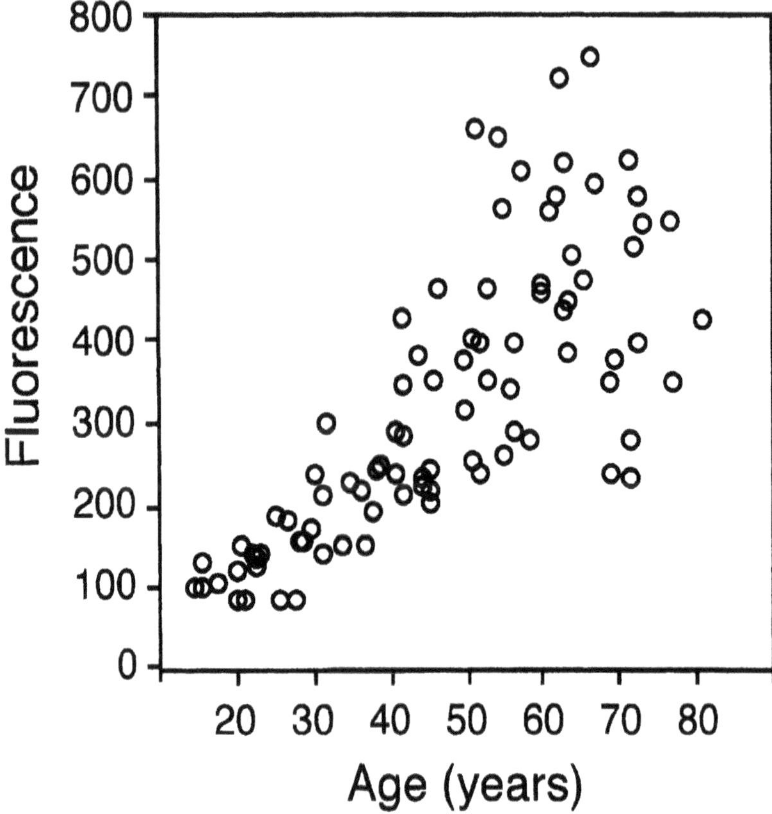

Fig. 2.   Fluorescence at 620 nm (excitation at 510 nm) in normal subjects ($n = 94$). The data are individually corrected for the absorption by the ocular media.

spectra have a remarkable constant shape for subjects below 60 years of age; the maximum is at 631 ± 4 nm (mean $\pm$ S.D) and the spectrum width at half height is 168 ± 5 nm.

Age-related macular degenerations

Fluorescence spectra in AMD, outside of areas of advanced pathology, are essentially similar to that of normal subjects. Fluorescence in areas of RPE atrophy is strongly attenuated, and the spectra are substantially distorted, often revealing absorption bands of choroidal blood superimposed on the weak fluorescence from choroidal collagen[23]. Fluorescence measurements over drusen show a shift of the emission spectrum towards shorter wavelengths. The magnitude of this shift increases significantly with the number of drusen present in the sampling field. It is, therefore, reasonable to conclude that lipofuscin fluorescence is augmented by fluorescence emanating from drusen (also observed in chemically fixed specimens from eyes subjects with AMD).

The contributions of lipofuscin and 'drusen' fluorescence can be separated by using template spectra (shapes) for the two fluorophores. The lipofuscin template was derived from spectra of normal subjects with high fluorescence (purest spectrum, minimally contaminated by minor fluorophores). The drusen template was derived from difference spectra obtained in two areas with many and few drusen. Templates for excitation at 510 nm are shown in Figure 3A, and an example of a spectral separation of a measured spectrum into its lipofuscin and 'drusen' components is shown in Figure 3B.

Lipofuscin and drusen fluorescence, derived from the total fluorescence by template analysis, are shown in Figure 4 as a function of age for the population of normal subjects and AMD patients. Lipofuscin fluorescence increases with age, and appears lower than normal in AMD. 'Drusen' fluorescence in normal subjects is relatively constant below the age of 60, and increases significantly above age 60. Drusen fluorescence in AMD is elevated, especially (and not surprisingly) when the measurement is made on drusen. These observations are confirmed by statistical analysis of the normal and AMD data in the age group 60–75 years (Fig. 5). Lipofuscin is reduced in AMD, the reduction increases with disease severity, and the changes are significant in all advanced AMD groups (IIIw, IV, and V; see legend of Fig. 5). Note that group IIIw, with more advanced AMD in the ipsilateral eye, have lower lipofuscin than in group IIIe. Drusen fluorescence is elevated in all AMD groups compared to normal subjects of the same ages.

There are several potential explanations for the decrease of lipofuscin in

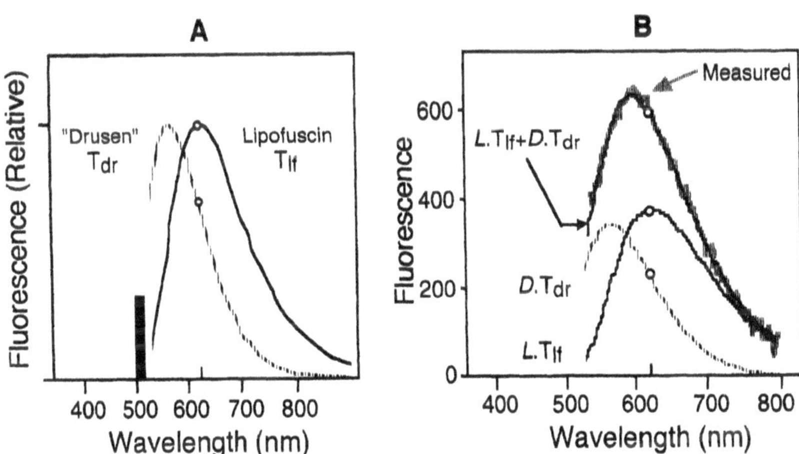

Fig. 3. A. Spectral templates for lipofuscin (T_{lf}) and 'drusen' (T_{dr}) fluorescence (excitation at 510 nm). B. Example of spectral separation of a measured spectrum into its lipofuscin and 'drusen' components. The measured spectrum is deconvolved into the sum of the 2 scaled templates; the scaling coefficients L and D are determined by fitting the sum ($LT_{lf} + D.T_{dr}$) to the measured spectrum. The fluorescence of lipofuscin and drusen at 620 nm is then calculated as $LT_{lf,620}$ and $D.T_{dr,620}$, respectively.

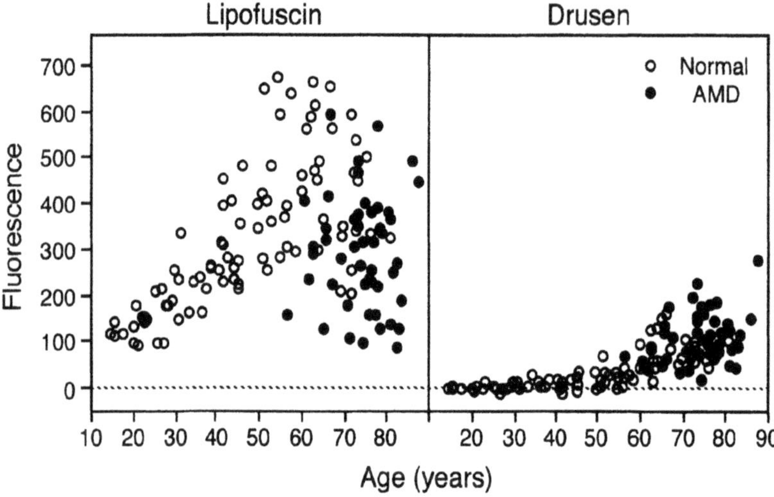

Fig. 4.   Fluorescence at 620 nm (excitation at 510 nm) of lipofuscin and of drusen for normal subjects ($n = 94$) and patients with AMD ($n = 48$).

advanced AMD. First, loss of cells in atrophy clearly lowers the detected fluorescence, but a study of donor eyes' RPE showed that intra-cellular lipofuscin is lower in AMD[5]. Second, fluorophore VIII (or A2-E), which is probably the dominant fluorophore detected *in vivo*, has been isolated and chemically characterized as a pyridinium bisretinoid[24]. This derivative has the potential to form micellar detergents and lyse the membrane enclosing the lipofuscin granule, releasing lipofuscin and lysosomal enzymes into the RPE cytoplasm, where they could cause cell death[25]. Third, loss of photoreceptors decreases the rate of formation of new lipofuscin, permitting turn-over to remove the accumulated lipofuscin from the cell. Finally, it is not possible to exclude the possibility that changes in the physical environment of the lipofuscin reduces its efficiency, therefore lowering the fluorescence, but not necessarily its mass. Each of the possible explanations listed above assume that the lipofuscin first reached some critical high level at which the disease started, and subsequently fell.

The fluorescence associated with drusen is inferred as it is increased at drusen sites and in AMD. This 'drusen' fluorescence is also evident in older normal individuals. This is consistent with this fluorescence originating from Bruch's membrane thickening and/or lipid deposits.

Conclusion

In vivo spectrofluorometry provides a rapid and sensitive measure of lipofuscin. Measurement of lipofuscin and drusen provides a useful tool to study

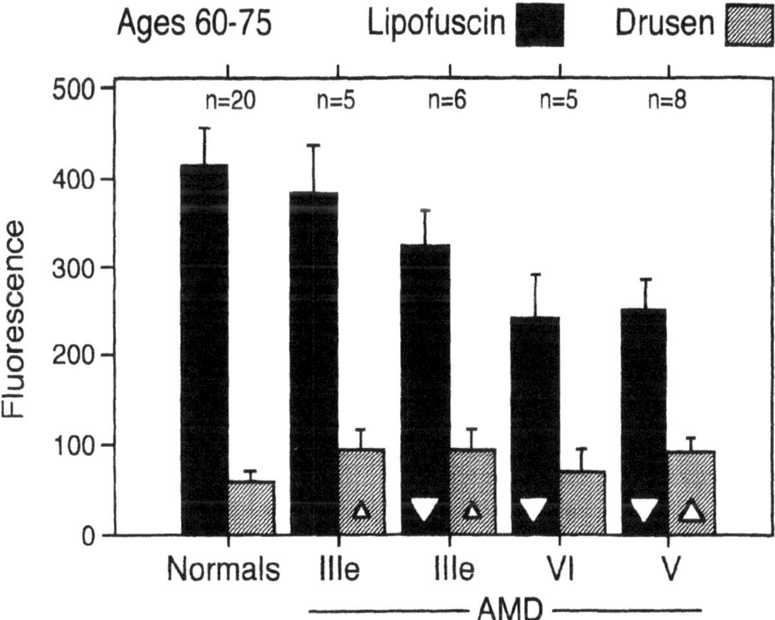

Fig. 5. Mean fluorescence of lipofuscin and of drusen for normal subjects and patients with AMD derived from statistical analysis (age adjusted) of the data of Fig. 4, for ages 60–75 years. AMD eyes are grouped as: IIIe: Eyes with initial AMD in both eyes (hard and soft drusen); IIIw: Eyes with initial AMD in tested eye, but advanced AMD in the other eye (IV, V); IV: Eyes with neovascular membranes, confluent drusen, and PE detachment; V: Eyes with any sign of atrophy but no neovascularization. Large triangles: statistical significance ($p < 0.05$), small triangles: tendency ($0.05 < p < 0.1$).

factors influencing lysosomal accumulation of lipofuscin in ageing, and to investigate relationships between lipofuscin and drusen fluorescence and the risk for development or progression of AMD. The recent introduction of techniques to image retinal autofluorescence[26,27] offers an opportunity to more tightly link progression at specific foci with changes in fluorescence. The combination of spectral and imaging techniques provide a powerful combination to investigate both basic and clinical aspects of the lipofuscin hypothesis.

Acknowledgements

The author thanks Dr Kathleen Dorey for her encouragement and collaboration throughout these studies, and Douglas Goger, B.S., for expert technical assistance. This work is supported by a Grant from the National Eye Institute (EY8511).

References

1. Feeney-Burns, L., Berman, E. R., Rothman, H. Lipofuscin of human retinal pigment epithelium. Am J Ophthalmol. 1980; 90: 783–791.
2. Boulton, M., Marshall, J. Effects of increasing numbers of phagocytic inclusions on human retinal pigment epithelial cells in culture: a model for ageing. Br J Ophthalmol 1986; 70: 808–815.
3. Weiter, J.J., Delori, F.C., Wing, G., Fitch, K.A. Retinal pigment epithelial lipofuscin and melanin and choroidal melanin in human eyes. Invest Ophthalmol Vis Sci. 1986; 27: 145–152.
4. Eldred, G.E. Questioning the nature of the fluorophores in age pigments. Adv Biosci. 1987; 64: 23–36.
5. Dorey, C.K., Staurenghi, G., Delori, F.C. Lipofuscin in aged and AMD eyes. In: Hollyfield, J.G., Anderson, R.E., LaVail, M.M. (eds.). Retinal degeneration. Clinical and laboratory application. New York: Plenum Press, 1993: 3–14.
6. Taylor, A., Jacques, P.F., Dorey, C.K. Oxidation and aging: impact on vision. J Toxicol Indust Health. 1993; 9: 349–371.
7. Dorey, C.K., Wu, G., Ebenstein, D., Garsd, A., Weiter, J.J. Cell loss in the aging retina: relationship to lipofuscin accumulation and macular degeneration. Invest Ophthalmol Vis Sci. 1989; 30: 1691–1699.
8. Eagle, R.C., Lucier, A.C., Bernadino, V.B., Janoff, M. Retinal pigment epithelial abnormalities in fundus flavimaculatus: a light and electron microscopic study. Ophthalmology. 1980; 87: 1189–1200.
9. Armstrong, D., Koppang, N., Rider, J. Ceroid Lipofuscinsosis (Batten's Disease). Amsterdam: Elsevier, 1982.
10. Eldred, G.E., Katz, M.L. Fluorophores of the human retinal pigment epithelium: separation and spectral characterization. Exp Eye Res. 1988; 47: 71–86.
11. Eldred, G. Questioning the nature of age pigment(lipofuscin) in the human retinal pigment epithelium and its relationship to age-related macular degeneration. In: Armstrong, D.A., Marmor, M.F., Ordy, J.M., (eds) The Effects of Aging and Environment on Vision. New York: Plenum Press, 1991: 133–142.
12. Boulton, M.D., Dayhaw-Barker, F., Ramponi, P., Cubeddu, R., Age-related changes in the morphology, absorption and fluoresence of melanosomes and lipofuscin granules of the retinal pigment epithelium. Vision Res. 1990; 30: 1291–1303.
13. Kitagawa, K., Nishida, S., Ogura, Y. In vivo quantification of autofluorescence in human retinal pigment epithelium. Ophthalmologica. 1989; 199: 116–121.
14. Delori, F.C. Spectrophotometer for noninvasive measurement of intrinsic fluorescence and reflectance of the ocular fundus. Appl Optics. 1994; 33: 7439–7452.
15. Delori, F.C., Burns, S.A. Fundus reflectance and the measurement of crystalline lens density. J Opt Soc Am. 1996; 13: 215–226.
16. Delori, F.C., Dorey, C.K., Staurenghi, G., Arend, O., Goger, D.G., Weiter, J.J. In vivo fluorescence of the ocular fundus exhibits retinal pigment epithelium lipofuscin characteristics. Invest Ophthalmol Vis Sci. 1995; 36: 718–729.
17. Delori, F.C., Staurenghi, G., Arend, O., Dorey, C.K., Goger, D.G., Weiter, J.J. In-vivo measurement of lipofuscin in Stargardt's disease/fundus flavimaculatus. Invest Ophthalmol Vis Sci. 1995; 36: 2337–2331.
18. Feeney-Burns, L., Hilderbrand, E.S., Eldridge, S. Aging human RPE: morphometric analysis of macular, equatorial, and peripheral cells. Invest Ophthalmol Vis Sci. 1984; 25: 195–200.
19. Delori, F.C. Macular pigment density measured by reflectometry and fluorophotometry. Noninvasive assessment of the visual system. OSA Tech Digest. 1993; 3: 240–243.
20. Gabel, V.P., Birngruber, R., Hillenkamp, F. Visible and near infrared light absorption in pigment epithelium and choroid. In: Shimuzu, K., Osterhuis, J.A. (eds) XXIII Concilium Ophthalmol Kyoto. Amsterdam-Oxford: Exerpta Medica, 1978: 658–662.
21. Wing, G.L., Blanchard, G.C., Weiter, J.J. The topography and age relationship of lipofuscin concentration in the retinal pigment epithelium. Invest Ophthalmol Vis Sci. 1978; 17: 601–607.

22. Okubo, A., Rosa, R.H., Fan, J.T., Luthert, P.J., Bunce, C.V., Bird, A.C. RPE residual body content, autofluorescence and aging. Invest Ophthalmol Vis Sci. (ARVO Suppl.). 1996; 37: 380.
23. Arend, O.A., Weiter, J.J., Goger, D.G., Delori, F.C. In-vivo fundus-fluoreszenz-messungen bei patienten mit alterabhangiger makulardegeneration. Ophthalmologie. 1995; 92: 647–653.
24. Sakai, N., Decatur, J., Nakanishi, K., Eldred, G.E., Ocular age pigment A2-E: an unprecedended pyridinium bisretinoid. J Am Chem Soc. 1996; 118: 1559–1560
25. Eldred, C.E., Laskey, M.R. Retinal age pigments generated by self-absorbing lysosomotropic detergents. Nature. 1993; 361: 724–726
26. von Ruckman, A., Fitzke, F.W., Bird, A.C. Distribution of fundus autofluorescence with a scanning laser ophthalmoscope. Br J Ophthalmol. 1995; 119: 543–562.
27. Hopkins, J., von Ruckmann, A., Fitzke, F.W., Bird, A.C. Fundus autofluorescence in age-related macular degeneration. Invest Ophthalmol Vis Sci. (ARVO Suppl.). 1996; 37: 115.

Schepens Eye Research Institute
and Harvard Medical School
Boston
MA
USA

8. Antioxidant functions of glutathione in human retinal pigment epithelium in relation to age-related macular degeneration

J.C. KURTZ, D.P. JONES, P. STERNBERG, JR., M.W. WU
and W. OLSEN
(Atlanta, GA, USA)

Introduction

Age-related macular degeneration (ARMD) is the leading cause of severe visual loss in the western world in people over 50 years of age[1-3]. Unfortunately, no effective preventive or treatment strategy for the disease exists. The mechanistic basis for development and progression of ARMD is not clearly understood but may involve degenerative changes to Bruch's membrane, damage to choroidal vasculature, or oxidative injury to the retinal pigment epithelial (RPE) photoreceptor complex[4,5].

Several observations support the interpretation that oxidative damage plays a key role in the occurrence and progression of ARMD. The RPE photoreceptor complex is exposed to oxidative stress as a consequence of daily light exposure with associated free radical formation and lipid peroxidation[4,5]. Photoreceptor outer segments contain a high concentration of fatty acids and are exposed to a high partial pressure of oxygen, a condition which predisposes the macular region to lipid peroxidation[4]. An age-related increase in retinal tissue peroxidation in this region has been reported[6]. Pathological studies show that the main source of vision loss is at the level of the photoreceptors; however, photoreceptor loss appears to be secondary to damage to the RPE cells, suggesting that the RPE cells are the site of primary injury[4].

Because oxidative injury appears to be a contributing factor to ARMD, protection of the RPE and retina may be achieved by enhancing antioxidant systems. We have investigated the potential role of the antioxidant, glutathione (GSH), in protecting RPE cells against oxidative injury. Glutathione is a naturally occurring tripeptide (γ-glu-cys-gly) which is the major nonprotein thiol compound present in RPE cells. GSH can function in several ways to protect against oxidative injury. Among the most important and well characterized functions is its role in reduction of hydrogen peroxide and lipid hydroperoxides. Peroxides generated during lipid peroxidation are normally metabolized by glutathione peroxidase (GSH Px), an enzyme dependent on GSH availability. GSH Px specifically uses GSH as a hydrogen donor to reduce hydroperoxides to their corresponding alcohols. GSH also functions

G. Coscas and F. Cardillo Piccolino (eds.), Retinal Pigment Epithelium and Macular Diseases, pp. 47–57.
© *1998 Kluwer Academic Publishers.*

in cellular protection by maintaining vitamin C (ascorbate) in its reduced form, which protects against free radical injury[7]. Because vitamin C maintains vitamin E (α-tocopherol) in its reduced and functional form, GSH indirectly can improve vitamin E-dependent antioxidant activities. In addition, GSH is used to detoxify reactive electrophiles, such as in 4-hydroxynonenol, a mutagenic product of lipid peroxidation[8].

Cultured human RPE cells as a model for oxidative injury

Oxidative cell injury in the human retina cannot be readily studied in humans *in vivo*; however, human RPE cells can be maintained in culture and they appear to offer a reasonable model for study of antioxidant defence mechanisms. In our studies, RPE cells were cultured from human donor eyes received from the Georgia Lions Eye Bank. Cells were isolated from autopsy eyes obtained within 72 h of death and grown to confluence. As a model for oxidative injury, we chose tert-butyl hydroperoxide (tBH), a relatively stable peroxide that is permeable to cell membranes. tBH is metabolized by GSH Px[9] and has been used extensively for *in vitro* studies of ocular injury. tBH induces oxidative damage in RPE cells in suspension (Fig. 1), in the range of 0.005–0.5 mM. Results showed that cell viability over 2-h decreased as the

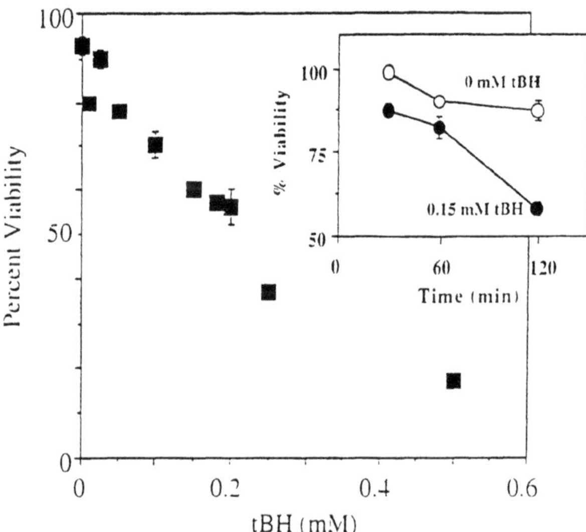

Fig. 1. Effect of varying concentrations of tBH on RPE viability in cultures prepared in suspension 2 h after treatment. The averages for experiments ($\pm$ SE) are given. The insert shows RPE viability as a function of time with or without 0.15 mM tBH ($n = 10$); RPE cells + 0.15 mM tBH ($n = 8$). Values for incubation with tBH were significantly different ($p < 0.05$) from control. Data from reference 22.

concentration of tBH increased. Further studies indicated that 0.15 mM tBH caused an approximate 50% loss of cell viability over 2-h. Thus, 0.15 mM tBH provided a reproducible model for cell injury due to peroxidation in cultured RPE cells prepared in suspension.

In similar RPE cell cultures grown in monolayer, a much higher concentration of peroxide was needed to elicit a measurable amount of loss in cell viability. Very little cell death was induced by 0.15 mM tBH; however, with 0.9 mM tBH, approximately 10% cell death was observed at 3 h (Fig. 2). By 24 and 48 h few dead cells were present, suggesting that the dead cells were phagocytosed by the remaining viable cells. This tBH-induced toxicity was exacerbated by inclusion of FeSO4 (0.68 mg/l) further supporting the interpretation that cell death was mediated by an oxidative mechanism.

Amino acid precursors of GSH protect RPE cell cultures from tBH-induced injury

The effect of precursor amino acids for GSH synthesis on tBH-induced cell death was evaluated in suspensions of RPE cells by adding a mixture of glutamate, cysteine and glycine 5 min before addition of tBH. Addition of this mixture at a concentration of 0.01 mM for each amino acid resulted in no detectable protection; addition of 0.1 and 1.0 mM demonstrated a concentration-dependent protective effect (Fig. 3). When cysteine was omitted from this mixture, no protection was observed at either 0.1 or 1.0 mM glutamate

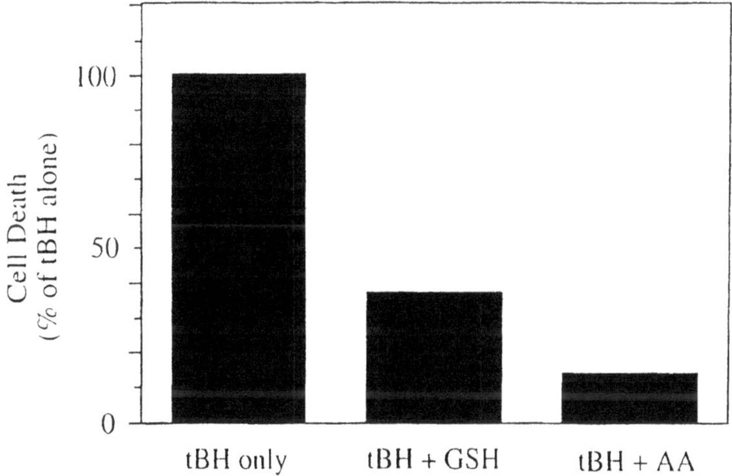

Fig. 2. Protective effect of GSH (0.5 mM) or the amino acid precursors (AA): glutamate, glycine and cysteine (0.5 mM) against tBH-induced (0.9 mM) injury to RPE cell cultures prepared in monolayer. Inclusion of either GSH or the amino acid precursors reduced cell death by 63% and 86% respectively ($n = 3$).

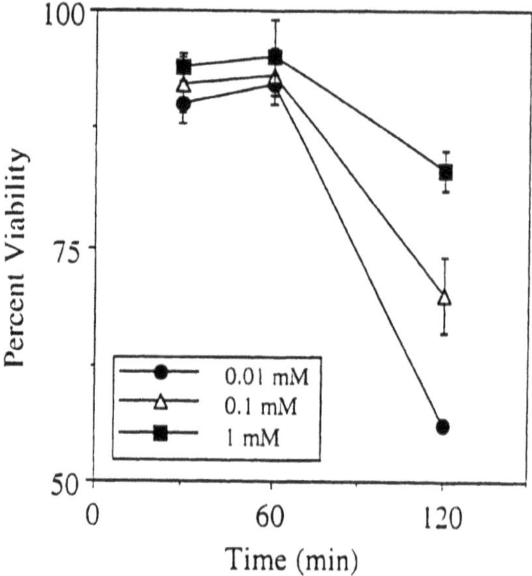

Fig. 3. Protection of RPE cultures prepared in suspension from 0.15 mM tBH-induced cell death by amino acid constituents of GSH. 0.01 mM glycine, glutamate, and cysteine ($n = 11$); 0.1 mM amino acid ($n = 11$); 1.0 mM amino acid ($n = 11$). Averages for experiments ($\pm$ SE) are given. Values for incubation with 0.1 and 1.0 mM amino acid were significantly different ($p < 0.05$) from 0.01 mM and control. In areas in which the error bar is missing the standard error is less than the size of the symbol. Data from reference 22.

and glycine. Similarly, cysteine alone did not provide protection. Therefore, the data showed that all three amino acid precursors must be present for protection against tBH-induced injury.

Similar experiments were performed on RPE cell cultures in monolayer (without resuspension). Results showed that inclusion of 0.5 mM of the amino acid precursors reduced cell death by 86%, demonstrating substantial protection against 0.9 mM tBH toxicity (Fig. 2). Compared with experiments with RPE cells in suspension, cells in monolayers required higher concentrations of peroxide to cause toxicity and higher concentrations of amino acids to provide protection. Thus both cells in suspension and cells remaining in a monolayer show the same pattern of response.

GSH synthesis from exogenously added amino acid precursors in RPE cells

To determine whether RPE cells can effectively synthesize GSH from the amino acid precursors, cell cultures were depleted of GSH by the addition of diethylmaleate (DEM)[10]. DEM causes this depletion by forming a covalent bond with cytoplasmic GSH. The depletion of GSH in turn relieves feedback inhibition of GSH on γ-glutamylcysteine synthetase, the rate-limiting enzyme for GSH synthesis.

Once cells were depleted of GSH and excess DEM was removed by washing with medium, the amino acids (1 mM each of glutamate, glycine and cysteine) were added to RPE cultures and incubated for up to 60 min. Results showed that the DEM treatment decreased cellular GSH by 84% and had no apparent effect on cysteine concentration or uptake. One hour after addition of amino acids, cellular GSH had recovered fully (Fig. 4). In two experiments, 0.2 mM BSO (an inhibitor of γ-glutamylcysteine synthetase)[11] was used to irreversibly inhibit GSH synthesis. Inclusion of BSO completely inhibited recovery of GSH.

Previous studies have shown that cysteine can be a limiting precursor in GSH synthesis[12]. In the blood, cysteine concentration is 10-fold lower than cystine (the oxidized form of cysteine). To determine whether RPE cells could take up and use cystine for the synthesis of GSH, we performed the same DEM pretreatment described previously and incubated cell cultures with 1 mM cystine, glutamate and glycine. Cellular cysteine was not increased, and a negligible increase in cellular GSH occurred during a 60 min incubation (data not shown). Thus cystine is not effectively taken up and used for GSH synthesis. These findings suggest that alterations in blood cysteine may be important in determining whether RPE cells are supplied with amounts of cysteine adequate for GSH synthesis.

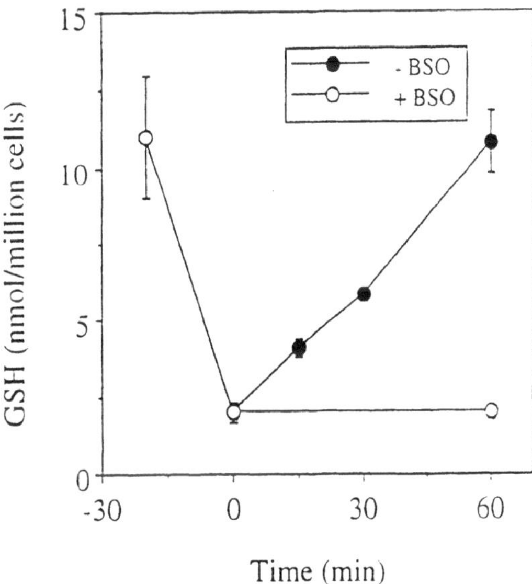

Fig. 4. GSH accumulation in RPE cultures prepared in suspension after depletion with diethylmaleate and incubation with amino acid precursors, in absence and presence of 0.2 mM buthionine sulfoximine. Data represent mean ($\pm$ SEM) ($n = 8$). Data from reference 23.

To determine whether the protection against tBH toxicity that occurred with amino acids was due to GSH synthesis, experiments were performed with DEM and BSO as described above. BSO blocked the ability of the amino acids to protect against tBH-induced toxicity (data not shown). Thus, the precursor amino acids protect against tBH-induced damage only if they are used for synthesis of GSH. This shows that maintenance of intracellular GSH in cultured human RPE cells is critical for protection against peroxide-induced cell death.

Exogenous GSH protects RPE cells

To assess whether the direct addition of GSH could protect against tBH-induced injury, suspensions of RPE cells that were not pretreated with DEM were preincubated with or without a near-physiological plasma GSH concentration (0.01 mM). tBH-treated cells without GSH showed an approximate 50% loss in cell viability at 2 h. Those cells pre-treated with 0.01 mM GSH showed little loss in cell viability and were protected significantly relative to cells without GSH (Fig. 5). Higher GSH concentration also provided protection, but at 0.001 mM the protective effect was only about 40% of that with 0.01 mM. Addition of BSO did not affect the ability of exogenous GSH to protect against tBH-induced injury. The lack of effect due to BSO and the

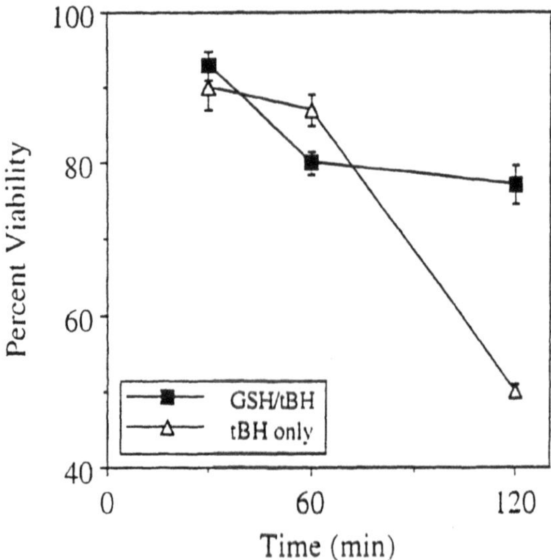

Fig. 5. Protection of RPE cultures prepared in suspension from tBH-induced injury by exogenous GSH. RPE cells + 0.15 mM tBH ($n = 34$); RPE cells + 0.01 mM GSH + 0.15 mM tBH ($n = 11$). Averages for experiments ($\pm$ SE) are given. Values for incubation with GSH were significantly different ($p < 0.05$) from those for incubation with tBH alone at 120 min. Data from reference 22.

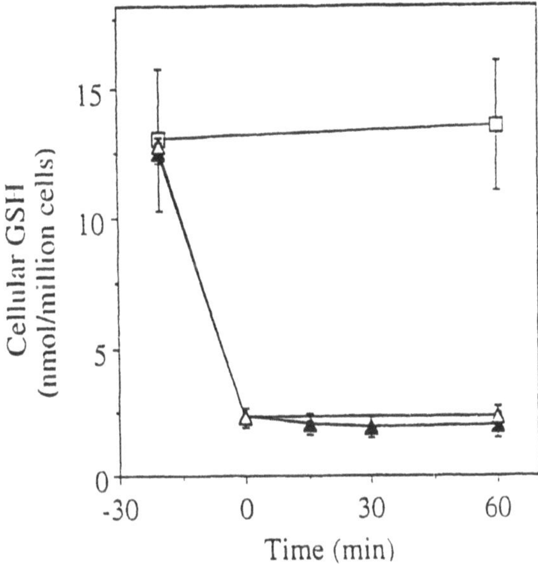

Fig. 6.   Effect of extracellular GSH concentration on intracellular GSH concentration. Control incubations were not treated with diethylmaleate but were incubated with 0.1 mM GSH (□). Cells treated with diethylmaleate and then without GSH showed no change in cellular GSH after depletion (△). Cells treated with diethylmaleate and then with 0.1 mM GSH showed no significant change from 0 min to 60 min (▲). Data represent mean ±SEM ($n = 6$). Data from reference 23.

protection by GSH at a 10-fold lower concentration than observed with the amino acid precursors, indicates that protection by exogenous GSH occurs by a different mechanism to that of the amino acids.

Similar experiments were performed in RPE cell cultures in monolayer. Results showed that inclusion of 0.5 mM GSH reduced cell death by 63%, demonstrating a similar pattern of responses but over a different concentration range (Fig. 2).

GSH transport and uptake

The above results show that a supply of amino acid precursors for GSH synthesis improved RPE cell resistance to oxidative injury by tBH. In addition, exogenous GSH offered protection but apparently did not depend upon GSH synthesis. These findings suggested that GSH may protect by being transported into RPE cells rather than undergoing degradation and supply of amino acid precursors. To determine whether net uptake of GSH occurs, cells were treated with DEM to deplete GSH and incubated with 0.1 mM GSH. No increase in cellular GSH occurred even after 60 min incubation (Fig. 5), indicating that net uptake does not occur at lower physiological concentrations of GSH. Thus, the results suggest that exogenously added GSH protects by a different mechanism than intracellular GSH. Such differences could occur if intracellular GSH is used to stimulate elimination of peroxides while extracellular GSH is used to protect cell surface proteins from oxidation.

Potential mechanisms of protection offered by amino acid precursors and intact GSH

In the experiments discussed, we imposed an oxidant load on RPE cells and showed that the amino acid precursors of GSH protect against oxidant-induced injury. Exogenously added GSH also protected against tBH-induced damage. Protection occurred at near-physiological concentrations (0.1 mM amino acids, 0.01 mM GSH), but the data suggested two different protective mechanisms. Protection by the amino acids is prevented by BSO, a known inhibitor of GSH synthesis. In contrast, protection by intact GSH was not inhibited by BSO. Thus, amino acid-dependent protection seems to involve intracellular GSH synthesis, whereas GSH-dependent protection does not. This conclusion is supported by the observation that a 10-fold lower concentration of GSH is needed for protection. Thus GSH degradation to its amino acids and subsequent intracellular resynthesis cannot account for the protection by exogenously added GSH.

The non-enzymatic reaction in the incubation medium of GSH with tBH is very slow (data not shown); thus extracellular metabolism of tBH does not appear to contribute significantly to the protection. Direct measurement of the GSH peroxidase-catalysed reduction of tBH in the cells and extracellular medium after 30 min incubation showed that $98.6 \pm 0.2\%$ ($n = 3$) of the activity was associated with cells, further supporting this interpretation[9]. In studies of effects of GSH on peroxide elimination by RPE cells, we detected no significant stimulation of peroxide elimination by exogenously added GSH (data not shown). We also examined whether GSH protects the Na^+/K^+ ATPase pump from oxidative damage and have found no protection. Thus, at present, we do not know whether the protection by GSH is due to a direct effect of GSH on specific enzymes or transport systems. An alternate possibility is that GSH could protect by maintaining cellular redox state thereby protecting against oxidant-induced apoptosis.

A model for light-induced toxicity of cultured human RPE cells

Recent studies indicate that an association exists between long-term exposure to visible light and the development of ARMD[13,14]. Retinas examined in both human and animal studies demonstrate that visible light damage involves both the photoreceptors and the RPE[15-19]. However, past *in vitro* studies have not included a strict thermal control and results may have been influenced by hyperthermic effects. By using an incubator that provides a precise temperature control at the level of the cell culture medium, we developed a model to evaluate photochemical injury to cultured human RPE cells that eliminates a potential cytotoxic-thermal effect.

RPE cells were exposed (under controlled temperature conditions) to white light for 24, 36 and 48 h, and using a 12 and 24 h exposure followed by 12 and 24 h of darkness. Constant light exposure for 36 and 48 h resulted in significant cytotoxicity, while exposure for 24 h did not induce a cytotoxic response. Cyclic exposures of either 12 or 24 h did not significantly increase cytotoxicity. The extent of cell death was decreased when light intensity was decreased with neutral density filters. The results suggest that this cell model may be suitable for studies of the role of antioxidants in protection against light-induced injury without complications due to hyperthermic effects.

Age-dependent change in plasma GSH levels: pathological, nutritional and demographic factors

To gain some insight into the potential role of GSH in ARMD, we studied GSH status *in vivo* in an attempt to correlate GSH levels in plasma with ageing and with age-related pathologies such as ARMD and non-insulin dependent diabetes mellitus (NIDDM). Literature studies show that plasma lipid peroxide levels are increased in patients with photooxidative damage to the retina[20], as well as in patients diagnosed with NIDDM[21]. These high peroxide levels may be associated with an altered GSH/GSSG redox potential or a variation in GSH concentration compared with disease-free individuals of similar age or younger control individuals. Similarly, patients with ARMD may have a more oxidized GSH status in the plasma which could reflect the disease process or an underlying vulnerability to disease development.

To address this issue, blood samples were analysed for GSH and redox status in 40 ARMD patients (>60 years), 33 diabetic patients without ARMD (>60 years), 27 similarly-aged non-ARMD and non-diabetic individuals (>60 years) and 19 younger individuals without ARMD or diabetes (<42 years). Results showed a significantly lower plasma GSH level in older individuals (ARMD, NIDDM and controls) than in younger individuals. Analyses of whole blood GSH showed that GSH was significantly lower in diabetic individuals compared to the other groups, but did not reveal differences associated with ageing or ARMD. However, GSSG was significantly higher in the older groups than in younger controls, suggesting that the cellular GSH antioxidant pool was decreased with ageing. Because ARMD subjects reported a higher consumption of antioxidant supplements, additional studies with a larger population and a control for vitamin consumption will be required to determine whether differences in GSH concentrations and redox status can be correlated to the onset and progression of ARMD.

Summary

The present studies are consistent with the hypothesis that an age-related decline in GSH antioxidant status could contribute to the susceptibility to ARMD. Human RPE cells are prone to oxidative injury; when studied *in vitro*, this injury can be decreased by addition of GSH and its constituent amino acids. However, at present, a causal link between oxidative injury and ARMD has not been established and the molecular targets of oxidative injury to the RPE and the specific mechanisms of protection remain to be identified. Nonetheless, the results provide reason for optimism that means to enhance antioxidant defences, perhaps by stimulating GSH levels, can provide an effective approach to prevent occurrence or delay progression of ARMD.

References

1. Kahn, H.A., Moorhead, H.B. Statistics on Blindness in the Model Reporting Area 1969–1970. United States Department of Health, Education and Welfare Publication Number (NIH) 73-427. Washington, DC: United States Government Printing Office, 1973.
2. Leibowitz, H., Kruger, D.E., Maunder, L.R. et al. The Framingham eye study monograph; an ophthalmological and epidemiological study of cataract, glaucoma, diabetic retinopathy, macular degeneration and visual acuity in a general population of 2,631 adults. 1973–1975. Surv Ophthalmol. 1980; 24 (Suppl): 335–610.
3. Sorsby, A. The incidence and causes of blindness in England and Wales, 1963–1968. Ministry of Health Reports on Public Health and Medical Subjects, Number 128. London, Her Majesty's Stationery Office, 1972.
4. Young, R.W. Pathophysiology of age-related macular degeneration. Surv Ophthalmol. 1987; 31: 291–306.
5. Tso, M. Pathogenic factors of aging macular degeneration. Ophthalmology. 1985; 92: 628–635.
6. De la Paz, M., Anderson, R.E. Region and age-dependent variation in susceptibility of the human retina to lipid peroxidation. Invest Ophthalmol Vis Sci. 1992; 33: 3497–3499.
7. Winkler, B.S. In vitro oxidation of ascorbic acid and its prevention by GSH. Biochem Biophys Acta. 1987; 925: 258–264.
8. Esterbauer, H. Lipid peroxidation products: formation, chemical properties, and biological activity. In: Poli, G., Cheeseman, K.H., Dianzani, M.U., Slater, T.F. (eds). Free Radicals in Liver Injury. Oxford: IRL Press; 1985: 29–47.
9. Wendel, A. Glutathione peroxidase. In: Jakoby, W.B. (ed). Methods in Enzymology Detoxifiction and Drug Metabolism: Conjugation and Related Systems. San Diego: Academic Press; 1981: 325–333.
10. Shan, X., Aw, T.Y., Shapira, R., Jones, D.P. Oxygen dependence of glutathione synthesis in hepatocytes. Toxicol Appl Pharmacol. 1989; 101: 261–270.
11. Griffith, O.W., Meister, A. Potent and specific inhibition of glutathione synthesis by buthionine sulfoximine (BSO: S-*n*-butyl homocysteine sulfoximine). J Biol Chem. 1979; 254: 7558–7560.
12. Bannai, S., Ishii, T., Takada, A., Tateishi, N. Regulation of glutathione levels by amino acid transport. In: Taniguchi, N., Higashi, T., Sakamoto, Y., Meister, A. (eds). Glutathione Centennial: Molecular Perspectives and Clinical Applications. San Diego: Academic Press; 1989: 407–421.
13. Cruickshanks, K.J., Klein, R., Klein, B. Sunlight and age-related macular degeneration, the Beaver Dam eye study. Arch Ophthalmol. 1993; 111: 514–518.

14. Taylor, H.R., West, S., Munoz, B. et al. The long-term effects of visible light on the eye. Arch Ophthalmol. 1992; 110: 99–104.
15. Friedman, E., Kuwabara, T. The retinal pigment epithelium, IV. The damaging effects of radiant energy. Arch Ophthalmol. 1968; 80: 265–279.
16. Green, W.R., Robertson, D.M. Pathologic findings of photic retinopathy in the human eye. Am J Ophthalmol. 1991; 112: 520–527.
17. Hansson, H.A. A histochemical study of cellular reactions in rat retina trasiently damaged by visible light. Exp Eye Res. 1971; 12: 270–274.
18. Noel, W.K., Walker, V.S., Kang, B.S. et al. Retinal damage by light in rats. Invest Ophthalmol. 1966; 5: 450–473.
19. Tso, M., Fine, B., Zimmerman, L. Photic maculopathy produced by the indirect ophthalmo-scope. 1. Clinical and histopathologic study. Am J Ophthalmol. 1972; 73: 686–699.
20. Delori, F.C., Dorey, C.K., Staurenghi, G., et al. In vivo fluorescence of the ocular fundus exhibits retinal pigment epithelium lipofuscin characteristics. Invest Ophthalmol Vis Sci. 1995; 36: 718–729.
21. Tsai, E.C., Hirsch, I.B., Brunzell, J.D., Chait, A. Reduced plasma peroxyl radical trapping capacity and increased susceptibility of LDL to oxidation in poorly controlled IDDM. Diabetes, 1993; 43: 1010–1014.
22. Sternberg, P., Jr., Davidson, P.C., Jones, D.P. et al. Protection of retinal pigment epithelium from oxidative injury by glutathione and precursors. Invest Ophthalmol Vis Sci. 1993; 34: 3661–3668.
23. Davidson, P.C., Sternberg, P., Jr., Jones, D.P. et al. Synthesis and transport of glutathione by cultured human retinal pigment epithelial cells. Invest Ophthalmol Vis Sci. 1994; 35: 2843–2849.

D.P. Jones Emory University School of Medicine
Department of Biochemistry
Atlanta
GA 30322, USA

9. Electrical activity of retinal pigment epithelium evaluated by EOG and c-wave

M. FIORETTO, C. ORIONE, C. CIURLO, E. VOLPI, C. BURTOLO
and G.P. FAVA

(Genoa, Italy)

Introduction

The c-wave was first defined by Einthoven and Jolly[1] as a slow cornea-positive component of the ERG that develops after the b-wave. c-waves have been described in a variety of animals[2], including mice and rats[3,4], rabbits[5], cats[6-9], sheep[10], monkeys[11,12], and humans[13,14]. The cornea-positive c-wave voltage is primarily generated by the pigment epithelium. This was demonstrated by Noell[5,15] in a series of experiments on the rabbit eye. First, he documented the 'azide reaction', comprising a sudden rise in the standing potential across the eye after an intravitreous injection of sodium azide. Then he demonstrated that the pigment epithelium was the site of the azide reaction. Evidence of the involvement of the pigment epithelium in the generation of the c-wave was obtained by Brown and Wiesel[16] and by Steinberg *et al.*[9], who recorded intracellularly from pigment epithelial cells of the cat and found responses that were similar in time course and relative amplitude to the c-waves of the local ERG. These findings have been confirmed in the perfused cat eye by Niemeyer[17].

As ordinarily recorded, the c-wave has the spectral sensitivity of rhodopsin[18,9] but, as one would expect, the c-wave cannot be generated by retina alone, separated from the pigment epithelium[19-22]. The form of the c-wave in human eyes, as in other vertebrate eyes, depends upon conditions of adaptation and stimulation and presumably upon a balance of the various slow potential generators in the eye. The c-wave may be elicited in man by brief flashes or by longer steps of light, and both the amplitude and time-to-peak increase with the log of stimulus intensity or stimulus duration[23-26]. The eyes must be dilated and dark-adapted in order to record c-waves in man. Taumer *et al.*[24] have confirmed that if no mydriatic is used, a large pupillary wave is recorded that is independent of the c-wave. Unfortunately, there is enormous variability in the amplitude and waveform of the c-wave among normal subjects.

In 1980 the first paper appeared dealing with the clinical evaluation of c-wave in vitelliruptive macular degeneration[27]. In 1983 Sasamori *et al.*[28] investigated the c-wave changes in early stages of diabetic retinopathy, while in 1985 Rover and Bach[29] evaluated the significance of c-wave in hereditary degenerations of the ocular fundus. The same authors[30] compared the c-wave

G. Coscas and F. Cardillo Piccolino (eds.), Retinal Pigment Epithelium and Macular Diseases, pp. 59–62.
© *1998 Kluwer Academic Publishers.*

and EOG in retinal pigment epithelium diseases. In 1989 Moschos *et al.*[13] reported c-wave changes in macular diseases. The aim of our work was to evaluate the clinical value of c-wave in early stages of retinitis pigmentosa, comparing its amplitude to the EOG Arden Index and to the amplitude of the computerized visual field.

Materials and methods

Recordings were made using pupils dilated by tropicamide 1%, after 20 min of adaptation at 2.5 lux ambient illumination. An active Ag/AgCl electrode was positioned on the inferior orbital margin, with reference electrodes at linked mastoids and a neutral electrode on the forehead. Gain was 500 μV/div, time of analysis, 5 s and sweep velocity 500 mm/s. The stimulus was a full field white flash of 300 asb intensity at the eye level every 10 min. Five responses were averaged for each trace.

We examined 98 patients with retinitis pigmentosa, and selected 12 in whom the ERG was still recordable and the amplitude of the visual field was wider than 20°. These patients (four males and eight females, aged 31–44 years; mean $\pm$S.D. 35.6 $\pm$2.8 years) underwent to a complete ophthalmological examination including fluoroangiography, computerized visual field (Octopus 2000R program G1), ERG, EOG and c-wave recording. fifteen healthy subjects (six males and nine females) aged between 23 and 49 years (32.3 $\pm$4.6) were tested as controls.

Results

The mean ($\pm$S.D.) amplitude of the c-wave in controls was 323 $\pm$76.3 μV (range 128–487 μV). The mean value of the c-wave implicit time was 2025 $\pm$195.6 ms. The c-wave was well recordable also in all patients, but the amplitude was significantly reduced (132 $\pm$46.1 μV, $p < 0.001$ vs. normal subjects) and the implicit time was slightly prolonged at 2106 $\pm$141.9 ms.

The amplitude of the c-wave was directly correlated to the Arden index of the EOG ($p < 0.005$) and to the amplitude of the visual field ($p < 0.01$), but the statistical correlation between EOG Arden index and the amplitude of the visual field was greater ($p < 0.001$).

Discussion

Alterations in the c-wave have been studied in several disease of the RPE, including retinitis pigmentosa and Best's disease[27,31,32], and in these cases the c-wave amplitude is reduced, whereas the implicit time is normal. On the contrary in cone dysfunction syndrome the c-wave implicit time is pro-longed[33]. Probably the implicit time reflects the functional ability of the RPE–photoreceptor complex and only in the advanced stages of retinitis pigmentosa (not tested in our study) will this be involved. A limit of clinical application of the c-wave is that 10–15% of normal subjects do not have recognizable c-waves. Probably in these individuals the balance between RPE and Muller cell signals is biased more towards the latter. The c-wave may be considered more useful than the EOG for studying the RPE activity in retinitis pigmentosa, since it requires less time to record and might be less dependent on the integrity of the inner retina, but any of the above can be considered as a simple index of pigment epithelium disease. Both examinations may be useful as an adjunct to other tests to evaluate retinal function.

In our results the statistical correlation between c-wave amplitude and computerized visual field shows that the c-wave may be a good electrophysio-logical examination to monitor retinitis pigmentosa in patients in which the perfect collaboration required to record EOG is not obtainable.

References

1. Einthoven, W., Jolly, W.A. The form and magnitude of the electrical response of the eye to stimulation by light at various intensities. Q J Exp Physiol. 1908; 1: 373–416.
2. Kikawada, N. Variation in the corneo-retinal standing potential of the vertebrate eye during light and dark adaptations. Jpn J Physiol. 1968; 18: 687–702.
3. Keeler, C., Sutcliffe, E., Chaffee, F.L. A description of the ontogenetic development of the retinal action currents in the house mouse. Proc Natl Acad Sci USA. 1928; 11: 811–815.
4. Pautler, E.L., Noell, W.K. The slow ERG potentials in hereditary retinal dystrophy of albino and pigmented rats. Exp Eye Res. 1976; 22: 493–503.
5. Noell, W.K. Studies on the electrophysiology and metabolism of the retina. U.S.A.F. School of Aviation Medicine, Randolph Field, Texas. 1953; Project Number 21-1201-0004.
6. Brucke, E.T., Garten, S. Zur vergleichenden Physiologie der Netzhautstrome. Pfluugers Arch. 1907; 120: 290–348.
7. Granit, R. The components of the retinal action potential in mammals and their relation to the discharge in the optic nerve. J Physiol. 1933; 77: 207–239.
8. Tamai, A. The c-wave of the cat ERG. Yonago Acta Med. 1965; 9: 199–205.
9. Steinberg, R., Schmidt, R., Brown, K.T. Intracellular responses to light from cat pigment epithelium: origin of the electroretinogram c-wave. Nature. 1970; 227: 728–730.
10. Knave, B., Moller, A., Persson, H.E. A component analysis of the electroretinogram. Vision Res. 1972; 12: 1669–1684.
11. Gouras, P., Carr, R.E. Light-induced DC responses of the monkey retina before and after central retinal artery interruption. Invest Ophthalmol. 1965; 4: 310–317.
12. Fujino, T., Hamasaki, D.I. The effect of the occluding the retinal and choroideal circulations on the electroretinogram of monkeys. J Physiol. 1965; 180: 837–845.
13. Moschos, M., Brouza, D., Panagakis, E. Onde-c et patologie maculaire. J Fr Ophtalmol. 1989; 12: 651–656.
14. Marmor, M.F. Clinical electrophysiology of the retinal pigment epithelium. Doc Ophthalmol. 1991; 76: 301–313.
15. Noell, W.K. The origin of the electroretinogram. Am J Ophthalmol. 1954; 38: 78–90.
16. Brown, K.T., Wiesel, T.N. Localization of origins of electroretinogram components by intraretinal recording in the intact cat eye. J Physiol. 1961; 158: 257–280.

17. Niemeyer, G. c-waves and intracellular responses from the pigment epithelium in the cat. Bibl Ophthalmol. 1976; 85: 68–64.
18. Granit, R., Munsterhjelm, A. The electrical responses of dark-adapted frogs'eyes to monocromatic stimuli. J Physiol. 1937; 88: 436–458.
19. Yamashita, E. Some analyses of slow potentials of toad's retina. Tohoku J Exp Med. 1959; 70: 221–233.
20. Ames, A., Gurian, B.S. Electrical recordings from isolated mammalian retina mounted as a membrane. Arch Ophthalmol. 1963; 70: 837–841.
21. Foulds, W.S., Ikeda, H. The effects of detachment of the retina on the induced and resting ocular potentials in the rabbit. Invest Ophthalmol. 1966; 5: 93–108.
22. Dowling, J.E., Ripps, H. Adaptation in shate photoreceptors. J Physiol. 1972; 60: 698–719.
23. Skoog, K.O., Nilsson, S.E.G. The c-wave of the human d.c. registered ERG. I. A quantitative study of the relationship between c-wave amplitude and stimulus intensity. Acta Ophthalmol. 1974; 52: 759–773.
24. Taumer, R., Rohde, N., Wichmann, W., Rover, J. Experiments concerning the human c-wave. Albrecht von Graefes Arch Klin Ophthalmol. 1976; 198: 139–153.
25. Textorius, O. The influence of stimulus duration on the human registered c-wave. Acta Ophthalmol. 1977; 55: 561–572.
26. Marmor, M.F., Lurie, M. Light-induced electrical responses of the pigment epithelium: physiological properties and clinical significance of the c-wave, standing potential changes (EOG) and melanin response. In: Zinn, K., Marmor, M.F. (eds). The Retinal Pigment Eepithelium. Cambridge: Harvard University Press, 1979: 226–246.
27. Nilsson, S.E.G., Skoog, K.O. The ERG c-wave in vitelliruptive macular degeneration. Acta Ophthalmol. 1980; 58: 659–666.
28. Sasamori, H., Takahashi, Y., Mori, T., Tazawa, Y. ERG c-wave at the early stages of diabetic retinopathy. Doc Ophthalmol Proc Series. 1983; 37: 169–174.
29. Rover, J., Bach, M. The c-wave in hereditary degenerations of the ocular fundus. Doc Ophthalmol. 1985; 60: 127–132.
30. Rover, J., Bach, M. C-wave versus electro-oculogram in the diseases of the retinal pigment epithelium. Doc Ophthalmol. 1987; 65: 385–391.
31. Weleber, R.G. Fast and slow oscillations of the electro-oculogram in Best's macular dystrophy and retinitis pigmentosa. Arch Ophthalmol. 1989; 107: 530–537.
32. Moschos, M., Brouza, D., Panagakis, E. c-wave changes in macular diseases. J Fr Ophtalmol. 1989; 12: 730–731.
33. Moschos, M., Brouzas, D., Papantonis, F., Chatzis, V. c-wave study in cone dysfunction syndrome. Ophthalmologica. 1993; 207: 37–41.

University Eye Clinic of Genoa
San Martino Hospital, Pad. 9
L.go Rosanna Benzi no 10
16132 Genoa, Italy

10. c-wave of ERG in carriers of Leber congenital amaurosis

M. MOSCHOS, D. BROUZAS, M. TSALOUKI, G. RELATOS
and G. PAPADOPOULOS

(Athens, Greece)

Introduction

Leber's congenital amaurosis is a congenital retinal dystrophy characterized by profound visual loss from birth, coarse nystagmus, extinct ERG and the appearance of degenerative and pigmentary changes from the fundus. In a high proportion of the presented cases there is history of parental consanguineous marriage.

In 1869, Theodore Leber described a disease which he called a 'pigmentary retinopathy with congenital amaurosis'[1]. In 1871 he emphasized the familial nature of the disease and the frequency of parental consanquinity[2]. Later he differentiated congenital and juvenile forms[3].

Patients and methods

We studied the parents of two patients with uncomplicated Leber congenital amaurosis[4]: namely, four subjects mean age 29 years (range 19–33 years). The investigation consisted of medical and ophthalmic history, visual acuity, biomicroscopy, fundus examination, flash and pattern ERG, c-wave of ERG.

Recording of the c-wave of ERG was performed as follows. After 20 min of adaptation under mesopic conditions (4 lux), a stimulus was applied with an intensity of 300 Abs, and duration 1250 ms. To standardize this protocol, registrations were recorded from 44 eyes of normal individuals with 10/10 S.C. visual acuity, and no family history of any ophthalmological abnormality, with ages ranging from 7 to 70 years (Table 1).

Results

The data obtained from our patients are given in Table 2. The best corrected visual acuity was 9/10–10/10 from both eyes; the fundus was normal, flash and pattern ERG recordings were within normal range. The c-wave of ERG was nearly extinct or severely affected in all cases, with a mean amplitude of

G. Coscas and F. Cardillo Piccolino (eds.), Retinal Pigment Epithelium and Macular Diseases, pp. 63–67.
© *1998 Kluwer Academic Publishers.*

Table 1. Data from normal controls.

Case no	Age (years)	c-wave amplitude (μV)	c-wave implicit time (ms)
1	47	367	2100
2	47	388	2100
3	50	338	2250
4	50	415	2150
5	57	431	1900
6	57	465	1950
7	26	611	1900
8	26	648	1900
9	15	784	1800
10	15	723	1800
11	29	644	1850
12	29	681	1900
13	38	689	1800
14	38	513	1750
15	28	685	1700
16	28	661	1750
17	32	596	2100
18	32	522	2000
19	38	563	2000
20	38	589	2000
21	7	736	2150
22	7	812	2100
23	24	444	1950
24	24	473	2000
25	54	526	2000
26	54	491	2000
27	18	588	1700
28	18	570	1650
29	51	429	2000
30	51	442	2000
31	62	371	2000
32	62	390	2000
33	15	705	1650
34	15	738	1650
35	23	580	1650
36	23	608	1700
37	41	520	1700
38	41	539	1800
39	65	278	2150
40	65	309	2200
41	70	265	2200
42	70	292	2200
43	19	689	1750
44	19	678	1800
Mean	36.773	540.590	1925
SD	17.886	145.530	177.023

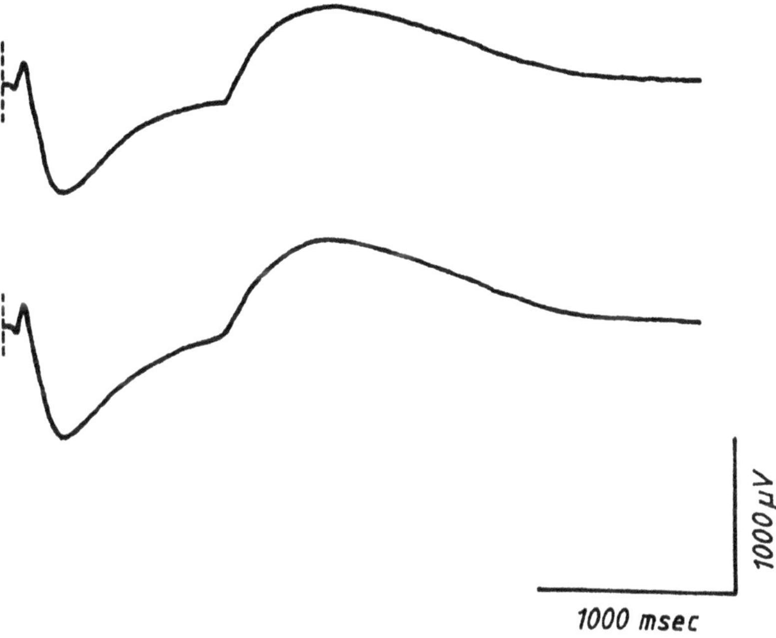

Fig. 1. c-wave of ERG recordings from a normal individual.

Table 2. Data from patients.

Case no	Age	Visual acuity	ERG	c-wave amplitude (μV)	c-wave implicit time (ms)
1	33	8/10	Normal	41.4	2350
2	33	9/10	Normal	35.5	2400
3	19	9/10	Normal	88.8	1550
4	19	9/10	Normal	100.6	1600
5	36	10/10	Normal	226.7	2150
6	36	10/10	Normal	189.8	2200
7	29	9/10	Normal	175.9	1730
8	29	9/10	Normal	221.5	1820
Mean	29.25			135.025	1975
SD	6.861			77.962	339.706

135.02 μV and mean implicit time of 1975 ms. In 22 normal individuals (44) eyes (mean age 36.77 years) mean amplitude was 540.59 μV (SD 145.53 μV) and mean implicit time was 1925 ms (SD 177.02 ms; Table 1).

Table 3 shows the statistical analysis between our patients and our normal sample. There is a significant difference between our patients and normals regarding the c-wave amplitude ($p < 0.001$), but no significant difference regarding the c-wave implicit time.

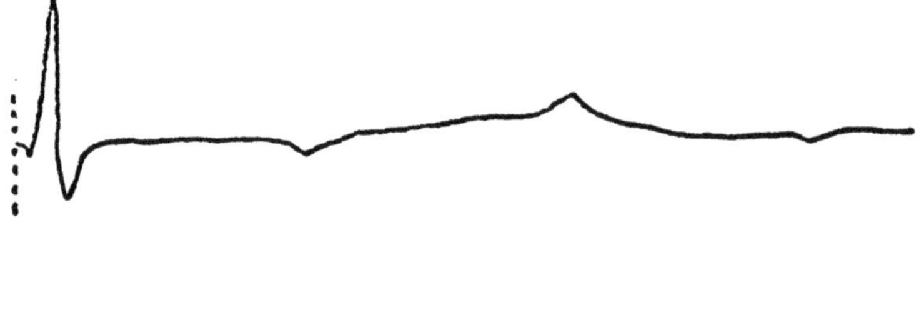

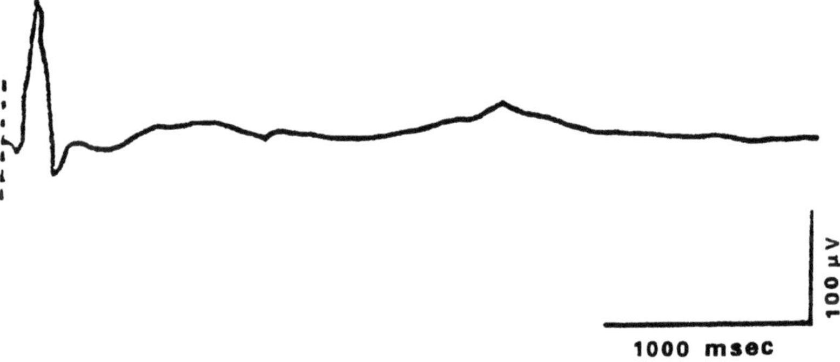

Fig. 2. c-wave of ERG recordings from our case 1.

Table 3. Statistical analysis, patients vs. normal controls.

	c-wave amplitude		c-wave implicit time	
	Patients	*Controls*	*Patients*	*Controls*
Mean	135.025	540.591	1975	1925
SD	77.962	145.530	339.706	177.023
Number of cases	8	44	8	44
SE	27.564	21.939	120.104	26.687
t-test (patients vs. controls)	7.642		0.627	
Fischer test	0.287		5.449	
z-test (patients vs. controls)	11.512		0.406	
F*	17.534		7.705	

*Modified degrees of freedom for the z-test to look on the tables of *t*-test.

Discussion

Up to now there has been no simple ophthalmoscopic or electrodiagnostic means to identify the carriers of the disease. In addition, it is impossible to record c-wave of ERG from a small proportion of normal subjects, and there is no reasonable explanation for this. The c-wave of ERG originates from the

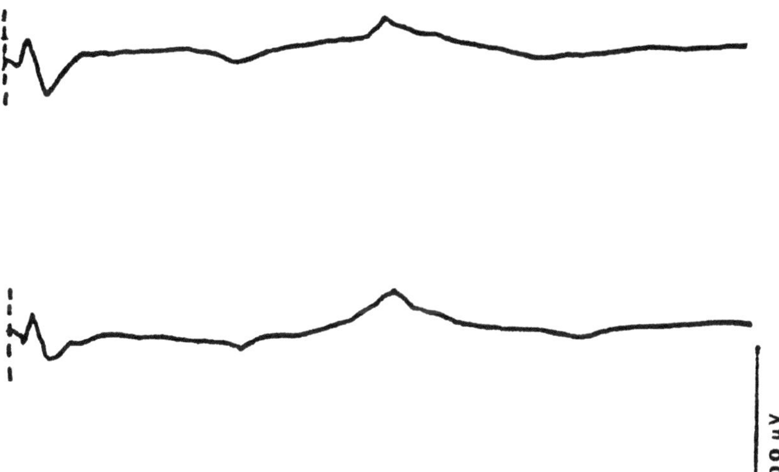

Fig. 3. c-wave of ERG recordings from case 4.

retinal pigment epithelium[5] and it has been suggested that the interactions between photoreceptors and the pigment epithelium play a role in the creation of the c-wave[6].

The above mentioned findings must be interpreted with some caution, given that the sample is very small and there is large variability of the normal data. A larger sample is required for conclusive evidence. However, in cases of consanguineous marriages an abnormal c-wave of ERG is highly suggestive of the disease.

References

1. Leber, T. Ueber Retinitis pigmentosa and angeborene Amaurose. Albrecht von Graefes Arch Ophthalmol. 1869; 15: 1–25.
2. Leber, T. Ueber anomale Formen der Retinitis pigmentosa. Albrecht von Graefes Arch Ophthalmol. 1871; 17: 314–340.
3. Leber, T. Die amaurosis durch Tapetoretinal-degeneration. In Graefe-Saemish Handbuch der Gesamten Augenheil kunde. II Aufl., Bd. 7, Teil 2, Kap. 10A. Die Krankheitem der Netzhaut, Leipzig: Engelmamm, 1916: 1025–1035.
4. Foxman, S.G., Heckenlively, J.R., Bateman, L.B. *et al.* A classification of congenital and early onset retinitis pigmentosa. Arch Ophthalmol. 1985; 108: 1502–1506.
5. Noell, C.K. The origin of electroretinogram. Am J Ophthalmol. 1954; 38: 78–93.
6. Heiling, P., Thaller, A., Bornschein, H. Slow potential of ERGin hemeralopia congenita. Doc Ophthalmol Proc Ser. 1973; 2: 219–224.

144 Kountouriotou Str,
18535 Piraeus
Greece

11. Congenital and acquired lesions of the retinal pigment epithelium

S. SCHNEIDER and W.R. GREEN

(Baltimore, MD, USA)

Introduction

The retinal pigment epithelium (RPE) is derived from neuroepithelium. At approximately the fifth week of gestation the primary optic vesicle invaginates to form the optic cup. The inner layer gives rise to the retina, non-pigmented ciliary epithelium, and iris pigment epithelium. The retinal pigment epithelium, the pigmented ciliary epithelium and iris muscles, are derived from the outer layer. The retinal pigment epithelium is the first tissue of the body to become pigmented, at about the fourth week of gestation[1].

The retinal pigment epithelium is a monolayer of hexagonal-shaped, low-cuboidal cells whose basement membrane forms the inner layer of Bruch's membrane. The apical villous processes of the epithelium closely appose the outer segments of the photoreceptors. The retinal pigment epithelium has many functions including absorption of light, metabolism of vitamin A, phago-cytosis of rod and cone outer segments, formation of an acid–mucopolysaccha-ride complex that surrounds the outer segments of the rods and cones and metabolite transport, and it is the site of the blood ocular barrier of the outer circulation.

The retinal pigment epithelium is a highly reactive tissue. Various responses include hypertrophy, hyperplasia, migration, membrane formation, hypopig-mentation, depigmentation, and degeneration[2]. Hypertrophic lesions of the RPE are sharply demarcated, flat, hyperpigmented areas that can be bordered by a thin rim of hypopigmented RPE and can contain hypopigmented lacunae. Microscopically, these lesions are composed of a single layer of enlarged cells with large, spherical, melanin pigment granules. Hyperplasia of the RPE, as opposed to hypertrophy, is an increase in the number of cells. Migration of the RPE and membrane formation can occur in two ways. One way is by passage of free desquamated cells or clusters of cells through the intraocular fluids or tissues. The other way is by proliferation to form continuous sheets along the surface of existing or newly formed surfaces. Hypopigmentation is due to reduced pigment and depigmentation represents complete absence or loss of melanin granules.

G. Coscas and F. Cardillo Piccolino (eds.), Retinal Pigment Epithelium and Macular Diseases, pp. 69–80.
© 1998 Kluwer Academic Publishers.

Congenital lesions of the retinal pigment epithelium

Lesions of the RPE can be classified as congenital or acquired. Congenital lesions include hypertrophy, hamartomas, combined RPE and retinal hamartoma, albinotic spots, albinism, and dystrophies.

Solitary hypertrophy of the retinal pigment epithelium (melanotic nevus)

These densely pigmented, solitary lesions are usually several millimeters in diameter and consist of variably enlarged RPE with large, spherical, melanin pigment granules (Figs 1 and 2). There may be central lacunae of depigmentation and a peripheral zone of less dense pigmentation. The lesions can have associated retinal vascular changes including capillary non-perfusion, microaneurysmal capillary dilatations and chorioretinal anastomosis[3]. There is variable degeneration of photoreceptor cells over the lesions and complete loss over areas of lacunar depigmentation. There may be thickening of the RPE basement membrane. Solitary hypertrophic lesions have, in the past, been confused with choroidal melanoma and led to unnecessary enucleation. This was the case in seven of 100 eyes reported by Ferry[4] and two of 41 eyes reported by Shields[5]. Solitary hypertrophy of the RPE may or may not be associated with familial adenomatous polyposis (FAP)[6]. In contrast to solitary hypertrophy of the RPE, the pigmented lesions seen in FAP are multifocal, bilateral, have an irregular border with a tail of depigmentation at one margin, are located more peripherally, have a haphazard distribution[7], and are of four types, one of which is solitary hypertrophy[7,8].

Congenital hypertrophy of the retinal pigment epithelium (CHRPE, bear tracks, grouped pigmentation)

These lesions are usually unilateral, non-progressive, discrete dark spots, that are uniformly pigmented with sharply defined edges. They usually number

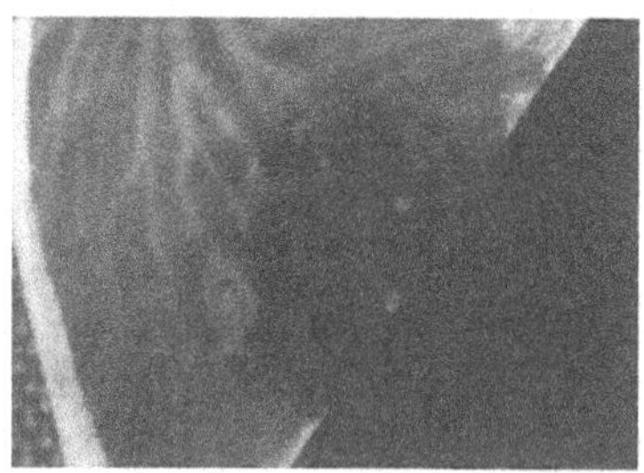

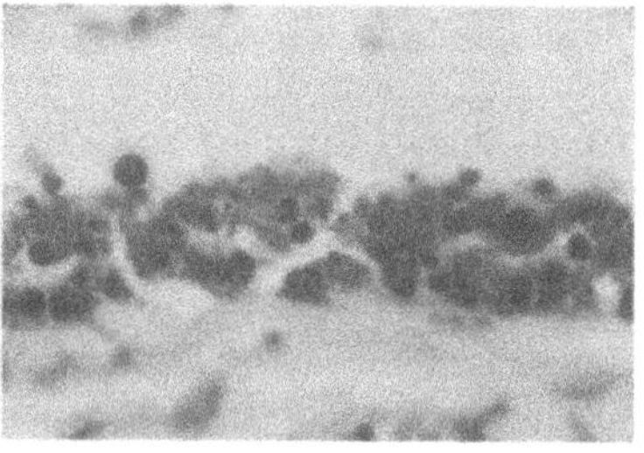

Fig. 1. Black appearance of a solitary area of hypertrophy of the RPE with a serrated margin.

Fig. 2. Lesion in Fig. 1 is composed of enlarged RPE cells with large spherical melanin pigment granules (partial bleached, haematoxylin and eosin, × 527).

between two and 30, with the largest spots located in the periphery (measuring up to 1 disc diameter) and the smaller spots located near the disc (measuring as little as 0.1 disc diameter). Typically, one sector of the retina is involved, usually temporally. Microscopically, there is an increased concentration of large spherical melanin pigment granules in the RPE cells in the affected area(s)[9]. The overlying photoreceptor cells are normal.

Familial adenomatous polyposis (FAP)

Familial adenomatous polyposis is inherited in an autosomal dominant trait. A single genetic defect has been localized to the long arm of chromosome 5[10,11]. This disorder is associated with the development of thousands of adenomatous colonic polyps in childhood or adolescence. If, in addition, extra-intestinal findings are present, the disorder is known as Gardner syndrome or FAP-EM. Extra-intestinal manifestations include desmoid tumours, benign soft tissue or bone (usually jaw) tumours, and/or extra-colonic cancers such as brain, thyroid, adnexal gland, and liver tumours. The presence of four or more patches of CHRPE-like lesions in children and young adults at risk for Gardner syndrome is a clinically useful predictor for the development of colorectal polyposis[11]. The RPE abnormality is in melanogenesis. Four types of RPE lesions have been described in patients with this syndrome[8,9]. In Type I there is a localized area of hypertrophic RPE, as seen with solitary and grouped CHRPE. In Type II a mound of pigmented cells is interposed between the thickened basement membrane of the RPE and the remainder of Bruch's membrane. Areas of nodular hyperplasia are present in Type III lesions while a mushroom-shaped mound of hyperplastic RPE occupies the full thickness of the retina in Type IV lesions.

Retinal pigment epithelial hamartoma.   RPE hamartoma, also known as congenital RPE adenoma or primary RPE hyperplasia, is a focal, nodular, jet black lesion measuring 0.5–1 disc diameter in size[12]. The lesion is usually located in the macula with full-thickness retinal involvement. The surrounding tissues are unaffected. The patient is usually asymptomatic and examination of the fellow eye is unremarkable.

Combined retinal pigment epithelial and retinal hamartoma.   Combined RPE and retinal hamartomas are slightly elevated, pigmented lesions with ill-defined borders. Most involve the optic nerve head and peripapillary retina. They may also be located in the retina away from the optic nerve head. Fluorescein angiographic findings include early hypofluorescence in the arterial phase and marked vascularity in the venous phase. Arteriovenous communications are sometimes seen. Leakage of fluorescein occurs from vessels within the hamartomas and not from the distorted, sometimes straightened, vessels peripheral to the lesions[13]. There may be an associated epiretinal membrane. These lesions are focal malformations composed of blood vessels and pigment epithelium that resemble neoplasms. These lesions usually occur in patients with no underlying systemic abnormalities. Because they are congenital lesions they may be an ophthalmic manifestation of the phakomatoses[14]. Some authors believe that these lesions are primarily a vascular lesion with secondary pigment epithelial hyperplasia[15]. Patients usually present with painless loss of vision. Depending on the patient's age, the differential diagnosis of combined RPE and retinal hamartoma includes choroidal melanoma, melanocytoma, reactive hyperplasia of the RPE, epiretinal membrane, glioma, capillary angioma, retinoblastoma and *Toxocara* larval infection. Two types of lesions are seen, papillary and non-papillary. Patients with the papillary type of lesion usually are young adults and complain of metamorphopsia.

Albinotic spots (amelanotic nevi of the retinal pigment epithelium).   In these congenital lesions the RPE is normal but lacking in pigment and the overlying retina and adjacent choriocapillaris are unremarkable[16]. Albinotic spots are usually solitary but rarely may occur in groups. The solitary lesion is round, sharply demarcated, measures 0.25–1 disc diameter in size, and is located in the mid-peripheral fundus. The grouped lesions, also referred to as polar bear tracks, are similar in size, shape, and distribution to congenital grouped pigmented lesions. These lesions can be unilateral or bilateral, are usually asymptomatic, and are seen in healthy children or adults[12].

Albinism

There are two main classes of albinism that affect pigmentation in the eye: oculocutaneous albinism (OCA) and ocular albinism. OCA is inherited in an autosomal recessive trait and is caused by the inadequate melanization of an apparently normal number of melanosomes. There are two forms of this disorder. One is tyrosinase negative and the other is tyrosinase positive. The tyrosinase negative form is associated with white hair, pale skin, photophobia, poor vision and nystagmus. There is a range of pigment variation and ocular findings associated with the tyrosinase positive form of the disorder. In ocular albinism, the pigmentary disorder is felt to be the result of a reduced number of melanosomes[17]. There is a high incidence of strabismus associated with ocular albinism, which is presumably due to aberrant visual pathway connections[18].

Ocular albinism can be inherited as an X-linked (XOA) or autosomal recessive (AROA) trait. One consistent finding in cases of XOA is the presence of giant pigment granules (macromelanosomes) in the pigmented epithelia of the eye and in keratinocytes and dermal melanocytes of both affected males and carrier females[19]. Giant pigment granules have also been described in the RPE of a fetus with XOA[20]. The presence of macromelanosomes in the RPE is a finding not unique to XOA. Other conditions in which giant pigment granules are present in the RPE include congenital and acquired hypertrophy, the Chédiak-Higashi syndrome, and Gardner syndrome. In AROA females are affected as severely as males. Biopsy specimens of hair and skin do not demonstrate the giant pigment granules found in XOA[21]. There is a range of pigment variation and ocular findings associated with ocular albinism.

Dystrophies of the retinal pigment epithelium

Ali *et al.*[22] list 15 macular dystrophies that principally involve the RPE: fundus flavimaculatus, Stargardt's disease, dominant foveal dystrophy, central areolar pigment epithelial dystrophy, North Carolina dystrophy, familial drusen, vitelliform dystrophy, pattern dystrophy of Marmor and Byers, foveomacular dystrophy (adult type), dominant slowly progressive macular dystrophy of Singerman-Berkow-Patz, butterfly-shaped dystrophy of fovea, macroreticular dystrophy of the RPE, Sjögren's reticular dystrophy of the RPE, pigment epithelial dystrophy of Noble-Carr-Siegel, and benign concentric annular dystrophy.

Dystrophies of the RPE fall into three morphological groups with atrophy, or at least hypopigmentation, of the RPE common to all[23]. The first group is characterized initially by predominantly whitish or yellowish lesions at the level of the RPE. Autosomal dominant drusen, fundus flavimaculatus, fundus albipunctatus and vitelliform dystrophy fall into this category. The second group is characterized initially by predominantly black, hyperpigmented RPE lesions and is further subdivided into autosomal recessive, autosomal dominant, and uncertain modes of inheritance. Sjögren's reticular dystrophy is inherited in an autosomal recessive pattern while fundus pulverulentus, reticular dystrophy of Benedikt and Werner, and 'pattern dystrophy' of Marmor and Byers are inherited in an autosomal dominant pattern. The mode of inheritance of macroreticular dystrophy is unknown. In the third morphological group of RPE dystrophies, the RPE is atrophic without any yellow, white or black lesions. Central areolar dystrophy and benign concentric annular dystrophy are included in this category.

Acquired lesions of the retinal pigment epithelium

Acquired hypertrophy of the retinal pigment epithelium

Acquired hypertrophy of the RPE occurs commonly in the peripapillary, and peripheral retina. Acquired RPE hypertrophy can be associated with choroidal lesions, serous RPE detachments, sub-RPE neovascularization, and at the margins of cobblestone degeneration, areolar RPE atrophy, and many other lesions.

Acquired hyperplasia of the retinal pigment epithelium

Acquired hyperplasia of the RPE may be seen in a localized or diffuse pattern. These lesions have a dark appearance and are usually associated with some other process. RPE hyperplasia can have a spiculate appearance due to the migration of pigmented cells into the retina in a perivascular location (Figs 3 and 4). Hyperplastic RPE always maintains polarity and this may give rise to a pseudoadenomatous appearance with the RPE arranged in double rows or in a tubuloacinar pattern (Fig. 5). Reactive hyperplasia of the RPE may occur over choroidal tumours. Hyperplasia with fibrous tissue and basement membrane production occasionally occurs over choroidal melanomas. Localized lesions of hyperplastic RPE can occur in association with healed chorioretinal scars, including multifocal choroiditis, toxoplasmosis and ocular histoplasmosis. RPE hyperplasia may rarely reach tumorous proportions, as reported in cases associated with lesions of ocular histoplasmosis and toxoplasmic retinochoroiditis[24]. Reactive RPE hyperplasia can simulate malignant melanoma and was the confirmed diagnosis in 4% of eyes enucleated for a presumed diagnosis of malignant melanoma in a study by Ferry[4] and in 6% of the eyes in a similar study by Shields[5]. Reactive hyperplasia, as opposed to neoplasia, usually contains evidence of previous ocular disease[25]. Microscopically, there is a conspicuous elaboration of basement membrane and collagen, no mitotic figures, and a lack of cellular pleomorphism.

Localized reactive hyperplasia of the RPE can also be seen in association with persistent hyperplastic primary vitreous choroidal infarction, macular

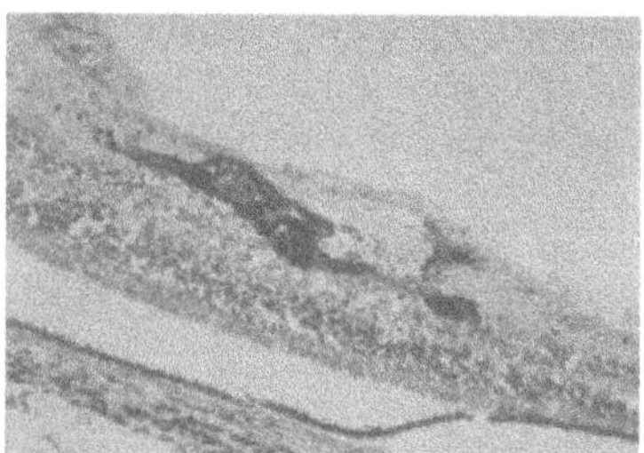

Fig. 3. Small area of hyperplasia of the RPE with migration into the retina in a perivascular location (haematoxylin and eosin, × 62).

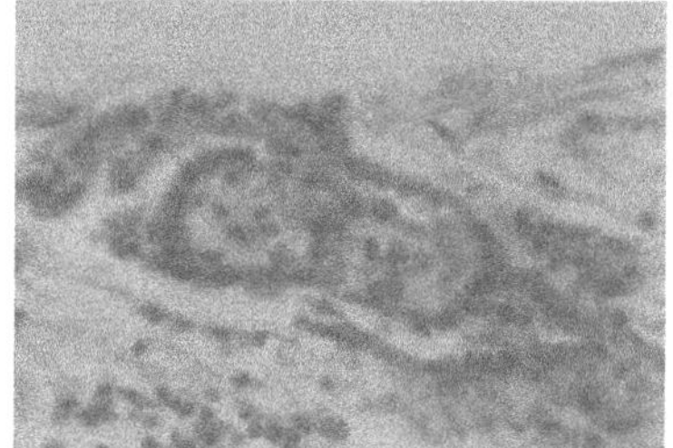

Fig. 4. Higher power view of lesion in Fig. 3 shows RPE surrounding retinal vessels (partial bleached, haematoxylin and eosin, × 248).

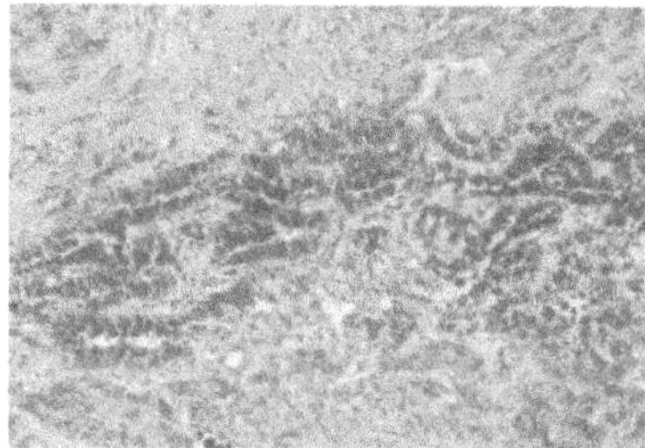

Fig. 5. Large nodule of hyperplastic retinal pigment epithelium arranged in a tubulo-acinar pattern (haematoxylin and eosin, × 155).

hole formation and experimental light toxicity. Examples of reactive RPE hyperplasia include Fuchs' spot and lacquer cracks in myopia, 'black sunburst' in sickle cell retinopathy, Verhoeff streaks in subsiding ciliochoroidal effusion, Siegrist's streaks in hypertension, angioid streaks and ringschwiele. Diffuse reactive RPE hyperplasia is a characteristic feature of retinitis pigmentosa and disorders with a retinitis pigmentosa-like picture. Diffuse hyperplasia also occurs in proliferative vitreoretinopathy with the formation of membranes on vitreous surfaces and on the retinal surface, usually following surgery for retinal detachment. RPE is also the principal cell seen in idiopathic epiretinal membranes[26].

Window defect of the retinal pigment epithelium

An RPE window defect is an area of depigmentation that lights up early but does not leak with fluorescein. These discrete areas of increased fluorescence appear early and disappear in the late phase of the study[27]. This lesion is also termed 'transmitted fluorescence'[28]. Microscopically, the RPE is intact but attenuated. There is partial or complete loss of melanin granules in the RPE cells, partial atrophy of the photoreceptor cells, and sclerosis of the choriocapillaris. Lesions with associated RPE window defects include vascular, inflammatory, and degenerative lesions of the choroid, disciform lesions, sub-RPE neovascularization, drusen, age-related macular degeneration, choroideremia, rubella and Best's macular degeneration. In addition, medications such as thioridazine can give rise to a chorioretinopathy and associated RPE window defects.

Inflammatory lesions of the retinal pigment epithelium

Presumed inflammatory lesions of the RPE include acute retinal pigment epitheliitis, acute posterior multifocal placoid pigment epitheliopathy (APMPPE) and diffuse posterior punctate pigment epitheliopathy.

Acute retinal pigment epitheliitis

Acute retinal pigment epitheliitis is marked by an acute onset and resolution in 6–12 weeks with total to near total visual recovery[29]. These lesions are typically dark, grey–black, circumscribed areas surrounded by a pale, yellow, halo-like zone with unremarkable intervening retina. The lesions appear in 2–4 clusters in the macular area and may change in visibility over time. Central serous choroidopathy may occur at a site of involvement[29]. There may be an association with hepatitis C[30].

Acute posterior multifocal placoid pigment epitheliopathy (APMPPE)

Acute posterior multifocal placoid pigment epitheliopathy is characterized by rapid loss of central vision secondary to multifocal yellowish-white placoid lesions at the level of the RPE[31]. There is minimal damage to the adjacent choroid and retina. Rapid resolution of the lesions occurs with permanent alteration of the RPE, and vision usually recovers or improves over months after apparent resolution of the acute lesions. This condition may be associated with a history of a preceding viral-like illness[32] and cerebral vasculitis[33,34]. Inflammatory signs associated with APMPPE include conjunctivitis, episcleritis, papillitis, iridocyclitis, uveitis, retinal vasculitis, retinal haemorrhage, retinal oedema and optic neuritis.

Diffuse posterior punctate pigment epitheliopathy

Diffuse posterior punctate pigment epitheliopathy was described by Blinder et al.[35]. These lesions are associated with a sudden loss of vision. They are bilateral, well circumscribed lesions present in the macula with progression into areas of RPE atrophy, hypertrophy and hyperplasia. Diffuse posterior punctate pigment epitheliopathy may have associated peripheral serous retinal detachment.

Detachment of the retinal pigment epithelium

Serous detachment of the RPE is a non-specific response of the RPE to choroidal diseases affecting the permeability of the choriocapillaris and adhesion of the RPE to Bruch's membrane. The lesions are dome-shaped elevations that are sharply demarcated with early and persistent staining with fluorescein. Serous detachment of the RPE is associated with age-related macular degeneration (ARMD), angioid streaks, ocular histoplasmosis syndrome (OHS), and central serous choroidopathy (ICSC).

Retinal pigment epithelial detachment (PED) often occurs in association with age-related macular degeneration. In histopathological studies[36,37] the cleavage in serous PED with ARMD is between basal laminar and basal linear deposits and the remainder of Bruch's membrane. In a study by Poliner et al.[38], 26% of these patients developed choroidal neovascular membranes (CNVM) by 1 year and 49% by 3 years. The risk of developing choroidal neovascular membranes in this setting is associated with older patient age, large detachment size, presence of subretinal fluid at initial presentation, disciform scar in the fellow eye and fluorescein angiogram showing a hot spot late filling, irregular filling and/or notching. Development of pigment epithelial atrophy and geographic atrophy occurs years after the pigment epithelial detachment. Factors associated with poor visual outcome include turbid or haemorrhagic PED, older patient age, large detachment size, and notched detachment shape. Scatter argon laser photocoagulation is of no benefit in the treatment of RPE detachments in the elderly as determined by the Moorfield's Macular Study Group in a prospective randomized trial[39].

Diagnosis of the idiopathic variant of RPE detachment is made in the absence of any other retinal or choroidal disease. This condition has a good prognosis. Because of the association with stress, male preponderance, and average age at occurrence of 44 years, this may be a variant of idiopathic central serous choroidopathy[40]. These lesions can be confused with multiple vitelliform lesions, a variant of Best's disease.

Other causes of RPE detachment include ocular B-cell lymphoma, leukemia, choroidal melanoma, multiple myeloma, and nocardiosis.

Tears of the retinal pigment epithelium

Tears of the RPE are most commonly associated with ARMD with choroidal neovascularization, and serous RPE detachment[41]. Most RPE tears are due to contraction of a fibrovascular membrane located between basal laminar deposit with RPE and the remainder of Bruch's membrane. Rarely, long-standing RPE detachment may lead to a tear of the RPE.

Tumours of the retinal pigment epithelium

Tumours of the RPE are often pigmented and may simulate melanoma. These lesions are typically seen in middle-aged patients. They can be benign or malignant and it is sometimes difficult to distinguish between the two.

Adenoma of the retinal pigment epithelium

Adenomas of the RPE are variably pigmented and are composed of large polyhedral cells containing intracellular vacuoles which stain positively for sialomucin. By electron microscopy, these cells have the characteristics of RPE cells which include basement membrane, junctional complexes, and microvilli[42]. Immature and mature melanosomes are also present in these tumours but not premelanosomes.

Adenocarcinoma of the retinal pigment epithelium

Adenocarcinomas of the RPE are extremely rare and are associated with an excellent prognosis. This tumour represents a true neoplasm of the RPE[43] and derives its name from the formation of gland-like structures. Criteria for neoplastic RPE have been defined by Tso and Albert[25] and include no history of or pathological evidence of previous ocular disease or injury, an otherwise normal eye with clear media, mitotic figures, cellular pleomorphism, no conspicuous elaboration of basement membrane material by the RPE, and various histological patterns. These histological patterns include mosaic, papillary, tubular, patternless with vacuolated cells, and patternless with anaplastic cells.

The mosaic pattern is the best differentiated and the patternless with anaplastic cells is the least. There is invasion of the retina and choroid but metastasis has not been observed.

Retinal pigment epithelial components in medulloepithelioma

Medulloepitheliomas are rare tumours that are composed of a variety of tissues including RPE.

Acknowledgements

Supported in part by: The International Order of Odd Fellows, Winston-Salem, North Carolina and Core Grant EYO 1765-21 form the National Eye Institute, Bethesda, Maryland.

References

1. Keeney, A.H. Chronology of Ophthalmic Development. Illinois: Charles C. Thomas, 1951.
2. Zinn, K.M., Marmor, M.E. The retinal pigment epithelium. Cambridge: Harvard Press, 1979: 3–6, 247–263.
3. Cohen, S.Y., Quentel, G., Quiberteau. B. *et al.* Retinal vascular changes in congenital hypertrophy of the retinal pigment epithelium. Ophthalmology. 1993; 199: 471–474.
4. Ferry, A.P. Lesions mistaken for malignant melanoma of the posterior uvea: A clinicopathologic analysis of 100 cases with ophthalmoscopically visible lesions. Arch Ophthalmol. 1964; 72: 463–469.
5. Shields, J.A., Zimmerman, L.E. Lesions simulating malignant melanoma of the posterior uvea. Arch Ophthalmol. 1973; 89: 466–471.
6. Shields, J.A., Shields, C.L., Shah, P.G. *et al.* Lack of association among typical congenital hypertrophy of the retinal pigment epithelium, adenomatous polyposis, and Gardner syndrome. Ophthalmology. 1992; 99: 1709–1713.
7. Traboulsi, E.I., Murphy, S.F., de la Cruz, Z.C., Maumenee, I.H., Green, W.R. A clinicopathologic study of familial adenomatous polyposis with extracolonic manifestations (Gardner's syndrome). Am J Ophthalmol. 1990; 110: 550–561.
8. Kasner, L., Traboulsi, E.I., de la Cruz, Z., Green, W.R. A histopathologic study of the pigmented fundus lesions in familial adenomatous polyposis. Retina. 1992; 12: 35–42.
9. Shields, J.A., Tso, M.O.M. Congenital grouped pigmentation of the retina. Histopathologic description and report of a case. Arch Ophthalmol. 1975; 93: 1153–1155.
10. Traboulsi, E.I., Maumenee, I.H., Krush, A.J. *et al.* Pigmented ocular fundus lesions in the inherited gastrointestinal polyposis syndromes and in hereditary nonpolyposis colorectal cancer. Ophthalmology. 1988; 95: 964–969.
11. Traboulsi, E.I., Maumenee, I.H., Krush, A.J. *et al.* Congenital hypertrophy of the retinal pigment epithelium predicts colorectal polyposis in Gardner's syndrome. Arch Ophthalmol. 1990; 108: 525–526.
12. Gass, J.D.M. Doyne lecture. Focal congenital anomalies of the retinal pigment epithelium. Eye. 1989; 3: 1–18.
13. Schachat, A.P., Shields, J.A., Fine, S. *et al.* Combined hamartomas of the retina and retinal pigment epithelium. Ophthalmology. 1984; 1: 1609–1619.
14. Palmer, M.L., Carney, M.D., Combs, J.L. Combined hamartomas of the retinal pigment epithelium and retina. Retina. 1990; 10: 33–36.

15. Green, W.R. Retina. In: Spencer, W.H. (ed.), Ophthalmic Pathology. An Atlas and Textbook, Vol. 3 (4th edn). Philadelphia: WB Saunders, 1996: 1302–1308.

16. Schlernitzauer, D.A., Green, W.R. Peripheral retinal albinotic spots. Am J Ophthalmol. 1971; 72: 729–732.

17. O'Donnell, F.E. Jr, Green, W.R. The eye in albinism. In: Duane, T.D. (ed.), Clinical Ophthalmology, Vol. 4. New York, Harper and Row, 1979: 1–23.

18. Wise, R.P., Lund, R.D. The retina and central projections of heterochromic rats. Exp Neurol. 1976; 51: 68–77.

19. O'Donnell, F.E., Hambrick, G.W., Green, W.R. *et al.* X-linked ocular albinism: An oculo-cutaneous macromelanosomal disorder. Arch Ophthalmol. 1976; 94: 1883.

20. Wong, L., O'Donnell, F.E., Green, W.R. Giant pigment granules in the retinal pigment epithelium of a fetus with X-linked ocular albinism. Ophthal Pediatr Genet. 1983; 2: 47–66

21. O'Donnell, F.E., King, R.A., Green, W.R. *et al.* Autosomal recessively inherited ocular albinism. Arch Ophthalmol. 1978; 96: 1621–1625.

22. Ai, E., Cavender, J.C., Lee, S. Hereditary macular dystrophies. Dept. Ophthalmol, California Pacific Medical Center, 2340 Clay Street, San Francisco, California.

23. O'Donnell, F.E., Schatz, H., Reid, P. *et al.* Autosomal dominant dystrophy of the retinal pigment epithelium. Arch Ophthalmol. 1979; 97: 680–683.

24. Jampel, H.D., Schachat, A.P., Conway, B. *et al.* Retinal pigment epithelial hyperplasia assuming tumor-like proportions. Report of 2 cases. Retina. 1986; 5: 105–112.

25. Tso, M.O.M., Albert, D.M. Pathologic conditions of the retinal pigment epithelium: Neoplasms and nodular non-neoplastic lesions. Arch Ophthalmol. 1972; 88: 27–38.

26. Smiddy, W.E., Maguire, A.M., Green, W.R. *et al.* Idiopathic epiretinal membranes: ultrastructural characteristics and clinicopathologic correlation. Ophthalmology. 1989; 96: 811–821.

27. Keno, D.D., Green, W.R. Retinal pigment epithelial window defect. Arch Ophthalmol. 1978; 96: 854–856.

28. Yannuzzi, L.A., Fisher, Y.L., Levy, J.H. A classification of abnormal fundus fluorescence. Ann Ophthalmol. 1971; 3: 711–718.

29. Krill, A.E., Deutman, A.F. Acute retinal pigment epitheliitis. Am J Ophthalmol. 1972; 74: 193–205.

30. Quillen, D.A., Zurlo, J.J., Cunningham, D. *et al.* Acute retinal pigment epitheliitis and hepatitis C. Am J Ophthalmol. 1994; 118: 120–121.

31. Gass, J.D.M. Acute posterior multifocal placoid pigment epitheliopathy. Arch Ophthalmol. 1968; 80: 177–185.

32. Ryan, S.J., Maumenee, E. Acute posterior multifocal placoid pigment epitheliopathy. Am J Ophthalmol. 1972; 274: 1066–1074.

33. Seigelman, J., Behrens, M., Hilal, S. Acute posterior multifocal placoid pigment epitheliopathy associated with cerebral vasculitis and homonymous hemianopsia. Am J Ophthalmol. 1979; 88: 919–924.

34. Wilson, C.A., Choromokos, E.A., Sheppard, R. Acute posterior multifocal placoid pigment epitheliopathy and cerebral vasculitis. Arch Ophthalmol. 1988; 106: 796–800.

35. Blinder, K.J., Peyman, G.A., Paris, C.L. Diffuse posterior punctate pigment epitheliopathy. Retina. 1994; 14: 31–35.

36. Green, W.R., Key, S.N. III. Senile macular degeneration: a histopathologic study. Trans Am Ophthalmol Soc. 1977; 75: 180–254.

37. Green, W.R., Enger, C. Age-related macular degeneration histopathologic studies. The 1993 Lorenz E. Zimmerman Lecture. Ophthalmology. 1993; 100: 1519–1535.

38. Poliner, L.S., Olk, R.J., Burgess, D. *et al.* Natural history of retinal pigment epithelial detachments in age-related macular degeneration. Ophthalmology. 1986; 93: 543–551.

39. Moorfield's Macular Study Group. Retinal pigment epithelial detachments in the elderly: A controlled trial of argon laser photocoagulation. Br J Ophthalmol. 1982; 66: 1–16.

40. Lewis, M.L. Idiopathic serous detachment of the retinal pigment epithelium. Arch Ophthalmol. 1978; 96: 620–624.

41. Green, W.R., McDonnell, P.J., Yeo, J.H. Pathologic features of senile macular degeneration. Ophthalmology. 1985; 92: 615–627.
42. Font, R.L., Zimmerman, L.E., Fine, B.S. Adenoma of the retinal pigment epithelium. Am J Ophthalmol. 1972; 73: 544–554.
43. Minckler, D., Allen, A.W. Adenocarcinoma of the retinal pigment epithelium. Arch Ophthalmol. 1978; 96: 2252–2254

Eye Pathology Laboratory
Johns Hopkins Hospital
600 N. Wolfe Street
Baltimore, MD 21287–9248
USA

12. The effects of UV-A light in indirect irradiation on cultures of bovine lens epithelium

U.M. MAYER, H. KLINGE and M. RADLMEIER

(Nürnberg, Germany)

Purpose

Conjunctivitis, keratitis actinica, retinal damage[1], and cataract formation[2] are consequences of excessive UV irradiation. As catalase activity has been found to be reduced in cataractuous lenses[3], we suggested a protective effect for catalase against UV irradiation. Using blue light of 400 nm, Radlmeier proved this in cultures of bovine lens epithelium[4,5] (Fig. 1). Showing that UV damage is a result of H_2O_2 stress. It is important determine whether addition of a 0.36% catalase solution can protect lens epithelial cells against morphological alterations and apoptosis by UV-A also. It remains unknown, whether indirect as well as direct irradiation can cause cell damage.

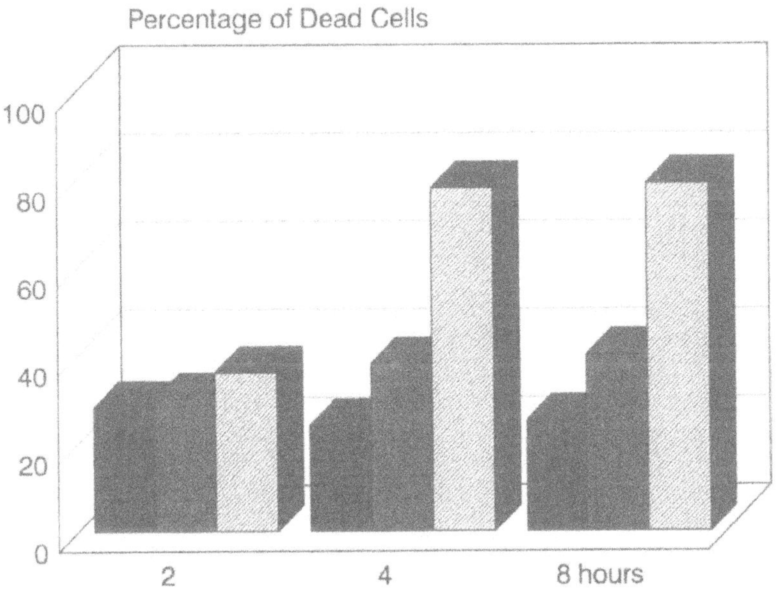

Fig. 1. Protective effect of catalase in direct irradiation by blue light (460 nm). ■ controls; ▦ irradiation + 0.36% catalase; ▨ irrradiation.

G. Coscas and F. Cardillo Piccolino (eds.), Retinal Pigment Epithelium and Macular Diseases, pp. 81–88.
© 1998 Kluwer Academic Publishers.

Materials and methods

The used culture medium was TCM 199, with the addition of 5% antibiotics (streptomycinsulphate 25 µg/ml, penicillin G 10 000 µg/ml, amphotericin B 0.85% in NaCl), 2% glutamine, 5% Hepes buffer and 20% FCS. It was exposed for 3 h to 100 mW/cm^2 direct UV-A irradiation (halogen vapour lamp as modified by Heller[6]). Normal monolayer grown lens epithelium (Fig. 2) was either exposed to UV-A light or fed by irradiated medium (Fig. 3). This latter method was called indirect irradiation of the cells. In a second experiment, the protective effect of catalase was examined. The surviving cells were counted and compared to those in non irradiated medium (Neubauer chamber, Mann-Whitney test). Morphologic evaluation as performed in 186 cultures by means of 665 slides (Leitz inverted microscope); parameters such as cell diameter, fibroblast-like growth, disconnection of the monolayer and formation of cellular inclusions were registered as a score, drawn in a diagram and compared with those of a control culture.

Results

The first cell alterations were observed after irradiation for 10 min; these were irreparable after an irradiation time of 30 min. After irradiation for 3 h, the

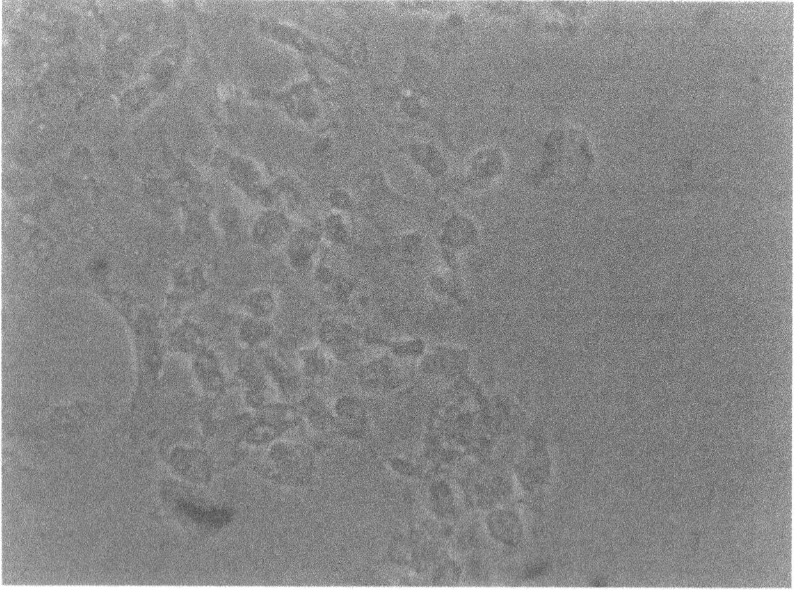

Fig. 2. Monolayer of lens epithelial cells, first subculture, third day.

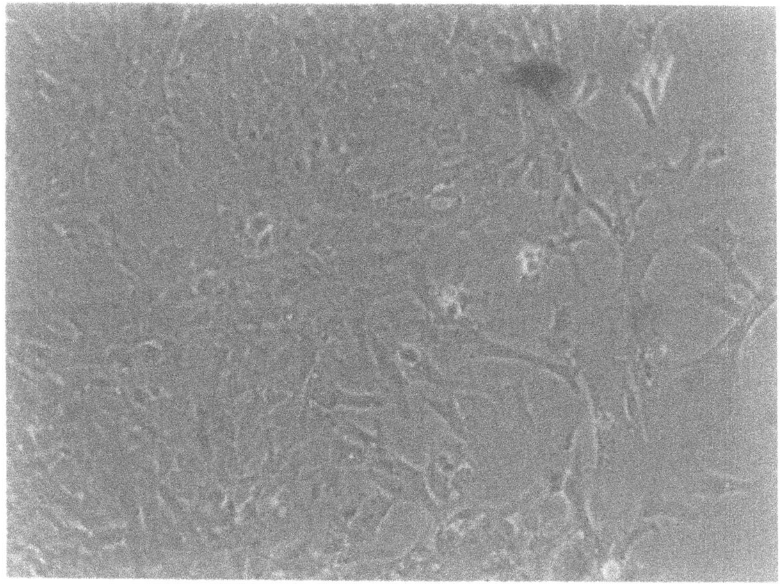

Fig. 3. Monolayer of lens epithelial cells, first subculture, third day in irradiated medium.

criterion of cell count proved to be the most reliable: indirect irradiation also inhibited cellular multiplication (Fig. 4). Catalase also protected the cells from the effects of indirect irradiation. Cell diameter, absence of fibroblast-like growth, formation of cellular inclusions and rupture of the monolayer were criteria for the evaluation of morphological differentiation. Cellular diameter was increased (Fig. 5a, b, c): in controls and in catalase-protected cells, it was 0.1 μm; while in cultures in irradiated medium (3 h), it was >0.16 μm. Monolayer disruption and fibroblast-like growth no longer occurred (Fig. 5d, e, f). The number of cellular inclusions was also increased in controls and after addition of catalase, but not in cultures in irradiated medium.

Discussion

This indirect UV-A damage could be explained by UV-A-induced alteration of Hepes buffer[7]. The question is, which other substances with similar toxic effect could play a comparable role. Since addition of catalase may eliminate this adverse effect, the damage should be due to H_2O_2 formation.

UV-A causes an increase in the diameter of cultivated lens epithelial cells, as seen in ageing cells[8] and in corneal cells. It also stops fibroblast-like growth. Even if cell multiplication can be repaired, some morphological alterations

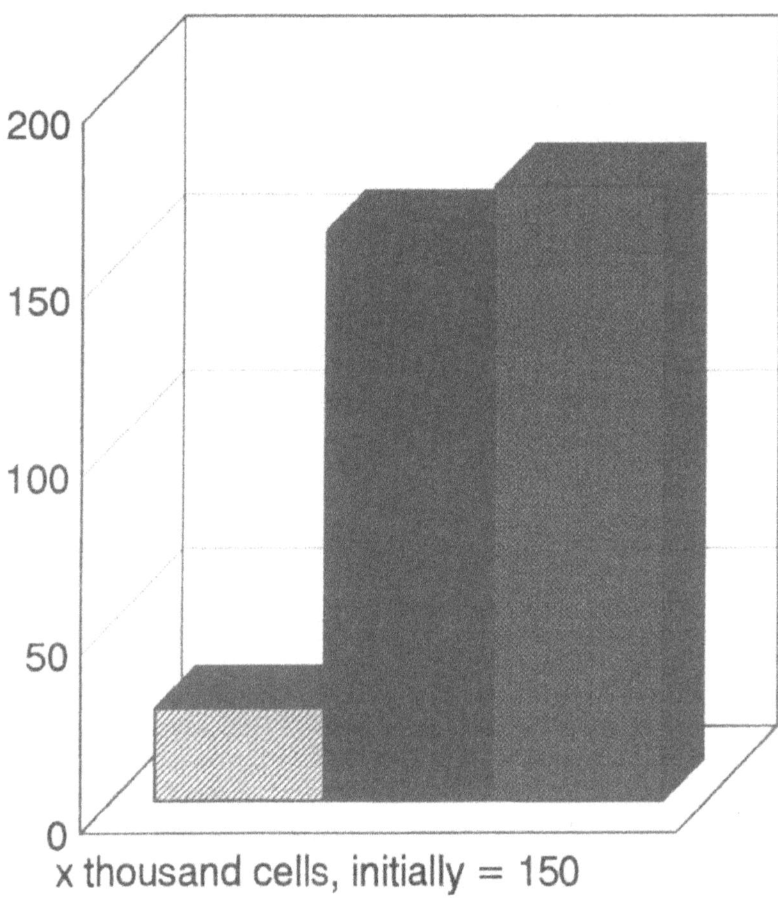

Fig. 4. Protection of 'indirectly' irradiated cells by catalase. ▨ irradiated (100 mW/cm^2, 3 h), 1 week in culture; ■ controls, 1 week in culture; ▦ controls + 0.06 mg/dl catalase, 1 week in culture.

such as fibroblast-like growth and formation of granules show a tendency to be affected. Such small effects may play a role in Hockwin's *Additionskataract*.

Similar phenomena may occur in the vitreous body. In 1980 Mayer found a relatively high concentration of catalase in the vitreous[9]. As the premacular area of the vitreous is permanently exposed to focused light, H_2O_2 production might be particularly high. Premacular vitreous is often destroyed in senile macular degeneration, and this might be one of the causes of age-related maculopathy. It should be possible to inject synthetic catalase and thus prevent macular degeneration.

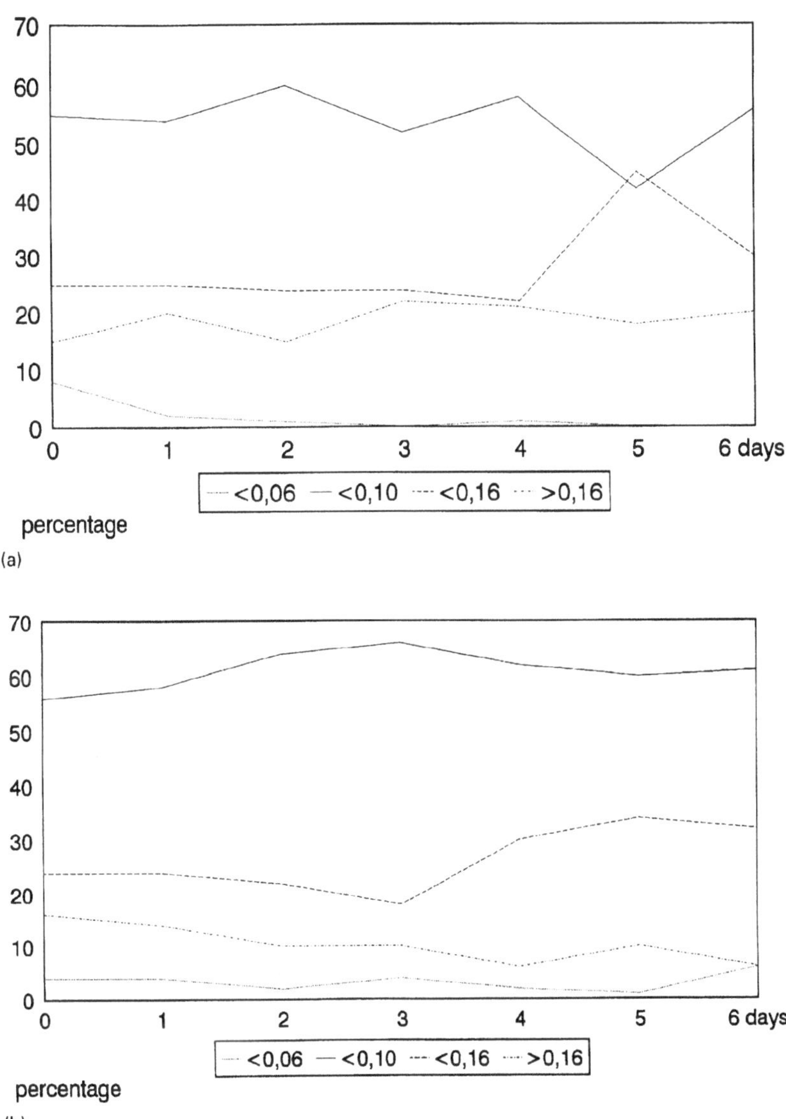

Fig. 5. Morphologic evaluation in 186 cell cultures by means of 665 slides. Cell diameter after 3 h in (a) controls, (b) cells irradiated with catalase, (c) after indirect irradiation. Fibroblast-like growth after 3 h in (d) controls, (e) cells irradiated with catalase and (f) after indirect irradiation. For details see text.

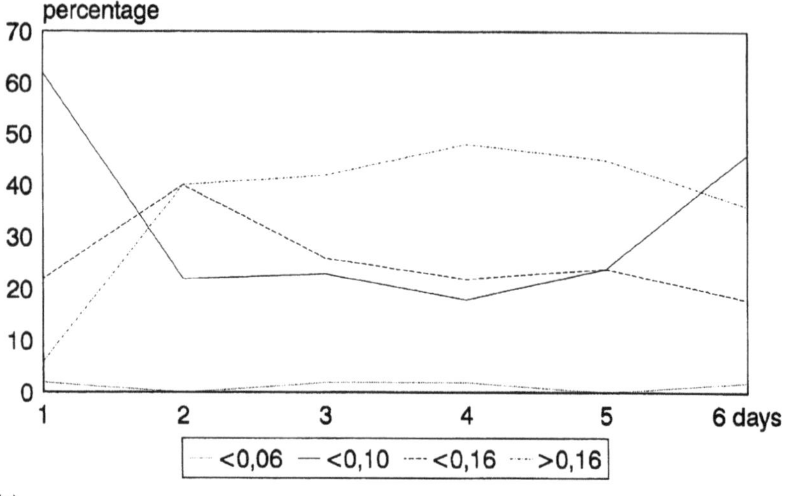

(c)

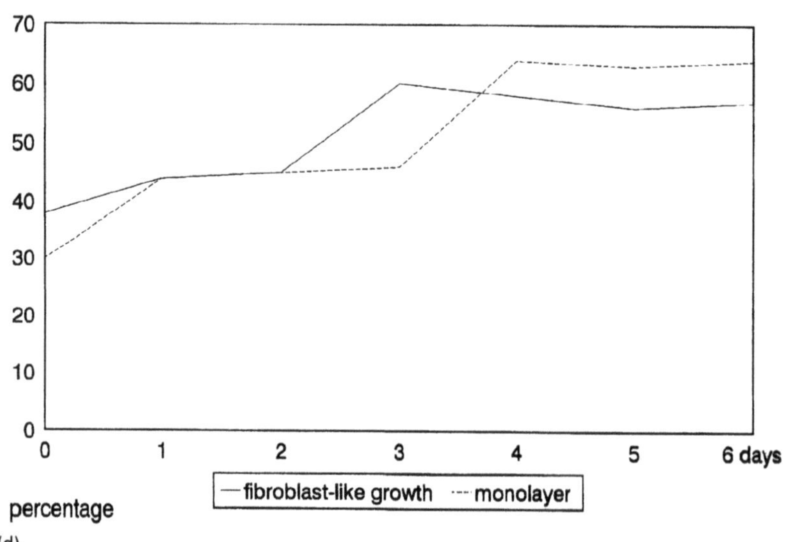

(d)

Fig. 5. (Continued.)

Conclusion

The unexpected result is that indirect irradiation may cause the same toxic effects to the cells as their direct exposure to the UV-A light, and that there exists the possibility of avoiding this effect by addition of catalase.

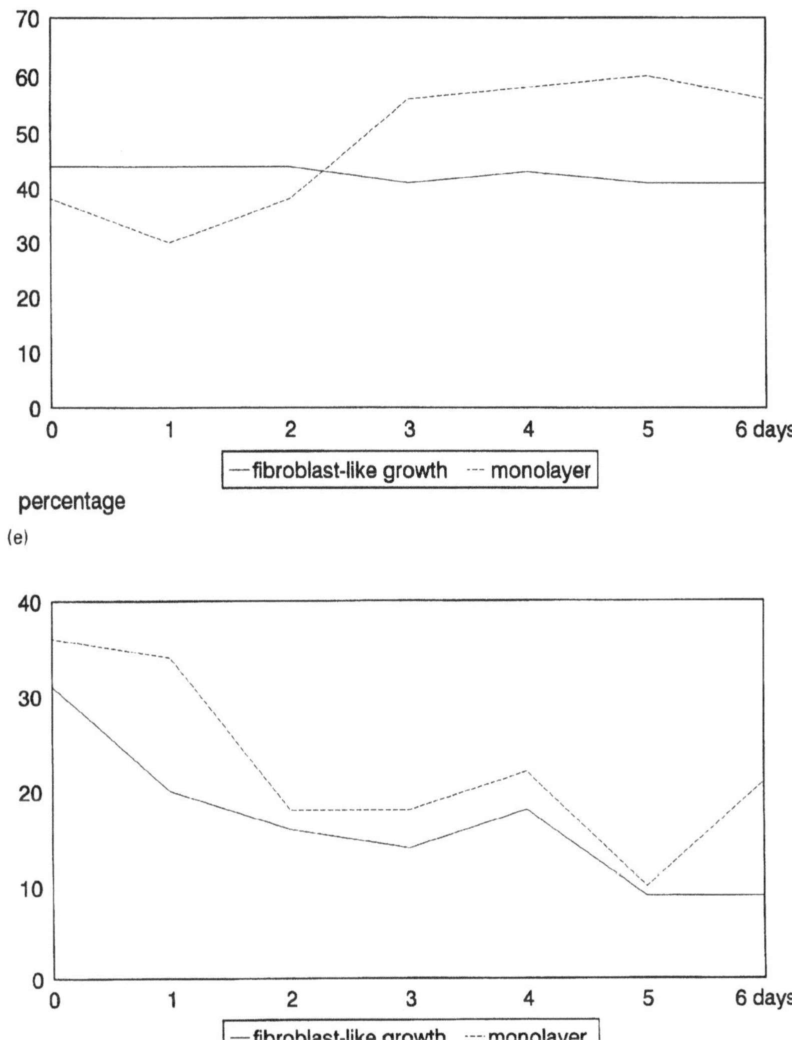

Fig. 5. (Continued.)

References

1. Ham, W.T. Jr, Mueller, H.A., Ruffolo, J.J., Guerry, D. III, Guerry, R.K. Action spectrum for retinal injury from near UV-violett radiation in the aphakic monkey. Am J Ophthalmol. 1982; 93: 299–306.
2. Taylor, H.R., West, S.K., Rosenthal, F.S. *et al.* Effect of ultraviolett irradiation on cataract formation. N Engl J Med. 1988; 319: 1429–1433.

3. Mayer, U.M., Schmidt-Götz, M.-L. Über die Aktivität der Katalase im menschlichen Auge und ihr Verhalten im Laufe des Lebens bei unterschiedlichen Trübungen der Linse. Ber Deutsch Ophthalmol Gesell 1977; 75: 432–434.
4. Radlmeier, M. Die Frage nach der Einwirkung von blauem Licht der Wellenlänge 420–430 auf Kulturen boviner Linsenepithelien. Thesis Med. University of Erlangen-Nürnberg (1994).
5. Mayer, U.M., Radlmeier, M., Gossler, B. Catalase protects from blue light. Invest Ophthalmol Vis Sci 1992; 33: 1039, n° 1740.
6. Heller, S., Mayer, U.M. Effect of UV-A light on the catalase activity in the vitreous body of calf eyes. German J Ophthalmol. 1994; 3: 445–446.
7. Lepe-Zuniga, J.L., Zigler, J.S. Jr, Gery, J. Toxicity of light exposed Hepes media. J Immunol Methods. 1987; 103: 145.
8. Bermbach, G., Mayer, U.M., Naumann, G.O.H. Human lens epithelial cells in tissue culture. Exp Eye Res. 1991: 52: 113–119.
9. Mayer, U.M. Comparative investigations of catalase activity in different ocular tissues of cattle and man. Albrecht von Graefe's Arch Klin Exp Ophthalmol. 1980; 213: 261–265.

Department of Ophthalmology
and Eye Clinic of the University
of Erlangen-Nürnberg

13. Localization of bFGF in wound healing process of RPE cell *in vitro*

H. YAMADA, N. OGATA, C. YAMAMOTO, M. MIYASHIRO,
M. UYAMA and A. DEL MONTE

(Osaka, Japan and Michigan, USA)

Introduction

Retinal pigment epithelium (RPE) plays a key role in forming choroidal neovascular membrane in age-related macular degeneration. Some growth factors, especially basic fibroblast growth factor, regulate wound healing mechanisms[1], and proliferation and regression of the choroidal neovascularization in experimental animal models[2,3]. There are few reports referring to the relationship between RPE and bFGF during this wound healing process.

This study attempted to determine the mechanism by which bFGF regulates RPE cell proliferation during wound healing. We analysed bFGF localization of RPE cells using immunohistochemical methods after laser injury *in vitro*.

Materials and methods

RPE cell culture

Cultured human RPE cells were a generous gift from Dr Del Monte and were cultured in a chamber slide (Cat. No. #177453, Nunc Inc., IL, USA). When they were confluent, direct laser photocoagulation was performed by Coherent 910A argon laser with power, 1 W; spot size, 100 µm; duration, 1 s. Ten spots were made per chamber slide.

Antibody

We used bFGF monochlonal antibody for human (Cat. No. #017-14281, Wako Junyaku, Japan).

Immunohistochemical study

RPE cells were fixed immediately and 12, 24 and 48 h after photocoagulation with chilled 100% acetone. Immunohistochemical staining was conducted according to the instructions of LSAB kit (DAKO A/S Denmark). This

G. Coscas and F. Cardillo Piccolino (eds.), Retinal Pigment Epithelium and Macular Diseases, pp. 89–93.
© *1998 Kluwer Academic Publishers.*

comprised neutralization with $3\%H_2O_2$ to block endogenous peroxidase, rinsing with 0.1%Triton-X100, followed by reaction with primary antibody for 20 min at room temperature. After washing with TBS, reaction with link solution and then with streptoavidin peroxidase was performed for 20 min each at room temperature. After washing with TBS immunoreactivity was visualized by DAB chromogen and was observed under a light microscope.

Results

Soon after laser treatment, a photocoagulation (PC) lesion was detected clearly as a round cellular defect in the centre of the spot (Fig. 1, top left).

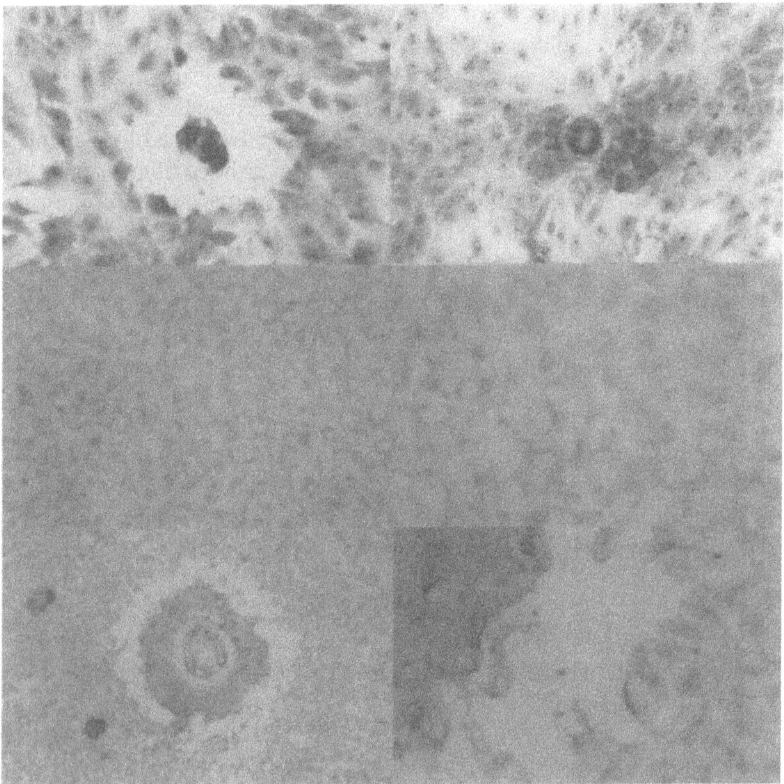

Fig. 1. Top left, immediately after laser treatment, stained by methylene blue; top right, 48 h after laser treatment, stained by methylene blue; middle left, bFGF staining before laser treatment (low magnification); middle right, bFGF staining before laser treatment (high magnification); bottom left, bFGF staining immediately after laser treatment (low magnification); bottom right, bFGF staining immediately after laser treatment (high magnification).

The entire spot closed by proliferation or sliding of the cells from the edge of the laser spot until 48 h after PC (Fig. 1, top right). As for control, bFGF immunohistochemical staining was performed before laser treatment (Fig. 1). Immunoreactivity for bFGF in the cytoplasm was weak before laser treatment. Immediately after PC, coagulated and damaged cells were detected in the centre of the PC lesion (Fig. 1, bottom left). At high magnification, the cytoplasm of the cells surrounding PC lesion showed comparatively strong immunoreactivity (Fig. 1, bottom right), but this was almost the same intensity as controls. Twelve hours after laser treatment immunoreactivity of PC lesion diminished (Fig. 2, top left, low magnification), but cytoplasm of the cells surrounding PC lesion showed stronger immunoreactivity than immediately after PC (Fig. 2, top right, high magnification). Twenty-four hours after laser

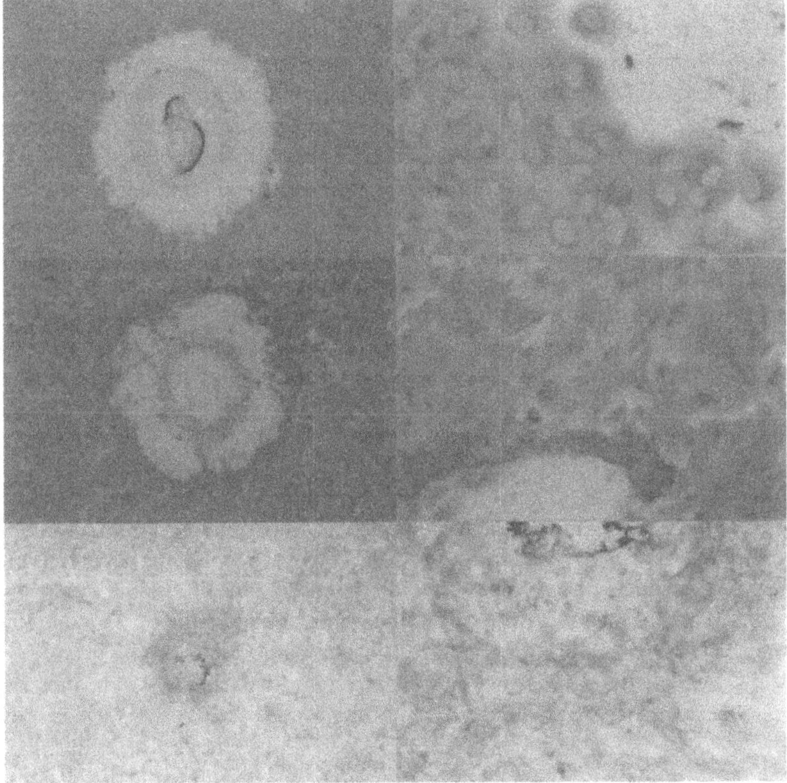

Fig. 2. Top left, bFGF staining 12 h after laser treatment (low magnification); top right, bFGF staining 12 h after laser treatment (high magnification); middle left, bFGF staining 24 h after laser treatment (low magnification); middle right, bFGF staining 24 h after laser treatment (high magnification); bottom left, bFGF staining 48 h after laser treatment (low magnification); bottom right, bFGF staining 48 h after laser treatment (high magnification).

treatment, immunoreactivity of the cells surrounding the PC lesion was strongest throughout all stages (Fig. 2, middle left, low magnification). At this stage in particular, strong immunoreactivity for bFGF was found in the nucleus of the cells surrounding PC lesion (Fig. 2, middle right, high magnification). By 48 h after laser treatment, the PC spot had been reconstructed by surrounding RPE cells (Fig. 2, bottom left, low magnification). Immunoreactivity became weaker than that seen at 24 h after laser treatment. There was no longer any strong immunoreactivity in the nucleus of the cells (Fig. 2, bottom right, high magnification).

Discussion

The bFGF family has been isolated from many kinds of organs and tissues since the 1970s. These factors regulate cell differentiation and proliferation[4]. Several studies have reported that bFGF promotes wound healing[5,6], and bFGF mRNA expression was detected during healing of wounds caused by laser photocoagulation in the rat eye[1]. In such models, however, it is impossible to exclude other factors which affect wound healing. In addition to RPE cells, other cells, such as macrophages and immune cells which are activated by inflammation, can also produce bFGF[7]. To distinguish which cell works mainly or cooperatively in wound healing process is very difficult in an *in vivo* model. In an *in vitro* model, we can isolate RPE cells from other cells and exclude the effect of other factors. The laser is an ideal device to use in a wound healing model, because it can make accurate size wounds easily and repeatedly. We believe, therefore, that this experimental system is suitable for evaluating how the growth factors affect cell proliferation and reconstruction.

bFGF showed immunoreactivity in the cytoplasm of control cells, indicating that the RPE cell contains or stores bFGF casually in its cytoplasm. Immediately after PC, weak immunoreactivity for bFGF was detected in cytoplasm of the cells surrounding the PC lesion. bFGF immunoreactivity became stronger at 12 h after PC. By 24 h after PC, immunoreactivity for bFGF was observed most intensely in the cells surrounding the PC lesion. It is supposed that RPE cell produces bFGF for tissue reconstruction and bFGF increases over this time course. By 48 h after PC, the PC lesion was reconstructed and at the same time, bFGF immunoreactivity reduced. This suggests that bFGF works during the stage of reconstruction and bFGF production stops when tissue reconstruction is completed. In particular, 24 h after PC, immunoreactivity for bFGF was remarkably observed in the nucleus compared to in the cytoplasm of the cells. It is very interesting that bFGF immunoreactivity attained its peak 24 h after PC and altered its localization. From this fact, we hypothesize that bFGF could have an intracellular transport mechanism from the cytoplasm to the nucleus of the cell during the process of cell reconstruction. Further study is necessary to analyse or to prove the relationship between intracellular localization of bFGF and the cell proliferation cycle.

Some studies[8,9] report that other growth factors can also play important roles in cell proliferation. For example, transforming growth factors[8], and platelet derived growth factors[9] are well known as regulators of RPE cell proliferation. We did not perform the experiment using other cytokines because good antibodies are not available. We are planning to perform immunohistochemical staining for other cytokines to unveil the cell proliferation mechanism and regulatory factors of RPE.

Acknowledgement

This study was supported in part by a grant from the Ministry of Education, Science, and Culture of Japan.

References

1. Yamamoto, C., Ogata, N., Matsushima, M. *et al.* Expression of basic fibroblast growth factor and its receptor in the process of wound healing of rat retina after laser photocoagulation. J Jpn Ophthalmol Soc. 1996; 100: 270–278.
2. Matsushima, M., Ogata, N., Takada, Y. *et al.* FGF receptor 1 expression in experimental choroidal neovascularization. J Jpn Ophthalmol Soc. 1996; 40: 329–338.
3. Ogata, N., Matsushima, M., Takada, Y. *et al.* Expression of basic fibroblast growth factor mRNA in developing choroidal neovascularization. Curr Eye Res. 1996; 15: 1008–1018.
4. Sato, Y., Shimada, T., Takaki, R. Autocrine activities of basic fibroblast growth factor: regulation of endothelial cell movement, plasminogen activator synthesis, and DNA synthesis. J Cell Biol. 1988; 107: 1199–1205.
5. McGee, G.S., Davidson, J.M., Buckley, A. *et al.* Recombinant basic fibroblast growth factor accelerates wound healing. J Surg Res. 1988; 45: 145–153.
6. Broadley, K.N., Aquino, A.M., Woodward, S.C. *et al.* Monospecific antibodies implicate basic fibroblast growth factor in normal wound repair. Lab Invest. 1989; 61: 571–575.
7. Baird, A., Monmede, P., Bohlen, P. Immunoreactive fibroblast growth factor in cells of peritoneal exudate suggest its identity with macrophage derived growth factor. Biochem Biophys Res Commun. 1985; 126: 358–364.
8. Tanihara, H., Yoshida, M., Matsumoto, M., Yoshimura, N. Identification of transforming growth factor-beta expressed in cultured human retinal pigment epithelial cells. Invest Ophthalmol Vis Sci. 1993; 34: 413–419.
9. Campochiaro, P.A., Sugg, R., Grotendorst, G., Hjelmeland, L.M. Retinal pigment epithelial cells produce PDGF-like proteins and secrete them into their media. Exp Eye Res. 1989; 49: 217–227.

Department of Ophthalmology
Kansai Medical University
10–15 Fumizonocho
Moriguchi, Osaka 570, Japan

14. Promotion of retinal pigment epithelial cell proliferation in experimental choroidal neovascularization by human interferon-beta

K. IWASHITA, K. TAKAHASHI, T. TOBE, H. YAMADA, M. UYAMA
and S. SONE

(Osaka and Kanagawa, Japan)

Introduction

Interferon (IFN) therapy for age-related macular degeneration is still controversial. We have already demonstrated that systemic administration of human IFN-β promotes proliferation of the retinal pigment epithelium (RPE) in experimental choroidal neovascularization (CNV) in monkey eyes[1]. We have now performed quantitative analysis regarding RPE proliferation in the regressive process associated with experimental CNV by IFN-β to clarify the effect of IFN-β *in vivo*.

Materials and methods

We used 12 eyes of six rhesus monkeys weighing 3.0—5.0 kg in this experiment. Under general anaesthesia induced by i.m. injection of ketamine hydrochloride (Ketalar), the pupil was dilated with Mydrin P, and photocoagulation was performed by krypton laser (Coherent Radiation model 900) in the posterior pole of the ocular fundus. Parameters of the photocoagulation were: spot size, 100 µm; duration, 0.1 s; power, 200 mW. Eight spots per eye were made around the fovea.

In the IFN-treated group (six eyes of three monkeys), IFN-β (Toray Industries), naturally occurring IFN derived from human fibroblasts, was administered systemically by i.v. injection for 28 days daily, at a dosage of 0.3 MIU/kg/day. Six eyes of three monkeys served as controls without IFN administration.

One week after photocoagulation, occurrence of choroidal neovascularization was confirmed by fluorescein angiography; fluorescein angiography was then performed weekly and clinical evaluation was performed at week 5. The eyes were then enucleated and the lesions were embedded in epoxy resin by routine methods for light and electron microscopy. Serial 1 µm sections were prepared with a microtome to examine the centre of the coagulated foci, and

G. Coscas and F. Cardillo Piccolino (eds.), Retinal Pigment Epithelium and Macular Diseases, pp. 95–100.
© *1998 Kluwer Academic Publishers.*

stained with toluidine blue. Using the light microscope, the number of RPE cells and macrophages on the section of centre of the lesion, indicated by the largest break of Bruch's membrane, was analysed.

As a standard of the size of the neovascular membrane (NVM), the histopathological diameter of between normal RPE cells were measured. The cell count was performed by two examiners, blinded according to the double masked method.

Results

Clinical finding

Thirty-one neovascular lesions were determined in both groups 5 weeks after photocoagulation by fluorescein angiography.

In the control group, only 29% of lesions showed regression of neovascularizations, which appeared as a decrease in diameter of the neovascular lesion and reduced fluorescein leakage. In the IFN-treated group, 61% of lesions showed regression. Clinical examination showed excellent regression rate of CNV in the IFN-treated group compared with the control group.

Histopathological findings

In 16 specimens from each group, the centre of the lesion was defined by serial sections. Morphometric study was performed in these lesions in both groups.

On light microscopy, control lesions showed CNV with relatively wide vascular lumen seen in the subretinal space. There was a continuous layer of RPE cells covering the neovascular tissue (Fig. 1A). IFN-treated lesions contained many cells in the neovascular tissue compared with the control group; most of these cells were RPE cells which vigorously proliferated in the subretinal space (Fig. 1B).

On electron microscopy, the control group showed abundant amorphous extracellular matrix around the CNV. The vascular lumen of CNV was wide and new vessels in the neovascular membrane showed thin endothelial cytoplasm and multiple fenestrations. Flat RPE cells with microvilli were observed around the CNV (Fig. 2A). The IFN-treated group showed vigorously proliferating cuboidal RPE cells with microvilli around the CNV. The vascular lumen of CNV was narrow due to compression by proliferating RPE cells. New vessels in the neovascular membrane showed thick endothelial cytoplasm and fewer fenestrations (Fig. 2B).

Morphometry

The mean diameter of the neovascular membrane in one lesion was $373.7 \pm 112.6\,\mu m$ in controls and $376.1 \pm 85.8\,\mu m$ in the IFN-treated group.

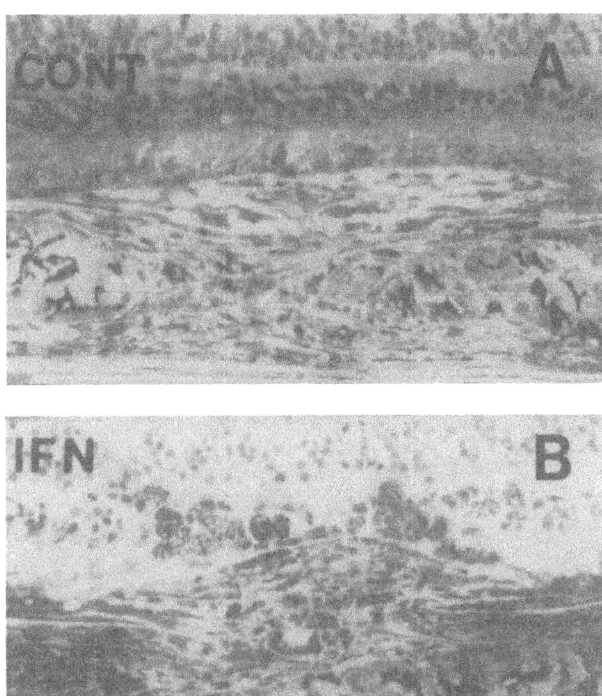

Fig. 1. (A) Light microscopy of control lesion. CNV was easily seen in the subretinal space and cells were sparse around new vessels. There was continuous layer of RPE cells covered the neovascular tissue. (B) Light microscopy of IFN-treated lesion. There were many cells in neovascular tissue compared with the control group. Most of these cells were RPE cells which proliferated vigorously around the new vessels.

This difference was not statistically significant ($p = 0.9850$; Fig. 3A).There was a mean of 52.7 ± 8.1 RPE cells in one lesion in the control group, compared with 91.5 ± 10.2 cells in the IFN-treated group. This difference was statistically significant ($p = 0.0059$; Fig. 3B). The mean number of macrophages in one lesion was 9.2 ± 1.2 cells in controls and 13.7 ± 1.7 in the IFN-treated group. This difference was not statistically significant ($p = 0.0899$; Fig. 3C).

Conclusion

Recently, the incidence of age-related macular degeneration has increased in Japan, and the disorder, which is a cause of blindness in aged people, has emerged as a social issue[2]. The development of drug treatment is necessary, especially for cases in which photocoagulation is difficult.

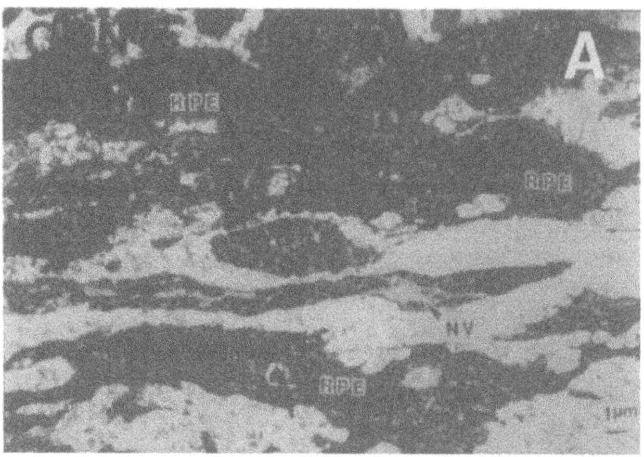

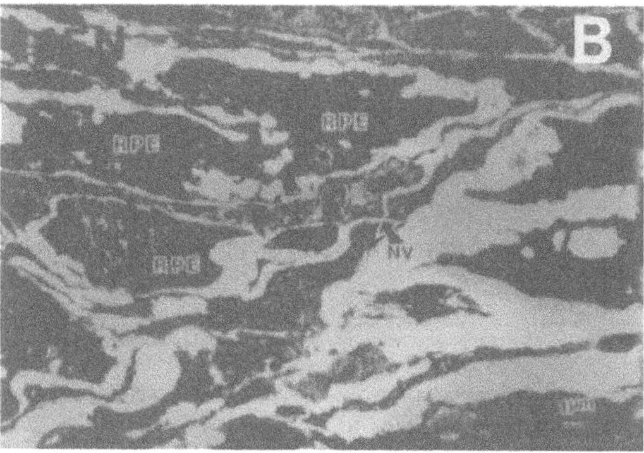

Fig. 2. (A) Electron microscopy of control lesion. The control group showed abundant amorphous extracellular matrix around the CNV. Vascular lumen of CNV was wide and new vessels in the neovascular membrane showed thin endothelial cytoplasm and multiple fenestrations. Flat RPE cells with microvilli were observed around the CNV. (B) Electron microscopy of IFN-treated lesion. The IFN-treated group showed vigorously proliferating cuboidal RPE cells with microvilli around the CNV. Vascular lumen of CNV was narrow due to compression by proliferating RPE cells. New vessels in the neovascular membrane showed thick endothelial cytoplasm and fewer fenestrations. RPE shows retinal pigment epithelial cell. Arrowhead and arrow show neovascular lumen. Scale represents 1 µm.

The basic mechanism of IFN against angiogenesis is thought to be inhibition of proliferation and migration of vascular endothelial cells[3-5] and regression of experimental iris neovascularization after treatment with IFN have been reported[6]. Treatment of age-related macular degeneration, which is caused by choroidal neovascularization, has been attempted using IFN[7-14].

Tobe *et al.*[1] reported that human IFN-β showed a regressive effect against

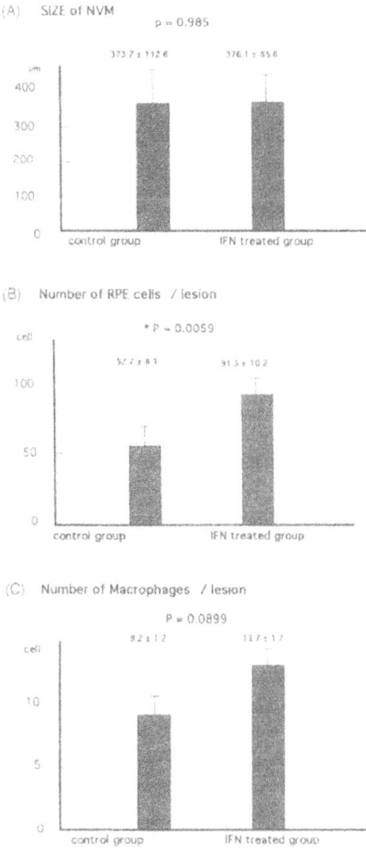

Fig. 3. (A) The difference in size of NVM was not statistically significant ($p = 0.9850$). (B) The difference in number of RPE cells was statistically significant ($p = 0.0059$). (C) The difference in number of macrophages was not statistically significant ($p = 0.0899$).

experimental choroidal neovascularization in monkey. They administered IFN-β (3.0–6.0 MIU) by intramuscular injection every day from day 8 until day 21 after intense laser photocoagulation. In this study, IFN-β (0.3 MIU/kg) was administered intravenously everyday from day 8 to day 35 after intense laser photocoagulation. The results of these two studies were almost equivalent to that in regard to the clinical and histopathological effects of IFN-β on experimental CNV.

We performed quantitative analysis regarding RPE proliferation in this regressive process of experimental CNV by IFN-β to clarify the effect of IFN-β *in vivo*. Promotion of RPE cell proliferation by IFN-β was quantitatively certified in this study. No significant difference in migration of the macrophages was detected between two groups. Histopathological examination showed vigorous proliferation of RPE cells around the new vessels, and RPE cells surrounded neovascular tissue completely. These are the characteristics of neovascular lesion regressing after treatment with IFN-β.

IFN-β is suggested to be beneficial against CNV by promoting the effect of RPE cell proliferation in addition to its direct inhibition of vascular endothelial proliferation.

Acknowledgement

This study was supported in part by a grant from the Ministry of Education, Science, and Culture of Japan.

References

1. Tobe, T., Takahashi, K., Ohkuma, H., Uyama, M. Inhibition of experimental choroidal neovascularization by interferon beta. Invest Ophthalmol Vis Sci. 1995; 36 (suppl): 552.
2. Uyama, M. Choroidal neovascularization, experimental and clinical study. Acta Soc Ophthalmol Jpn. 1991; 95: 1145–1180.
3. Brouty-Boye, D., Zetter, B.R. Inhibition of cell motility by interferon. Science. 1980; 208: 516–518.
4. Friesel, R., Komoriya, A., Maciag, T. Inhibition of endotherial cell proliferation by gamma-interferon. J Cell Biol. 1987; 104: 689–696.
5. Tsuruoka, N., Sugiyama, M., Tawaragi, Y. et al. Inhibition of *in vitro* angiogenesis by lymphotoxin and interferon-γ. Biochem Biophys Res Commun. 1988; 155: 429–435.
6. Miller, J.W., Stinson, W.G., Fojkman, J. Regression of experimental iris neovascularization with systemic alpha-interferon. Ophthalmology. 1993; 100: 9–14.
7. Fung, W.E. Interferon alpha 2a for treatment of age-related macular degeneration. Am J Ophthalmol. 1991; 112: 349–350.
8. Engler, C.B., Sander, B., Koefoed, P., Larsen, M., Vinding, T., Lund-Anderse, H. Interferon alpha-2a treatment of patients with subretinal neovascular macular degeneration. A pilot investigation. Acta Ophthalmol. 1993; 71: 27–31.
9. Gilies, M.C., Sarks, J.P., Beaumont, P.E et al. Treatment of choroidal neovascularization in age-related macular degeneration with interferon alfa-2a and alfa-2b. Br J Ophthalmol. 1993; 77: 759–765.
10. Kirkpatrick, J.N.P., Dick, A.D., Forrester, J.V. Clinical experience with interferon alfa-2a for exudative age-related macular degeneration. Br J Ophthalmol. 1993; 77: 766–770.
11. Poliner, L.S,. Tornambe, P.E., Michelson, P.E., Heitzmann, J.G. Interferon alpha-2a for subfoveal neovascularization in age-related macular degeneration. Ophthalmology. 1993; 100: 1417–1424.
12. Thomas, M.A., Ibanez, H.E. Interferon alpha-2a in the treatment of subfoveal choroidal neovascularization. Am J Ophthalmol. 1993; 115: 563–568.
13. Matsui, M. Senile disciform macular degeneration. Jpn J Clin Ophthalmol. 1994; 48: 163–170.
14. Matsui, M. Applications of interferon in ophthalmological field and its ocular complications. Acta Soc Ophthalmol Jpn. 1994; 98: 511–512.

Department of Ophthalmology
10–15 Fumizono-cho
Moriguchi, Osaka 570, Japan

15. Local administration of interferon-beta promotes proliferation of retinal pigment epithelial cells in repairing process after laser photocoagulation

T. KIMOTO, K. TAKAHASHI, T. TOBE, M. UYAMA and S. SONE

(Osaka, Japan)

Introduction

Trials of systemic administration of interferon (IFN) for treatment of choroidal neovascularization (CNV) have been widely adapted[1,2]. We have demonstrated that IFN has a stimulating effect on retinal pigment epithelium (RPE) proliferation in an experimental model of choroidal neovascularization[3]. Systemic administration of IFN, however, remains a problem with respect to side effects and a high cost. We therefore performed animal experiments to clarify the effect of local administration of human IFN-β on repair of the RPE after laser photocoagulation (PC).

Materials and methods

We designed following two experiments using human IFN-β (Toray Industries), naturally derived from human fibroblasts.

Interferon levels in intraocular tissue after local administration

We measured IFN-β levels in ocular tissues after local administration to 20 adult albino rabbits (3.25 kg). The right eye was used for IFN-β administration and the left eye served as a control with no IFN-β administration. Subtenon injection of 5 MIU IFN-β per eye was performed with a 26-gauge needle. The eyes were enucleated at 15 min and 1, 6, 24 and 48 h after injection and the iris/ciliary body, vitreous body, retina and choroid were dissected. IFN-β levels in each tissue was measured by means of ELISA at each time point.

Effects of local administration of interferon

We observed effects of local administration of IFN-β on repair of the RPE after PC histopathologically. Twelve eyes of six adult pigmented rabbits weighing 2.7–3.0 kg were examined. Photocoagulation was performed on

G. Coscas and F. Cardillo Piccolino (eds.), Retinal Pigment Epithelium and Macular Diseases, pp. 101–105.
© *1998 Kluwer Academic Publishers.*

ocular fundus using a dye laser system (Dye Laser System 920, Coherent Radiation), orange wavelength (595 nm). The conditions of coagulation were 200 µm in diameter, 0.2 s in duration, and 50 mW power (moderate coagulation). Photocoagulation was performed at 8–10 sites each time on days 4 and 8. Five animals (10 eyes, IFN group) were injected subtenon with IFN-β at 1.0×10^6 (two rabbits, group 1), 0.1×10^6 (two rabbits, group 2), 0.01×10^6 (one rabbit, group 3) on 10 consecutive days. In control eyes (one rabbit), placebo (albumin + lactose) was administered in the same manner.

Results

Interferon levels in intraocular tissue after local administration

Locally administrated IFN diffused into the intraocular tissues. The highest IFN level was detected in the choroid (Fig. 1).

Effect of local administration of interferon

In the control group, effects of PC were observed in the RPE, outer nuclear layer and superficial layer of choroid at 3 days. The cells in the lesion were necrotic due to coagulation. Around the coagulated area, RPE cells began to

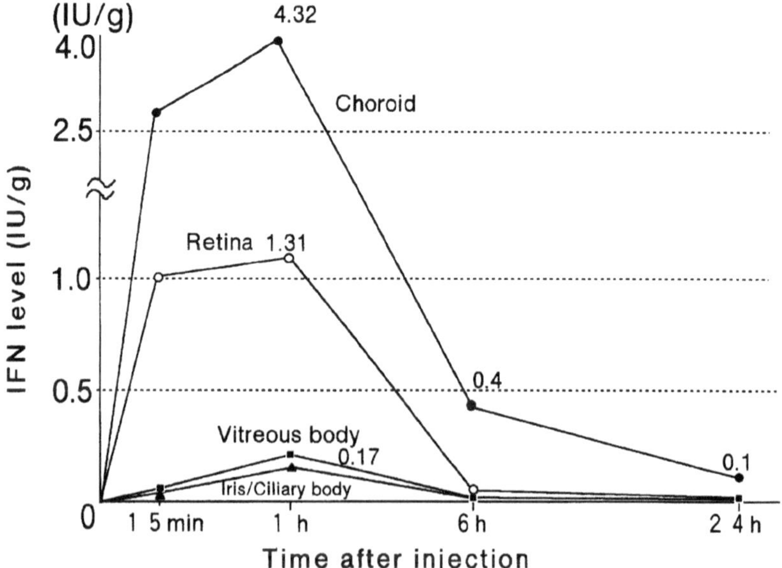

Fig. 1. IFN-β level in intraocular tissues after local administration. Locally administrated IFN spread in diffusion into the intraocular tissues. The highest IFN level was detected in the choroid comparing any other intraocular tissues.

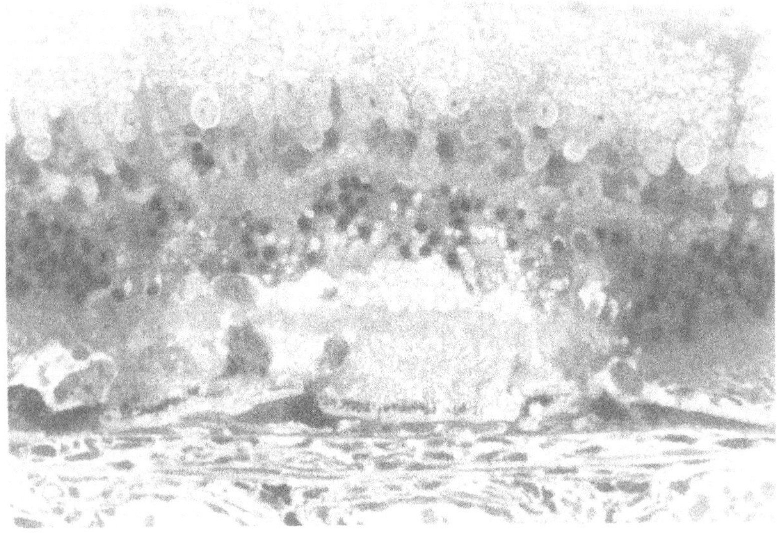

Fig. 2. Control lesion 3 days after photocoagulation. Effects of PC were observed in the RPE, outer nuclear layer and superficial layer of choroid. The cells in the lesion were necrotic due to coagulation. Around the coagulated area, RPE cells began to proliferate from margin of PC lesion, however proliferation were slight.

proliferate from margin of PC lesion; however, proliferation were slight (Fig. 2). Seven days after PC, no remnants of necrotic cells were found in the coagulated area. RPE incompletely repaired the coagulated area.

In IFN group, RPE cells had proliferated markedly by 3 days, spreading to the centre of the PC lesion. A large part of necrotic tissue was already cleared (Fig. 3). Seven days after PC, light microscopy revealed a monolayer of RPE covering Bruch's membrane whic had completely repaired the coagulated area. Many pigment-laden macrophages were observed in the subretinal space.

Electron microscopy revealed that the cells, which had microvilli and cellular polarity, had markedly proliferated in the subretinal space and were seen over Bruch's membrane. A few intercellular junctions were observed between cells, showing characteristics of RPE cells.

Following administration of a low dose of IFN (groups 2 and 3), there was no significant difference in histopathology compared with control groups.

Discussion

Lincoff *et al.* detected IFN-α 2a in the choroid of rabbits after retrobulbar administration of IFN-α 2a and suggested that it provided a significant

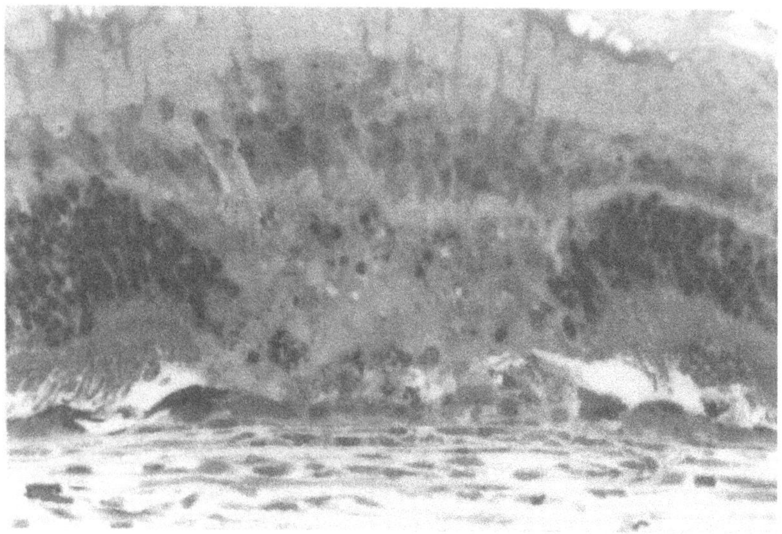

Fig. 3. IFN-treated lesion 3 days after photocoagulation. RPE cells have already proliferated markedly to spread to the centre of the PC lesion. A large part of necrotic tissue is already clear.

concentration of IFN-α 2a within the choroid with minimum systemic effect[3]. In our study, subtenon injection of IFN-β also showed the highest IFN level in the choroid. There were low IFN levels in the other intraocular tissues.

Tobe *et al.* demonstrated regression of experimental CNV in the monkey eye following systemic administration of IFN-β[4]. They suggested that enhanced proliferation of RPE might be important for regression of experimental CNV. In our study, RPE cells proliferated remarkably and rapidly in INF-treated eyes. Local injection of IFN-β also promoted proliferation of RPE cells in the repair process after laser PC when administered systemically.

IFN shows species specificity. The activity of human IFN-β is equivalent to 12% for monkey[5], and about 1% for rabbit. IFN levels in choroid are estimated at about 8000 IU after subtenon administration of 1 MIU IFN-β in this study. This is equivalent to 10 000 IU for human and is an efficient dose for the regression of CNV in human eyes. Subtenon administration of IFN-β provided sufficient IFN-β to the choroid and promoted proliferation of RPE cells in repairing process after laser PC. Local administration of IFN-β might be an ideal treatment for age-related macular degeneration with minimum systemic side effects.

Acknowledgement

This study was supported in part by a grant from the Ministry of Education, Science and Culture of Japan.

References

1. Fung, W.E. Interferon alpha 2a for treatment of age-related macular degeneration. Am J Ophthalmol. 1991; 112: 349–50.
2. Poliner, L.S., Tornambe P.E., Michelson, P.E., Heitzmann, J.G. Interferon alpha-2a for subfoveal neovascularization in age-related macular degeneration. Ophthalmology. 1993; 100: 1417–1424.
3. Lincoff, H., Movshovich, A., Palleroni, A., Rivera, R. Delivery of interferon across the posterior sclera by means of retrobulbar injections. Invest Ophthalmol Vis Sci. 1993; 34 (suppl): 1160.
4. Tobe, T., Takahashi, K., Ohkuma, H., Uyama, M. Inhibition of experimental choroidal neovascularization by interferon beta. Invest Ophthalmol Vis Sci. 1995; 36 (suppl): 552.
5. Bannnai, H., Tatsumi, M., Kohase, M., Ohnishi, E.,Yamazaki, S. Pharmacokinetic study of a human recombinant interferon (RE-IFN-aA) in cynomolgus monkey by 2′-5 oligoadenylate synthetase assay. Jpn J Med Sci Biol. 1985; 38: 113–124.

Department of Ophthalmology
Kansai Medical University
10–15 Fumizonocho
Moriguchi, Osaka 570, Japan

16. Transdifferentiation of cultured retinal pigment epithelial cells

S. GRISANTI, C. GUIDRY and K. HEIMANN

(Cologne, Germany, and Birmingham, AL, USA)

Introduction

Tractional retinal detachment is a common final pathway to a number of different pathological entities, including trauma, rhegmatogenous retinal detachment and diabetic retinopathy[1]. Fundamentally, the various stages of this peculiar process can be characterized as wound healing or response mechanisms. Triggered by an inciting event which disturbs the physioanatomy of the posterior segment, the subsequent breakdown of the vitreo- and blood–retinal barrier leads to the dispersion, migration and proliferation of ocular and non-ocular cells in the vitreous cavity[2]. The development of a contractile scar-like tissue ultimately results in deleterious vitreoretinal traction[3].

The contraction of proliferative vitreoretinal membranes is a cell-mediated event[4]. Immunohistological and light and electron microscopic studies of vitreoretinal membranes have identified many different cells, including inflammatory cells, retinal pigment epithelial cells (RPEC), glia and a mesenchymal-like cell type described as a myofibroblast[5-15]. This latter cell type has been suggested to play a critical role in extracellular matrix contraction associated with wound healing in general, as well as vitreoretinal membranes. Myofibroblasts are so named because these cells have features which are common to both fibroblasts and smooth-muscle cells[16-18]. Although their origin in vitreoretinal membranes has not yet been clarified, it has been suggested that they might be derived from RPEC. The retinal pigment epithelium is a highly specialized monolayer, but its characteristics are dependent on appropriate external signals. Environmental alterations can, therefore, result in metaplastic changes[6,14,19-24]. In the present study we demonstrate that transdifferentiating RPEC *in vitro* not only undergo a morphologic shift but also display cytoskeletal and behavioural changes which result in an ambiguous role of RPEC both to promote and to exert tractional forces. The pathological relevance to the pathogenesis of proliferative vitreoretinal disorders is discussed.

Materials and methods

Cells and culture conditions

Primary cultures of RPEC were established from porcine eyes. The methods used for securing animal tissue were humane and complied with the ARVO

G. Coscas and F. Cardillo Piccolino (eds.), Retinal Pigment Epithelium and Macular Diseases, pp. 107–123.
© *1998 Kluwer Academic Publishers.*

Statement for the Use of Animals in Ophthalmic and Vision research. Freshly enucleated porcine eyes were transported to the laboratory in ice-cold normal saline and processed using a modification of the method of Flood[25] as described previously[26]. Briefly, cells were released from posterior eyecups by treatment with trypsin 0.25% and ethylenediaminetetraacetic acid (EDTA) 0.02% (GibCo, Grand Island, NY). To avoid contamination with other cells we performed a density gradient centrifugation through a cushion composed of Percol 40% (Pharmacia Biotech Inc., Piscataway, NJ) with 0.01 mol/l Na_2PO_4 and 0.15 mol/l NaCl, pH 7.4. After centrifugation at room temperature, the pigmented cells were recovered in the pellet, while other cells remained near the top of the cushion. All cells were harvested for subculture or experimentation using trypsin 0.05% and EDTA 0.02%. For experimentation we routinely used cultures at 70–80% confluence. The isolated cells were defined as a pure population by ascertaining cytokeratin expression and according to their intact epithelial morphology and growth characteristics.

Human dermal fibroblasts (HDF) were established from foreskins obtained at circumcisions as previously described[27] Cells between passage numbers 5–10 were used for these experiments. The tenets of the Declaration of Helsinki were followed for the collection and use of human material. The human material utilized was normally discarded surgical specimens.

Cells were maintained in Dulbecco's modified Eagle's medium (GibCo) supplemented with 20 mM HEPES (Sigma, St. Louis, MO) (DMEM) and 10% fetal bovine serum (GibCo). Cultures were incubated at 37°C in a humidified atmosphere of 5% CO_2/95% air with medium changes three times per week. Morphological changes occurring during culture were documented using an inverted phase-contrast microscope (Nikon TMS, Garden City, NY).

Indirect immunofluorescence

RPEC at different transdifferentiation stages were plated on sterile glass coverslips (Fisher Scientific, Atlanta, GA) in 35-mm tissue culture dishes (Corning) and incubated in growth medium. Specimens were washed in PBS and consequently fixed with methanol/acetone (1:1) for 15 min at −24°C. Coverslips were rinsed with PBS, and then incubated with blocking buffer (PBS) containing 20% normal serum from rabbit or goat (Sigma) and 5% bovine serum albumin for 1 h in a moist chamber at room temperature. Washes with PBS (3 × 10 min) were followed by incubation (overnight at 4°C) with the primary antibodies. These consisted of a monoclonal mouse anti-alpha smooth muscle actin (clone 1A4, Sigma) and a monoclonal anti-pan-cytokeratin from mouse (Sigma, C-2931) diluted in PBS containing 1% normal rabbit serum and 3% bovine serum albumin. After repeated washes the coverslips were incubated for an additional 45 min with fluorescein-conjugated rabbit anti-mouse IgG (Sigma) or rhodamine-conjugated goat anti-mouse IgG (Sigma). The slides were finally mounted onto slides with fluoromount G (Fisher Scientific). Staining was visualized using a Nikon

Optiphot-2 microscope (Nikon) equipped with epifluorescence and phase contrast optics and appropriate filters. In control incubations, the primary antibody was omitted.

Production of cell conditioned media

For the production of cell-conditioned media we used porcine RPEC at passages 1, 7 and 15, grown under routine conditions in 75 cm^2 tissue culture flasks[24]. Different populations were tested. When confluent, the flasks were washed extensively and incubated with serum-free media for 24 h at 37°C. Thereafter, the cultures were rinsed again and replaced with serum-free DMEM (10 ml/flask) containing 1mg/ml BSA. After the second 24 h incubation the conditioned medium was collected and the cells released with trypsin/EDTA and counted electronically. The conditioned media were centrifuged to remove any cellular debris and stored at -20°C until use. Using these same techniques we demonstrated previously, using an enzyme-linked immunosorbent assay to detect BSA, that contamination of conditioned media by serum proteins is less than 0.001%[26].

Assay of collagen gel contraction

Native type I collagen gels were prepared as described previously[27]. Vitrogen 100 (Celltrix, Palo Alto, CA) was adjusted to physiological ionic strength, pH and a concentration of 1.5 mg/ml with 10% of 10 × PBS (0.1 M Na_2HPO_4/1.5 M NaCl) and 0.1 M NaOH while maintained at 4°C. Aliquots (200 µl) of this solution were added to the center of a 12 mm circular score on the bottom of a 24-well tissue culture plate (Corning Glass Works) and polymerized at 37°C for 90 min. The resulting hemispherical gels are approximately 2 mm thick and attached only to the bottom surface of the well.

Cells released by trypsin/EDTA treatment were washed once with growth medium (containing serum) and again with serum-free medium before they were placed in the appropriate number on the top of the polymerized collagen gels in 50 µl serum-free medium. These were incubated for an additional 30 min at 37°C to allow cell adhesion. After incubation each well was flooded with DMEM containing 1.0 mg/ml BSA, with the appropriate experimental additives, to a final volume of 1.0 ml/well (Fig. 1A).

Gel contraction was observed as a function of reduced gel thickness (Fig. 1B). The gel height was measured using an inverted phase-contrast microscope (Nikon) equipped with a Z-axis digitizer (LaSico, Los Angeles, CA) by adjusting the plane of focus from a central reference point on the bottom to the cell layer on the top of the gel and recording the distance of stage movement. For kinetic studies, the gel thicknesses were measured after well flooding and re-measured after appropriate incubation times at 37°C. Percentage contraction was determined by dividing the remaining height by

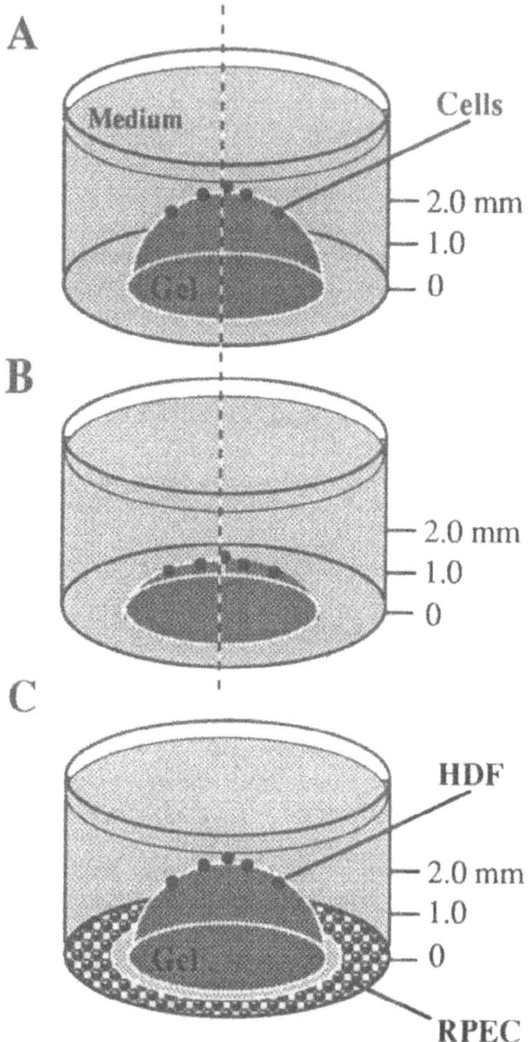

Fig. 1. Contraction assay model. (A) A polymerizing solution of type I collagen (0.2 ml) is placed within circular scores on the bottom of wells. Cells suspended in media are placed on top of the polymerized gel and allowed to attach before the well is flooded with medium. (B) Gel contraction is measured as reduced gel thickness in the center of the gel, at a mark applied during scoring. (C) Modified assay containing both the secretory, contraction promoting (RPEC) cells and the contractile target (HDF) cells.

the original height and then subtracting this from 100. All assays were performed in triplicate and each experiment was repeated at least three times, with different cell populations and included negative and positive control wells containing serum-free medium and wells with medium containing 100 ml (10%) FBS, respectively. The mean extent of contraction was determined for each incubation time and the standard deviation calculated.

Co-culture experiments including both secretory and contractile target cells (Fig. 1C) were prepared using a modification of the previously described technique[26]. The cells acting as the secretory component were released with trypsin/EDTA treatment, washed once with growth medium (containing serum) and again with serum-free medium. These cells were placed in the appropriate number outside the 12 mm circular score on the bottom of a 24-well tissue culture plate in 50 µl serum-free medium. They were then incubated for 6 h to allow cell adhesion, after which the collagen aliquots were prepared and placed within the circular score as normal. After polymerization, target cells were placed on the gel surface. The influence of the secretory cells on the collagen gel was excluded since omission of the contractile target cells resulted in non-contraction of the collagen gels, light microscopic analysis of the wells showed no contact between secretory cells and hemispherical gels, and using 35 mm 6-well plates with secretory cells placed in the concentric ring area surrounding a 24 mm circular score and the gels within the 12 mm circular internal score we obtained similar results.

Materials

Cell culture reagents, including DMEM, FBS and trypsin-EDTA were purchased from Gibco Laboratories (Grand Island, NY). BSA, HEPES and other general chemicals were obtained from Sigma Chemical Co. (St. Louis, MO) and Fisher Scientific (Atlanta, GA).

Results

Cultured RPEC undergo morphological transdifferentiation

The homogeneity of the RPEC cultures isolated from porcine eyes was assessed by light and fluorescence microscopy. Within 1 week after seeding the proliferating cells formed a confluent monolayer which appeared homogenous. All cells examined possessed the characteristic epithelial morphology (Fig. 2A), cobblestone configuration, were pigmented and dysplayed cytokeratin filaments. With continuous subcultivation, the cells transdifferentiated to a mesenchymal cell-like phenotype. The transdifferentiation was associated with cell spreading, loss of pigmentation and cobblestone configuration, the development of cytoplasmic extensions and resulted in a more fusiform, fibroblastic morphology (Fig. 2B).

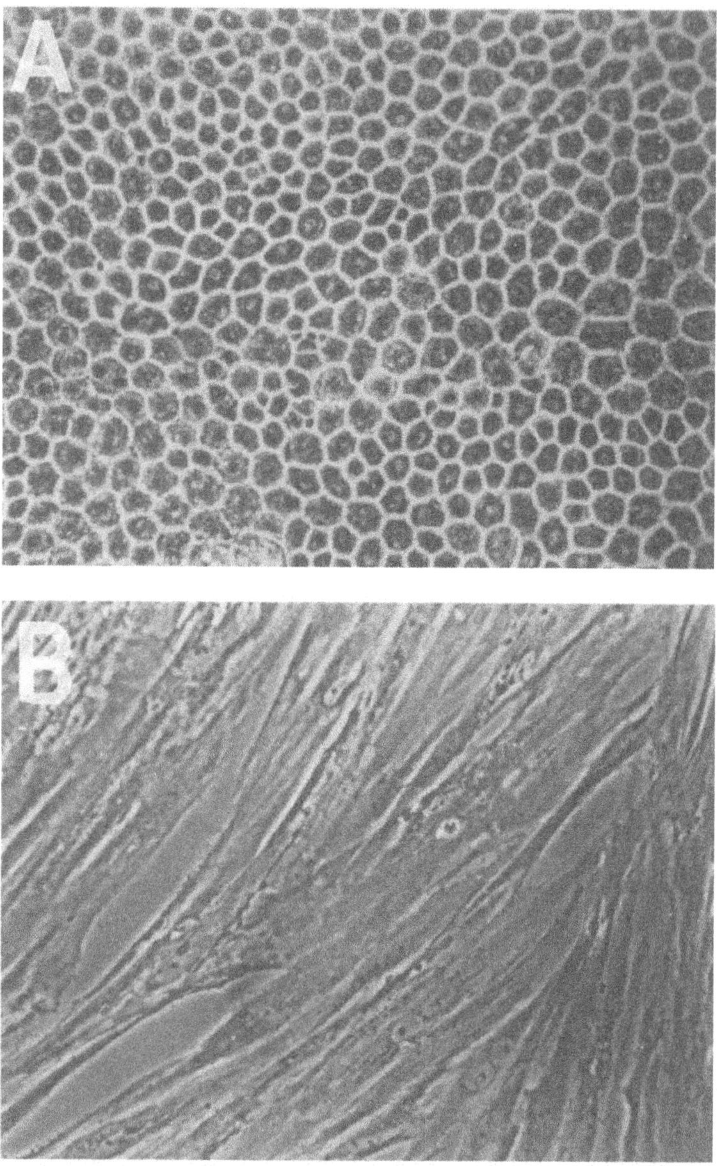

Fig. 2. Morphologies of retinal pigment epithelium cells (RPEC) cultured under routine conditions. Primary culture (A) and passage 15 (E) RPEC from the same animal.

Transdifferentiated RPEC have an altered actin cytoskeleton and exhibit de novo expression of alpha-smooth muscle actin

As reported previously[24], transdifferentiation includes the shift from the differentiated cicumferential actin ring to a linearly arranged cytoskeleton composed of numerous stress fibers. Similarly the newly expressed alpha-smooth muscle actin filaments also span through the cytoplasm (Fig. 3).

Transdifferentiation of RPEC is coincident with enhanced serum-stimulated matrix contraction

Morphological transdifferentiation of RPEC is associated with increased contraction potentials. During the course of a 48 h incubation, differentiated, first passage RPEC seeded at a density of 25 000 cells/gel were not able to produce significant changes in gel thickness (Fig. 4A) and remained rounded (Fig. 5A). In contrast, the same number of seventh passage cells, which we termed transitional cells because of their incomplete transdifferentiation, reduced the gel thickness by nearly 60% after 24 h (Fig. 4B). The same extent of reduction of the gel thickness was produced by fully transdifferentiated RPEC after only 6 h. These cells extended robust pseudopodia and produced visible striations of the underlying collagen matrix (Fig. 5B). Incubation for 48 h resulted in an 80% reduction in gel thickness (Fig. 4C).

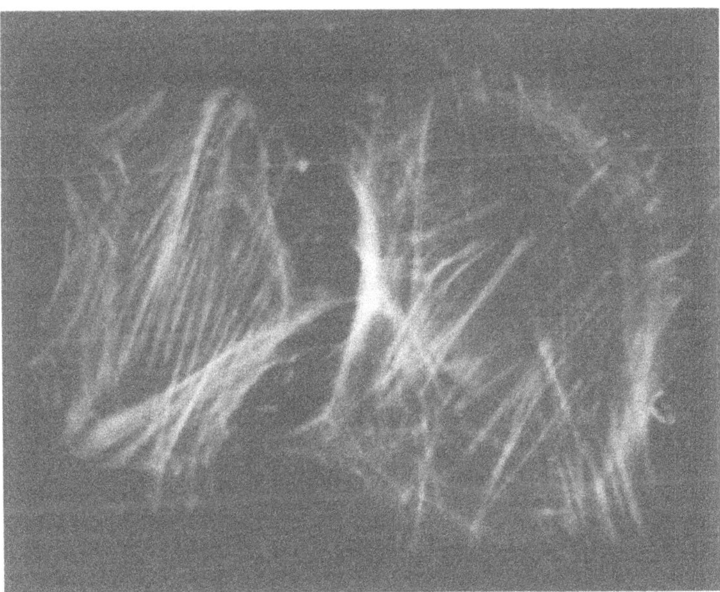

Fig. 3. Immunolocalization of alpha-smooth muscle actin filaments expressed by transdifferentiated retinal pigment epithelial cells (RPEC).

 S. Grisanti et al.

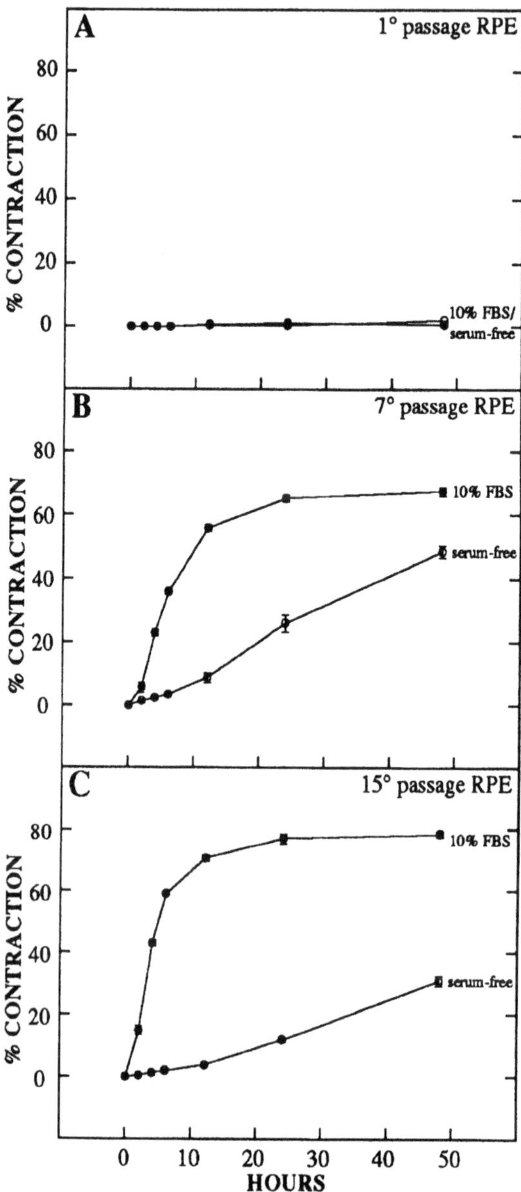

Fig. 4. Kinetics of collagen gel contraction by differentiated and transdifferentiated retinal pigment epithelial cells (RPEC). Primary culture (A), passage 7 (B) and passage 15 (C) RPEC were attached to collagen gels (25 000 cells/gel) and incubated in medium with (●) or without 10% FBS (○). At the times indicated, gel thickness was measured and the percent contraction was determined. Data represent the averages ± S.D. from triplicate cultures.

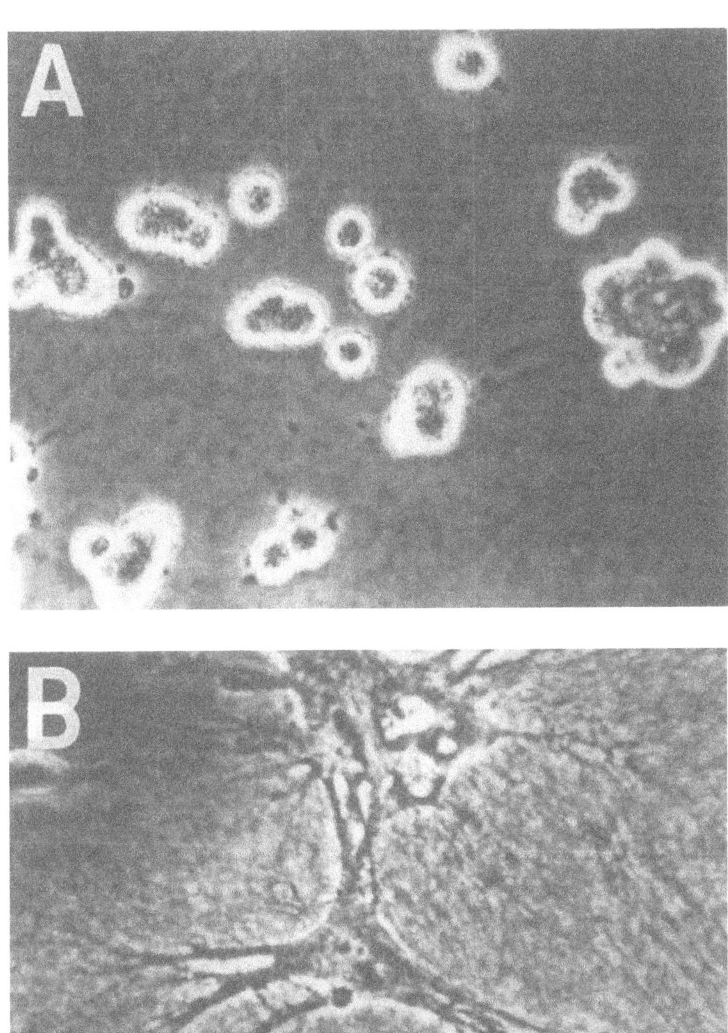

Fig. 5. Morphologies of differentiated (primary culture, A) and transdifferentiated (passage 15, B) retinal pigment epithelial cells (RPEC) attached to collagen gels and incubated in medium containing serum (10%) for 24 h (A) and 6 h (B), respectively.

Transitional RPEC generate tractional forces under serum-free conditions but lose this ability with progressive transdifferentiation

We also examined the ability of cells to generate tractional forces while incubated in serum-free medium. As expected, highly differentiated RPEC, lacking the ability to exert serum-promoted tractional forces, were not able to produce a significant change in gel thickness within 48 h (Fig. 4A). The same number of transitional seventh passage cells, however, reduced the gel thickness by 35% after 24 h and by nearly 50% after a 48 h incubation (Fig. 4B). Although fully transdifferentiated RPEC displayed the highest serum-promoted traction potentials, their ability to contract the collagenous matrix under serum-free conditions was somewhat lower, 10% and 30% after 24 and 48 h, respectively (Fig. 4C).

RPEC contraction under serum-free conditions is dependent on endogenous factors

We have demonstrated previously[26] that RPEC secrete soluble factor(s) which stimulate human dermal fibroblasts to generate tractional forces. To examine whether this observation was related to the enhanced ability of RPEC to contract under serum-free condition we examined the responsiveness of highly contractile 15th passage RPEC to serum-free medium conditioned by noncontractile first passage cells (Fig. 6). Passage 15 RPEC were seeded on collagen gels (25 000 cells/gel) and incubated with DMEM alone, plus serum (10% FBS) or plus RPEC-conditioned media. Cells incubated in DMEM containing serum were highly contractile and reduced the gel thickness by 75% and 85% after a 12 and 24 h incubation, respectively. Matrix contraction promoted by conditioned media caused the reduction of the gel thickness by 33% and 67% after 12 and 24 h of incubation, respectively. In contrast, cells incubated in serum-free medium did not induce substantial collagen matrix contraction after 12 h and reduced the gel thickness by only 19% after 24 h of incubation.

Transdifferentiating RPEC progressively lose the ability to secrete contraction-promoting factors

Having demonstrated that RPEC contraction is enhanced by endogenously produced contraction-stimulating factors, we next examined whether the reduced contraction by fully transdifferentiated RPEC, under serum-free conditions, is related to diminished production of the same. For this we examined the secretory products of cells at different stages of transdifferentiation, collected as conditioned media. To accurately compare the secretory activities, we counted the conditioning cells and used a volume equivalent to the secretory product of 10 000 cells/gel diluted to the final total volume of 1 ml/well. The response profile of the medium based on numerically standardized cell numbers is shown in Fig. 7. Fibroblasts incubated in medium conditioned by first passage RPEC reduced gel thickness

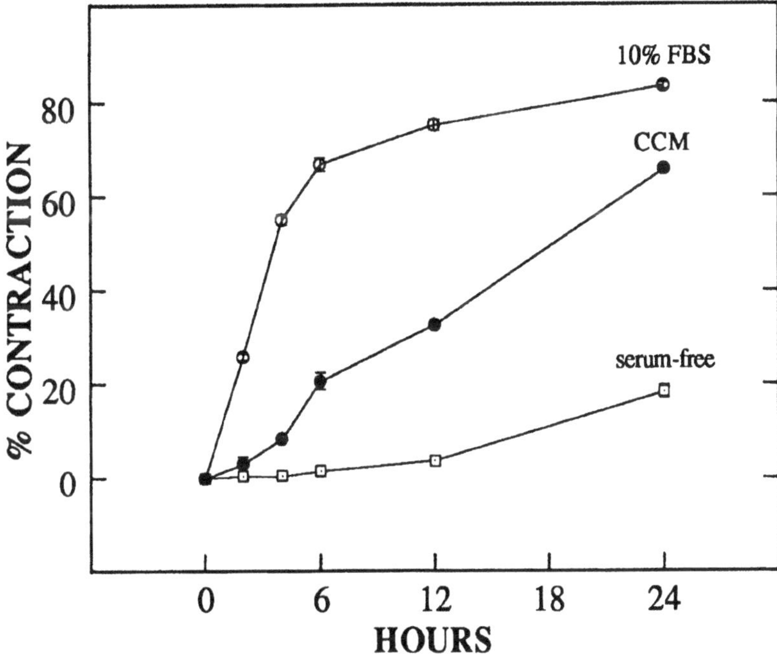

Fig. 6. Factor(s) released by differentiated retinal pigment epithelial cells (RPEC) induce contraction of transdifferentiated RPEC. Passage 15 RPEC attached to collagen gels (25 000 cells/gel) were incubated in serum-free medium (□), DMEM plus 10% FBS (○) or medium conditioned by primary passage RPEC (CCM; ●). At the times indicated gel thickness was measured and the percent contraction was determined. These data represent the averages ± S.D. from triplicate cultures.

by a maximum of 52% after 24 h of incubation. Similarly the secretory product of seventh passage cells induced a gel thickness reduction of approximately 45% after 24 h of incubation. The lowest cell-contraction promoting activity was displayed by media exposed to fully transdifferentiated RPEC.

RPEC in a closed system continuously release cell contraction promoter(s) affecting the activity of distinct target cells

In order to examine whether the contraction exerted by transitional RPEC under serum free conditions is promoted by continuously released factors through a paracrine mechanism, we modified our routine contraction assay model. We placed the potential secretory cells in the periphery of the well where they could not have a direct effect on the collagen gel dimensions and placed 25 000 HDF on the top of the gels to serve as target cells. Differentiated RPEC derived from the first passage induced HDF gel contraction of approximately 50% after a 25 h incubation (Fig. 8A). A similar result could be

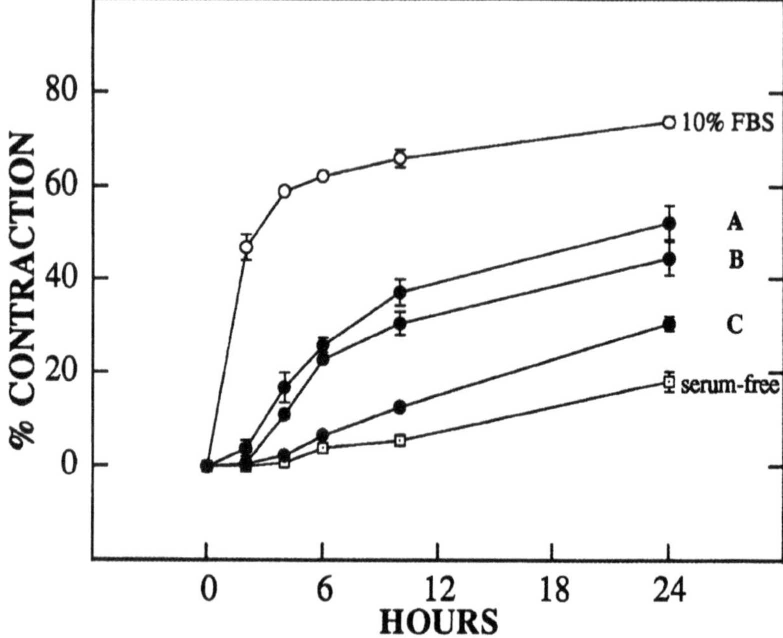

Fig. 7. Fibroblast contraction stimulated by factor(s) secreted by differentiated and trans-differentiated RPEC. Human dermal fibroblasts attached to collagen gels (25 000 cells/gel) were incubated in DMEM containing 1.0 mg/ml bovine serum albumin without serum (□) or plus 10% FBS (○) as negative and positive control. Kinetics of collagen gel contraction promoted by factor(s) released by equivalent numbers of RPEC at passage 1 (A), passage 7 (B) and passage 15 (C). Data represent the averages ± S.D. from triplicate cultures.

achieved by using seventh passage, transitional RPEC (Fig. 8B). In contrast, the thickness of gels incubated for 25 h with passage 15, transdifferentiated RPEC were reduced by 30% (Fig. 8C).

Discussion

Retinal pigment epithelial cells (RPEC) are highly specialized cells with well defined characteristics[28–31]. However, certain environmental signals associated with disease induce a morphological and biological transdifferentiation in these cells, characterized by a gradual shift from the differentiated pigment-filled epithelial cell to the transdifferentiated phenotype with a fibroblastic appearance. RPEC *in vitro* undergo a similar phenotypic modulation and transdifferentiate from an epithelial cell (Fig. 2A) into a cell with mesenchyme-like appearance (Fig. 2B). This study presents evidence that retinal pigment epithelial cell metaplasia includes a gradual transition from a secretory cell with prostrate traction potentials to an highly contractile phenotype with

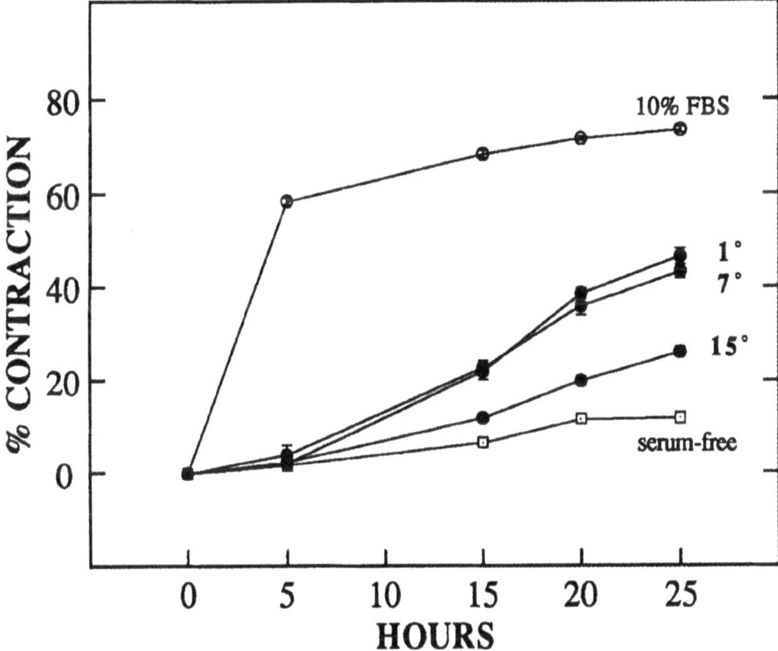

Fig. 8. Kinetics of collagen gel contraction by human dermal fibroblasts cocultured with RPEC of different passages. Fibroblasts seeded on the top of collagen gels (25 000 cells/gel) were incubated in DMEM containing 1 mg/ml bovine serum albumin without (□) and plus 10% FBS (○) as negative and positive control. RPEC from passage 1 (1°), passage 7 (7°) and passage 15 (15°) were seeded on the well bottom (25 000 and 50 000 per well) apart from the hemispherical collagen gel. Changes in gel thickness were measured at the times indicated and the percent contraction was determined. The results shown are the means ± S.D. as calculated from triplicate cultures under each condition. Other details are described in Methods.

modest secretory activities. With the capacity to function both as a promoter and target cell, it appears likely that these cells play a pivotal role in the development of tractional forces in vitreoretinal membranes[14,20,24,26]. The transdifferentiation process, hereby, seems to be crucially dependent on proliferation and cell spreading[24].

Highly differentiated RPEC have been shown to contain a contractile cytoskeleton. Nevertheless, differentiated RPEC stimulated by FBS are not able to generate sufficient tractional forces to reduce the thickness of a collagenous matrix (Fig. 4A). Transdifferentiated cells, however, incubated under the same conditions reduce the gel thickness by approximately 80% within 24 h (Fig. 4C). Interestingly, increased contraction potentials correlate with the expression of alpha-smooth muscle actin, a myoid marker which is up-regulated in fibrocontractive tissues and implicated as a functional component of cell contraction[15-18].

We also observed that the magnitude of the FBS response was inversely related to the ability of the cells to generate tractional forces without exogenous stimulation. RPEC which are not fully transdifferentiated had lower serum-stimulated responses than fully transdifferentiated cells, but contracted the gel thickness to an higher extent when incubated under serum-free conditions (Fig. 4B, C). In light of the previous report that RPEC are able to synthesize and secrete contraction-promoting factor(s)[26] we considered whether cellular contraction under serum-free conditions might be mediated by an autocrine mechanism and that this capacity declines with continuous transdifferentiation as a consequence of reduced synthesis and/or release of the relevant factor(s).

To examine these theories we first demonstrated that RPEC conditioned media did indeed contain factor(s) which induce matrix contraction by responsive cells (Fig. 6). Therefore, autocrine stimulation should be possible. To compare the relative amounts of contraction-stimulating activity secreted by the distinct RPEC types at different stages of transdifferentiation, we used human dermal fibroblasts as the target cell. Media conditioned by differentiated RPEC possessed the highest activity, in contrast to fully transdifferentiated cells which promoted substantially lower amounts of activity (Fig. 7). We found it intriguing that RPEC, which were not fully transdifferentiated, but were already capable of generating significant tractional force (Fig. 4B), were also able to secrete large amounts of contraction-stimulating activity (Fig. 6). These cells, which we called transitional cells, also had the highest capacity to contract in the absence of exogenous stimulation (Fig. 4).

A previous study has already demonstrated that the RPEC-secreted contraction promoter(s) is a soluble, released factor(s)[26]. However, we performed an experiment to better mimic the circumstances of a paracrine-type stimulatory event which might occur in a semi-closed system like the vitreal cavity. This included the coculture of both a promoter (RPEC) and a responder cell (HDF; Fig. 1C). The results shown in Fig. 8 demonstrate the potential of this mechanism. Furthermore, these results are consistent with the contraction-promoting activity in media derived from different RPEC passages (Fig. 6). Both differentiated and transitional RPEC release factor(s) capable of inducing significant cell-mediated contraction. Fully transdifferentia ted RPEC retain only a fraction of this ability.

A number of studies have reported that cultured RPEC synthesize and release several factors which induce mitosis, chemotaxis, affect angiogenesis and retinal cell survival[32–40]. Some of these factors have been identified including transforming growth factor-β[41–43], basic fibroblast growth factor[44,45], insulin-like growth factor (IGF)[46–49], interleukin-6[50–52], platelet derived growth factor (PDGF) and PDGF-like molecules[40,53,54]. The presence of related receptors, such as IGF binding-proteins[46–49] and PDGF receptors[54] on RPEC supports the suggested autocrine mechanisms. Further studies to determine the contraction-promoting factors in RPEC conditioned media should confirm this hypothesis.

In summary, our results confirm that differentiated RPEC synthesize and release soluble mediators able to induce tractional forces in other cell types. The ability of RPEC to elaborate and release contraction promoters decreases with progressive transdifferentiation and is negatively correlated with the ability of the cells to generate tractional forces. The released factors may have a paracrine effect both on distinct contractile target cells and transdifferentiated, highly contractile RPEC. Autocrine and autostimulatory mechanisms enable transitional RPEC to play a bivalent and autonomous role. The contraction-promoting activity induced by RPEC-conditioned media probably reflects the aggregate effect of several factors. The precise nature of the produced cell contraction-promoting factors remains to be elucidated. The understanding of the mechanisms accounting for the development of membrane contraction and vitreoretinal traction may provide relevant insights and reveal itself as beneficial in envisioning a future therapy for patients with tractional retinal detachments.

Acknowledgements

This study was supported by the Deutsche Forschungsgemeinschaft (GR 1354/1-1); National Eye Institute (EYO9536); the Juvenile Diabetes Foundation, International, New York, NY.

References

1. Hilton, G., Machemer, R., Michels, R., Okun, E., Schepens, C., Schwartz, A. The Retina Society Terminology Committee: The classification of retinal detachment with Proliferative Vitreorctinopathy. Ophthalmology. 1983; 90: 121–125.
2. Weller, M., Heimann, K., Wiedemann, P. Proliferative vitreoretinopathy – is it anything more than wound healing at the wrong place? Int Ophthalmol. 1990; 14: 105–117.
3. Wiedemann, P., Weller, M. The pathophysiology of proliferative vitreoretinopathy. Acta Ophthalmol. 1988; 189: 3–15.
4. Glaser, B.M., Cardin, A. and Biscoe, B. Proliferative vitreoretinopathy: the mechanism of development of vitreoretinal traction. Ophthalmology. 1987; 94: 327–332.
5. Laqua, H., Machemer, R. Glial cell proliferation in retinal detachment (massive periretinal proliferation). Am J Ophthalmol. 1975; 80: 602–618.
6. Machemer, R., Lacqua, H. Pigment epithelium proliferation in retinal detachment (massive periretinal proliferation). Am J Ophthalmol. 1975; 80: 1–23.
7. Van Horn, D.L., Aaberg, T.M., Machemer, R., Fenzl, R.F. Glial cell proliferation in human retinal detachment with massive periretinal proliferation. Am J Ophthalmol. 1977; 84: 383–395.
8. Kampik, A., Kenyon, K., Michels, R., Green, W., de la Cruz, Z. Epiretinal and vitreous membranes: comparative study of 56 cases. Arch Ophthalmol. 1981; 99: 1445–1454.
9. Hiscott, P., Grierson, I., McLeod, D. Retinal pigment epithelial cells in epiretinal membranes. An immunohistochemical study. Br J Ophthalmol. 1984; 68: 708–715
10. Hiscott, P., Grierson, I., McLeod, D. Natural history of fibrocellular epiretinal membranes. A quantitative, autoradiographic and immunohistochemical study. Br J Ophthalmol. 1985; 69: 810–823.

11. Jerdan, J.A., Pepose, J.S., Michels, R.G. *et al.* Proliferative vitreoretinopathy membranes: An immunohistochemical study. Ophthalmology. 1989; 96: 801–811.
12. Guerin, C.J., Wolfshagen, R.W., Eifrig, D.E., Anderson, D.H. Immunocytochemical identification of Muller's glia as a component of human epiretinal membranes. Invest Ophthalmol Vis Sci. 1990; 31: 1483–1491.
13. Vinores, S., Campochiaro, P., Conway, B. Ultrastructural and electron-immunocytochemical characterization of cells in epiretinal membranes. Invest Ophthalmol Vis Sci. 1990; 31: 14–28.
14. Fuchs, U., Kivelä, T., Tarkkanen, A. Cytoskeleton in normal and reactive human retinal pigment epithelial cells. Invest Ophthlamol Vis Sci. 1991; 32: 3178–3186.
15. Walshe, R., Esser, P., Wiedemann, P., Heimann, K. Proliferative retinal diseases: myofibroblasts cause chronic vitreoretinal traction. Br J Ophthalmol. 1992; 76: 550–552.
16. Gabbiani, G., Hirschel, B.J., Ryan, G.B., Statkov, P.R., Majno, G. Granulation tissues as a contractile organ: a study of structure and function. J Exp Med. 1972; 135: 719–734.
17. Gabbiani, G. The myofibroblast. A key cell in wound healing and in fibrocontractive diseases of the connective tissue. Schweiz Rundsch Med Prax. 1984; 73: 939–941.
18. Darby, I., Skalli, O., Gabbiani, G. α-Smooth muscle actin is transiently expressed by myofibroblasts during experimental wound healing. Lab Invest. 1990; 63: 21–29.
19. Mueller-Jensen, K., Machemer, R., Roobik, A. Autotransplantation of retinal pigment epithelium in intravitreal diffusion chamber. Am J Ophthalmol. 1975; 80: 530–537.
20. Mandelcorn, M., Machemer, R., Fineberg, E., Hersch, S. Proliferation and metaplasia of intravitreal retinal pigment epithelium cell autotransplants. Am J Ophthalmol. 1975; 80: 227–237.
21. Newsome, D., Rodrigues, M., Machemer, R. Human massive periretinal proliferation: *in vitro* characteristics of cellular components. Arch Ophthalmol. 1981; 99: 873–880.
22. Radtke, N., Tano, Y., Chandler, D., Machemer, R. Simulation of massive periretinal proliferation by autotransplantation of retinal pigment epithelial cells in rabbits. Am J Ophthalmol. 1981; 91: 76–87.
23. Heriot, W., Machemer, R. Pigment epithelial repair. Graefe's Arch Clin Exp Ophthalmol. 1992; 230: 91–100.
24. Grisanti, S., Guidry, C. Transdifferentiation of retinal pigment epithelial cells from epithelial to mesenchymal phenotype. Invest Ophthalmol Vis Sci. 1995; 36: 391–405.
25. Flood, M., Gouras, P., Kjeldbye, H. Growth characteristics and ultrastructure of human retinal pigment epithelium *in vitro*. Invest Ophthalmol Vis Sci. 1980; 19: 1309–1320.
26. Guidry, C., McFarland, R., Morris, R., Witherspoon, C., Hook, M. Collagen gel contraction by cells associated with proliferative vitreoretinopathy. Invest Ophthalmol Vis Sci. 1992; 33: 2429–2435.
27. Guidry, C., Grinnel, F. Studies on the mechanism of hydrated collagen gel reorganization by human skin fibroblasts. J Cell Sci. 1985; 79: 67–81.
28. Young, R., Bok, D. Participation of the retinal pigment epithelium in the rod outer segment renewal process. J Cell Biol. 1969; 42: 392–403.
29. Zinn, K., Marmor, M. The Pigment Epithelium. Cambridge: Harvard University Press, 1979.
30. Owaribe, K. The cytoskeleton of retinal pigment epithelial cells. Prog Ret Eye Res. 1989; 8: 23–49.
31. Hunt, R. Intermediate filaments and other cytoskeletal structures in retinal pigment epithelial cells. Prog Ret Eye Res. 1994; 13: 125–145.
32. Glaser, B.M., Campochiaro, P.A., Davis, J.L., Sato, M. Retinal pigment epithelial cells release an inhibitor of neovascularization. Arch Ophthalmol. 1985; 103: 1870–1875.
33. Rosenbaum, J.T., O'Rourke, L., Davies, G., Wenger, C., David, L., Robertson, J.E. Retinal pigment epithelial cells secrete substances that are chemotactic for monocytes. Curr Eye Res. 1987; 6: 793–800.
34. Bryan, J.A., Campochiaro, P.A. A retinal pigment epithelial cell-derived growth factor(s). Arch Ophthalmol. 1986; 104: 422–425.
35. Wong, H.C., Boulton, M., McLeod, D., Bayly, M., Clark, P., Marshall, J. Retinal pigment epithelial cells in culture produce retinal vascular mitogens. Arch Ophthalmol. 1988; 106: 1439–1443.

36. Morse, L.S., Terrell, J., Sidikaro, Y. Bovine retinal pigment epithelial cells promotes proliferation of choroidal endothelium *in vitro*. Arch Ophthalmol. 1989; 107: 1659–1663.
37. Tombran Tink, J., Johnson, I.V. Neuronal differentiation of retinoblastoma cells induced by medium conditioned by human RPE cells. Invest Ophthalmol Vis Sci. 1989; 30: 1700–1707.
38. Liu, Y., Gaur, V., Turner, J.E. Photoreceptor cell survival and differentiation stimulated by rat retinal pigment epithelium conditioned medium in tissue culture. Invest Ophthalmol Vis Sci. 1990; 31: 75.
39. Adamis, A.P., Shima, D.T., Yeo, K.T. *et al.* Synthesis and secretion of vascular permeability factor/vascular endothelial growth factor by human retinal pigment epithelial cells. Biochem Biophys Res Commun. 1993; 193: 631–638.
40. Campochiaro, P.A. Cytokine production by retinal pigment epithelial cell. Int Rev Cytol. 1993; 146: 75–82.
41. Connor, T., Roberts, A., Sporn, M., Davis, J., Glaser, B. RPE cells synthesize and release transforming growth factor-beta, a modulator of endothelial cell growth and wound healing. Invest Ophthalmol Vis Sci. 1988; 29: 307.
42. Tanihara, H., Yoshida, M., Matsumoto, M., Yoshimura, N. Identification of transforming growth factor-β expressed in cultured human retinal pigment epithelial cells. Invest Ophthalmol Vis Sci. 1993; 34; 413–419.
43. Masumoto, M., Yoshimura, N., Honda, Y. Increased production of transforming growth factor-$\beta2$ from cultured human retinal pigment epithelial cells by photocoagulation. Invest Ophthalmol Vis Sci. 1994; 35: 4245–4252.
44. Schweigerer, L., Malerstein, B., Neufeld, G., Gospodarowicz, D. Basic fibroblast growth factor is synthesized in cultured retinal pigment epithelial cells. Biochem Biophys Res Commun. 1987; 143: 934–940.
45. Gao, H., Hollyfield, J.G. Basic fibroblast growth factor (bFGF) immunolocalization in the rodent outer retina demonstrated with an anti-rodent bFGF antibody. Brain Res. 1992; 585: 355–360.
46. Ocrant, I., Fay, C.T., Parmelee, J.T. Expression of insulin and insulin-like growth factor receptors and binding proteins by retinal pigment epithelium. Curr Eye Res. 1991; 52: 581–589.
47. Randolph, A., Yee, D., Feldman, E.L. Insulin-like growth factor binding protein expression in human retinal pigment epithelial cells. Ann NY Acad Sci. 1993; 692: 265–267.
48. Moriarty, P., Boulton, M., Dickson, A., McLeod, D. Production of IGF-1 and IGF binding proteins by retinal cells *in vitro*. Br J Ophthalmol. 1994; 78: 638–642.
49. Tagaki, H., Yoshimura, N., Tanihara, H., Honda, Y. Insulin-like growth factor-related genes, receptors, and binding proteins in cultured human retinal pigment epithelial cells. Invest Ophthalmol Vis Sci. 1994; 35: 916–923.
50. Elner, V.M., Scales, W., Elner, S.G., Danforth, J., Kunkel, S.L., Strieter, R.M. Interleukin-6 (IL-6) gene expression and secretion by cytokine-stimulated human retinal pigment epithelial cells. Exp Eye Res. 1992; 54: 361–368.
51. Benson, M.T., Shepherd, L., Rees, R.C., Rennie, I.G. Production of interleukin-6 by human retinal pigment epithelium *in vitro* and its regulation by other cytokines. Curr Eye Res. 1992; 11: 173–179.
52. Chiba, K., Inada, K., Sakamoto, S. Human cultured retinal pigment epithelial cells produce interleukin-6. Nippon Ganka Gakkai Zasshi. 1993; 97: 29–35.
53. Campochiaro, P.A., Sugg, R., Grotendorst, G., Hjeleland, L.M. Retinal pigment epithelial cells produce PDGF-like proteins and secrete them into their media. Exp Eye Res. 1989; 49: 217–227.
54. Campochiaro, P.A., Hackett, S.F., Vinores, S.A. *et al.* Platelet-derived growth factor is an autocrine growth stimulator in retinal pigment epithelial cells. J Cell Sci. 1994; 107: 2459–2469.

University Eye Clinic Cologne
Joseph-Stelzmann-Strasse 9
50931 Cologne, Germany

17. Retinal pigment epithelial transplantation in exudative age-related macular degeneration: what do *in vivo* and *in vitro* studies teach us?

L.V. DEL PRIORE, T.H. TEZEL, T.C. HO and H.J. KAPLAN

(St Louis, MO, USA and Taipei, Taiwan)

Introduction

Subfoveal choroidal neovascularization remains a leading cause of severe visual loss in patients with age-related macular degeneration (AMD)[1-4]. Unfortunately, most patients who develop choroidal neovascularization in AMD have subfoveal choroidal neovascularization at the time of presentation, or ill-defined choroidal neovascularization which is not readily amenable to laser treatment. Studies of the natural history of subfoveal choroidal neovascularization in AMD indicate that 70% of eyes achieve a visual acuity of 20/200 (6/60) or worse within 2 years of presentation[1]. In 1991, the Macular Photocoagulation Study group demonstrated a treatment benefit of laser photocoagulation compared with no treatment for a select subgroup of eyes with subfoveal choroidal neovascularization associated with AMD[3,4], but there is a significant postoperative reduction in visual acuity which is an unavoidable consequence of subfoveal laser photocoagulation. In addition, 51% of eyes with subfoveal membranes in AMD demonstrate persistent or recurrent choroidal neovascularization by 24 months after treatment[3].

Because of these limitations, several workers have developed and refined the techniques necessary for surgical excision of subfoveal choroidal neovascular membranes in AMD, presumed ocular histoplasmosis syndrome (POHS), and other miscellaneous disorders[5-11]. In 1991, Thomas and Kaplan reported two patients with subfoveal neovascular membranes and POHS who improved dramatically to 20/20 and 20/40 vision after surgical excision of subfoveal choroidal neovascularization[5]. Extension of these techniques to patients with choroidal neovascularization secondary to AMD has met with more limited success[6-9].

Although atrophy of the subfoveal choriocapillaris may occur as part of the natural history of AMD, clinical studies suggest that the development of postoperative atrophy of the subfoveal choriocapillaris is an important factor which limits visual recovery after surgery for subfoveal choroidal neovascularization. Clinical studies and evidence from animal studies suggest that removal of the RPE with the choroidal neovascular complex may induce secondary atrophy of the subfoveal choriocapillaris in some eyes. In view of these

G. Coscas and F. Cardillo Piccolino (eds.), Retinal Pigment Epithelium and Macular Diseases, pp. 125–134.
© *1998 Kluwer Academic Publishers.*

findings, RPE transplantation at the time of submacular surgery, or stimulation of migration and proliferation of adjacent residual RPE, is the next logical step in the management of this condition. Transplantation of RPE may prevent postoperative atrophy of the subfoveal choriocapillaris, and thus improve the visual prognosis after submacular surgery[12]. In this chapter we review the rationale for RPE transplantation at the time of submacular surgery in exudative AMD, and examine the effects of the condition of the underlying Bruch's membrane on subsequent reattachment and survival of the transplant.

Rationale for RPE transplantation in exudative AMD

At the American Academy of Ophthalmology meeting in 1993, we reported eight patients with AMD who demonstrated atrophy of the subfoveal choriocapillaris after surgical excision of subfoveal choroidal neovascularization[13]. Histological examination of the excised specimens revealed that the choriocapillaris was not removed at the time of surgery, but RPE was removed with the choroidal neovascular membrane. At the same meeting, Zarbin and Nasir showed several examples of AMD patients in whom the subfoveal choriocapillaris was perfused 1–2 weeks after submacular surgery, but then became nonperfused without further surgery or laser photocoagulation[14]. We subsequently reported a patient with POHS who developed choriocapillaris atrophy after excision of a subfoveal choroidal neovascular membrane[15]. Two weeks after surgery, the choriocapillaris was perfused under the area of the excised membrane, but 2 months later, there was nonperfusion or atrophy of the choriocapillaris in this area[15]. These observations suggested that postoperative atrophy of the subfoveal choriocapillaris can develop after surgery for subfoveal neovascularization.

Preservation of the subfoveal choriocapillaris after surgery is important because patients who develop atrophy of the subfoveal choriocapillaris have a worse visual prognosis than those who do not. Over 90% of AMD eyes and 37% of POHS eyes demonstrate postoperative atrophy of the subfoveal choriocapillaris after submacular surgery, and the visual prognosis is worse in AMD eyes than POHS eyes[16,17]. Thus, when AMD eyes were compared to POHS eyes, the postoperative perfusion status of the subfoveal choriocapillaris correlated with the final visual result. We then examined the incidence of postoperative atrophy of the subfoveal choriocapillaris within the POHS subgroup alone, and determined the relationship between the final visual result and perfusion of the subfoveal choriocapillaris after surgical excision of subfoveal neovascularization in POHS. We retrospectively reviewed the records of 38 eyes of 37 patients with gradable postoperative fluorescein angiograms and color photographs after surgical excision of a subfoveal neovascular membrane in POHS[17]. The postoperative photographs and fluorescein angiograms were graded in a masked fashion for the presence of perfusion of the subfoveal choriocapillaris. We used preoperative and postoperative best-corrected visual acuities to determine the correlation between postoperative perfusion of the subfoveal choriocapillaris and both the final visual acuity and visual improvement after surgery. After surgery, the subfoveal choriocapillaris of the 38 eyes was perfused in 24 (63%) eyes and nonperfused in 14 (37%) eyes. Best-corrected visual acuity improved by at least two lines in 17 of 24 (71%) perfused eyes and 2 of 14 (14%) non-perfused eyes ($p = 0.0089$). Additionally, a best-corrected vision of 20/100 or better was achieved in 18 (75%) of the perfused eyes and only four (29%) of the non-perfused eyes ($p < 0.05$). Thus, both the final visual acuity and improvement in visual acuity correlated with postoperative perfusion of the subfoveal choriocapillaris in patients with POHS.

Why does the subfoveal choriocapillaris undergo atrophy after submacular surgery? Korte *et al.* have previously suggested that atrophy of the choriocapillaris may occur after loss of the RPE[18]. Subfoveal membranes in AMD are intimately associated with the RPE, so that removal of the subfoveal neovascular complex is necessarily associated with debridement of the RPE beneath the fovea in these eyes. Histopathological examination of an eye from a patient who died postoperatively and who had undergone surgical excision of a choroidal neovascular membrane in AMD revealed incomplete resurfacing of the RPE defect after surgery[19]. Thus, AMD patients are likely to have an area of Bruch's membrane that is bare of RPE after surgery, and the RPE defect is likely to persist after surgery in these eyes.

We have developed an animal model to investigate the effects of RPE removal on the overlying retina and underlying choriocapillaris[20-22]. We removed the RPE from Bruch's membrane in one eye of 6-month-old domestic farm pigs. In most regions, Bruch's membrane was completely covered with regenerated RPE 1 month after surgical debridement of the RPE. In areas of regenerated RPE, the outer nuclear layer and outer limiting membrane remained intact, and the choriocapillaris was perfused. We occasionally observed areas where the RPE did not heal on Bruch's membrane 1 month after surgery, and there was extensive disruption of the outer retina in these areas, with atrophy of the choriocapillaris. Pharmacological inhibition of RPE healing with mitomycin-c at the time of RPE debridement resulted in large, geographic patches of Bruch's membrane remaining bare of RPE, with choriocapillaris atrophy throughout the debridement zone. The sequence of changes that occurs after surgical removal of the RPE in our animal model, and in patients in whom RPE is removed at the time of surgical excision of the subfoveal choroidal neovascularization in AMD, is summarized in Figures 1 and 2.

On the basis of these observations, it is clear that a logical step in the management of exudative AMD is to transplant RPE at the time of surgical excision of the choroidal neovascular membrane[12]. To date, RPE transplantation has been attempted in a handful of patients with subfoveal neovascularization in exudative AMD[23]. In the first five patients, scanning laser

RPE REMOVAL WITH HEALING

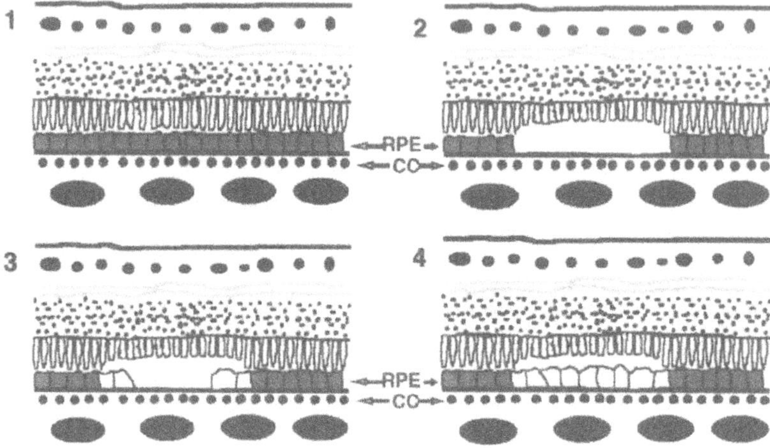

Fig. 1. Effects of RPE removal on the choriocapillaris and overlying retina. RPE regeneration after debridement. 1. Normal anatomy of outer retina. 2. An RPE defect is present under the fovea in many eyes after surgical excision of choroidal neovascularization. There may be some shortening of photoreceptor outer segments. 3. In a younger, healthier eye, Bruch's membrane becomes repopulated by migration and proliferation of the RPE from the margins of the epithelial defect. The proliferating cells are hypopigmented. 4. Bruch's membrane is covered by hypopigmented RPE. There are no changes in the subjacent choriocapillaris. The photoreceptor outer segments are shortened after surgery, but regenerate to normal length within 1–3 months after surgery. Reprinted with permission from Ref. 22.

ophthalmoscopic microperimetry demonstrated that all were able to fixate over the area of the RPE graft immediately after surgery, but an absolute scotoma developed in this region several months later. There are several possible explanations for these observations, including the fact that the transplanted RPE may have been rejected, since the patients were not immunologically suppressed[24,25].

RPE must reattach to diseased Bruch's membrane to survive after transplantation

Another explanation for loss of function over the RPE graft after transplantation is that the transplant may have not survived because of the status of the underlying Bruch's membrane. It is critically important that RPE cells which are harvested for transplantation reattach to a substrate, and this fact has not been emphasized in the RPE transplant literature. We have demonstrated that reattachment of harvested, dissociated human RPE to a substrate is necessary to prevent apoptosis[26]. This property is not unique to RPE cells,

RPE REMOVAL WITHOUT HEALING

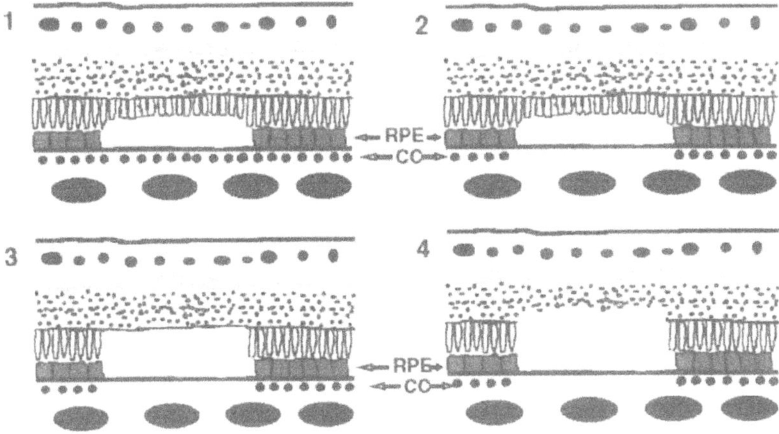

Fig. 2. RPE debridement without healing. 1. An RPE defect is present under the fovea in many eyes after surgical excision of choroidal neovascularization. 2. Bruch's membrane remains bare in an eye with older RPE, or a very large epithelial defect. Portions of Bruch's membrane do not become repopulated by migration and proliferation of adjacent RPE. The choriocapillaris becomes atrophic. 3. The outer segments do not regenerate, and continue to atrophy because of absence of RPE and choriocapillaris. 4. Atrophy of the outer nuclear layer develops secondary to nonperfusion of the choriocapillaris. Reprinted with permission from Ref. 22.

but is a general property of epithelial cells. In our experiments, second passage human RPE cells were plated onto tissue culture plastic precoated with either ECM, fibronectin, laminin, uncoated tissue culture plastic, untreated plastic, or untreated plastic coated with 4% agarose. Reattachment rates were determined for each substrate 24 h after plating. The TUNEL technique was used to determine apoptosis rates in attached cells, unattached cells, and the entire cell population. Apoptotic rates for the entire cell population increased as the RPE cell attachment rate decreased, and the proportion of apoptotic cells in the entire population was inversely related to the cell reattachment rate ($r = -0.95$). These results have important clinical implications in the interpretation of RPE transplantation studies, because they imply that harvesting RPE from its substrate as cell suspensions can initiate apoptosis, and that RPE harvested for transplantation must reattach rapidly to a substrate to prevent apoptosis. We are currently investigating whether RPE sheets harvested as an organized monolayer must also reattach to a substrate to prevent apoptosis.

How do harvested RPE reattach to Bruch's membrane? The basal surface of RPE cells contain the β_1-subunit of integrin[27,28], and the inner aspect of Bruch's membrane contains laminin, fibronectin, heparan sulfate, collagen and vitronectin[29]. Several studies suggest that the attachment of RPE to Petri dishes coated with laminin and fibronectin can be mediated by an interaction between the β_1-subunit of integrin and known ECM molecules[28-30]. For example, RPE cells bind to Petri dishes coated with laminin or fibronectin, but do not attach to bare Petri dishes[28]. The synthetic tetrapeptide RGDS (arginine-glycine-aspartate-serine), which is derived from the cell binding domain of fibronectin, will decrease RPE binding to laminin-coated or fibronectin-coated dishes[30]. When added simultaneously with the cells, the binding of RPE to fibronectin-coated dishes and laminin-coated dishes can be blocked by an antibody to the β_1-subunit of integrin. In contrast, RPE cell binding to charged tissue culture plastic is not affect by the antibody[28]. When RPE are initially allowed to attach and spread on fibronectin or laminin-coated petri dishes, addition of antibodies to fibronectin or laminin causes the attached cells to detach from the surface and round up[28]. These *in vitro* binding studies suggest that RPE attachment to plastic surfaces coated with laminin or fibronectin can be mediated partially by an interaction between the β_1-integrin subunit and laminin and fibronectin coating the surface.

We have determined the role of integrin subunits and ECM molecules in RPE reattachment to native ECM and Bruch's membrane by plating suspensions of passage 3 human RPE onto RPE-derived ECM on tissue culture plastic or human Bruch's membrane exoplants denuded of cells by treatment with 0.02 N ammonium hydroxide[31]. We measured RPE reattachment to uncoated surfaces or surfaces precoated with ECM proteins (fibronectin, laminin, vitronectin or type IV collagen), antibodies to ECM proteins, or the synthetic peptide RGDS. Some RPE were pretreated with anti-β_1 integrin antibodies prior to plating onto either substrate. Coating the surface of either tissue culture plastic dishes covered with RPE-derived ECM or Bruch's membrane with ECM proteins (fibronectin, laminin, vitronectin, or type IV collagen) increased the RPE attachment rate. Exposing RPE to anti-β_1 integrin antibodies or RGDS, or precoating the surface with antibodies to fibronectin, laminin, vitronectin or type IV collagen, decreased the RPE attachment rate to both surfaces. These experiments demonstrate that the attachment of human RPE to human Bruch's membrane or to RPE-derived ECM proteins is mediated by an interaction between the β_1-subunit of integrin on the RPE surface and ligands in the ECM that include laminin, fibronectin, vitronectin and type IV collagen[31].

We have also demonstrated that RPE reattachment to Bruch's membrane derived from the macular region of human eye bank eyes depends on the age of the recipient[31]. The reattachment rate of RPE to Bruch's membrane harvested from the macula of younger individuals was significantly higher than the reattachment rate of RPE to Bruch's membrane harvested from older individuals ($64.3 \pm 2.5\%$ vs. $52.4 \pm 3.6\%$; $p < 0.05$). Interestingly, the simultaneous addition of fibronectin, laminin, vitronectin and collagen IV increased the attachment rates to $75.5 + 4.1\%$ and $76.5 + 4.8\%$ ($p < 0.05$ for each compared to uncoated Bruch's membrane) for younger and older Bruch's membrane, respectively, and eliminated the difference in the attachment rates between young and old Bruch's membranes ($p > 0.05$). The simultaneous addition of anti-extracellular matrix proteins antibodies decreased the attachment rate of RPE cells to young and old Bruch's membrane to $32.6 + 6.5\%$ and $34.6 + 2.5\%$, respectively ($p < 0.05$ for each compared to uncoated Bruch's membrane), and again eliminated the difference in attachment rates to young and older Bruch's membrane ($p > 0.05$). The reasons for the age-dependent difference in RPE reattachment were not explored in our study, but our data suggests that there may be an age-related decline in the number of binding sites for RPE to ECM proteins within Bruch's membrane.

It is interesting to note that the age-related difference in RPE binding to macular Bruch's membrane is present despite the fact that we excluded eyes that had submacular pathology visible with the dissecting microscope, such as blood, scars or visible choroidal neovascularization[31]. Since these disorders are likely to degrade the integrity of the inner aspects of Bruch's membrane, it is likely that RPE reattachment to Bruch's membrane may be reduced further in these disease states. We are currently determining the RPE reattachment rate as a function of the disease status of the host macula. A complete understanding of the factors involved in RPE reattachment to normal and diseased human Bruch's membrane is necessary in order to maximize the chances of successful transplantation of RPE into the subretinal space, and ultimately improve the visual prognosis after surgical excision of subfoveal choroidal neovascularization.

Harvesting and transfer of RPE-derived extracellular matrix

Since transplanted RPE may not reattach to diseased Bruch's membrane and survive in the subretinal space, the question arises as to whether transplantation of ECM before or at the same time as RPE transplantation will improve the survival, attachment and subsequent proliferation of transplanted RPE[32]. We have developed a technique to harvest and transfer native ECM produced by bovine, porcine and human cell lines. Briefly, ECM was harvested by treating a confluent monolayer of cells with 0.02 N ammonium hydroxide. The ECM was then coated with a thin 100 μm layer of 12% gelatin and cooled to 4°C. Patches of the ECM were isolated and transferred to another culture plate. The transferred ECM was characterized by immunohistochemistry, and we determined the ability of cultured RPE to reattach to the harvested ECM, and the ability of the harvested ECM to inhibit RPE apoptosis.

Our results demonstrate that ECM can be transferred to another location *en bloc* with this technique[32]. Immunohistochemistry demonstrated that the transferred ECM contained fibronectin, laminin and collagen IV. The reattachment rate of human RPE cell suspensions to transferred ECM was higher ($83.6 \pm 2.8\%$) than RPE reattachment to bare tissue culture plastic ($57.6 \pm 9.8\%$). The apoptotic rate of attached RPE cells on transferred bovine corneal endothelial ECM (4.3 ± 1.4%) was lower than their apoptotic rate on bare plastic (69.3 ± 4.1%). The apoptotic rates of unattached cells was 80.3 ± 4.4% on transferred bovine corneal endothelial ECM and 79.2 ± 3.4% on bare plastic. Thus, ECM produced by various cell lines can be harvested and transferred by this technique, and the transferred ECM promotes cell reattachment and inhibited RPE cell apoptosis. Harvesting and transfer of ECM at the time of RPE transplantation may inhibit apoptosis and promote survival of the transplant.

Summary

The development of techniques to surgically excise choroidal neovascular membranes introduces the possibility of surgically reconstructing the RPE monolayer and inner lamellae of Bruch's membrane in patients who have subfoveal choroidal neovascularization in AMD, POHS, and other disorders. Simple surgical excision of a choroidal neovascular membrane can be accompanied by good visual results if the subfoveal RPE is not removed at the time of surgery, or if the RPE is removed and adjacent RPE then repopulates the subfoveal area of Bruch's membrane rapidly after surgery. The presence of native or regenerated RPE is required to prevent postoperative atrophy of the subfoveal choriocapillaris, because the subfoveal choriocapillaris will undergo atrophy if Bruch's membrane remains devoid of RPE for 3–7 days after subfoveal surgery. Persistent bare areas of Bruch's membrane will be present in patients who have large defects in the RPE monolayer, or in whom advanced patient age or disease to the inner aspects of Bruch's membrane prevents complete RPE resurfacing by migration and proliferation of adjacent RPE. The next challenge in submacular surgery is to deliver RPE into the subretinal space as an organized monolayer, ensure the rapid reattachment of these cells to Bruch's membrane, and prevent immunological rejection. Cell survival immediately after transplantation is important to prevent secondary atrophy of the subfoveal choriocapillaris. Future efforts should be directed to characterizing the ECM molecules remaining on Bruch's membrane after the excision of subretinal choroidal neovascularization, and identifying the molecular components of Bruch's membrane that are responsible for the reattachment of transplanted RPE to diseased Bruch's membrane.

Acknowledgements

Supported in part by the Foundation Fighting Blindness, the National Eye Institute core grant EY02687 and individual grant EY10311 (Dr. Del Priore), the Foundation Fighting Blindness, and unrestricted funds from Research to Prevent Blindness.

References

1. Bressler, S.B., Bressler, N.M., Fine, S.L. et al. Natural course of choroidal neovascular membranes within the foveal avascular zone in senile macular degeneration. Am J Ophthalmol. 1982; 93: 157–163.
2. Olk, R.J., Burgess, D.B., McCormick, P.A. Subfoveal and juxtafoveal subretinal neovascularization in the presumed ocular histoplasmosis syndrome: visual prognosis. Ophthalmology. 1984; 91: 1592–1602.
3. Macular Photocoagulation Study Group. Laser photocoagulation of subfoveal neovascular lesions in age-related macular degeneration. Results of a randomized clinical trial. Arch Ophthalmol. 1991; 109: 1220–1231.
4. Macular Photocoagulation Study Group. Laser photocoagulation of subfoveal recurrent neovascular lesions in age-related macular degeneration. Results of a randomized clinical trial. Arch Ophthalmol. 1991; 109: 1232–1241.
5. Thomas, M.A., Kaplan, H.J. Surgical removal of subfoveal neovascularization in the presumed ocular histoplasmosis syndrome. Am J Ophthalmol. 1991; 111: 1–7.
6. Berger, A.S., Kaplan, H.J. Clinical experience with the surgical removal of subfoveal neovascular membranes. Ophthalmology. 1992; 99: 969–976.
7. Thomas, M.A., Grand, M.G., Williams, D.F. et al. Surgical management of subfoveal choroidal neovascularization. Ophthalmology. 1992; 99: 952–968.
8. Lopez, P.F., Grossniklaus, H.E., Lambert, H.M. et al. Pathologic features of surgically excised subretinal neovascular membranes in age-related macular degeneration. Am J Ophthalmol. 1991; 112: 647–656.
9. Lambert, H.M., Capone, A. Jr, Aaberg, T.M., Sternberg, P. Jr, Mandell, B.A., Lopez, P.F. Surgical excision of subfoveal neovascular membranes in age-related macular degeneration. Am J Ophthalmol. 1991; 113: 257–262.
10. deJuan E. Jr, Machemer, R. Vitreous surgery for hemorrhagic and fibrous complications of age-related macular degeneration. Am J Ophthalmol. 1989; 105: 25–29.
11. Adelberg, D.A., Del Priore, L.V., Kaplan, H.J. Surgery for subfoveal membranes in myopia, angioid streaks, and other disorders. Retina. 1995; 15: 198–205.
12. Del Priore, L.V., Kaplan, H.J., Silverman, M.S., Valentino, T.L., Mason, G., Hornbeck, R. Experimental and surgical aspects of retinal pigment epithelial cell transplantation. Eur J Implant Ref Surg. 1993; 5: 128–132.
13. Pollack, J.S., Kaplan, H.J., Del Priore, L.V., Smith, M.S. Choriocapillaris atrophy following subfoveal membrane excision in exudative age-related macular degeneration. Ophthalmology. 1993; 100: 122.
14. Zarbin, M.A., Nasir, M. Impaired choriocapillaris perfusion following subfoveal surgery for macular degeneration. Ophthalmology. 1993; 100: 97.
15. Desai, V.N., Del Priore, L.V., Pollack, J.S., Kaplan, H.J. Choriocapillaris atrophy after submacular surgery in the presumed ocular histoplasmosis syndrome. Arch Ophthalmol. 1995; 113: 409–410.
16. Pollack, J.S., Del Priore, L.V., Smith, M.E., Feiner, M.A., Kaplan, H.J. Postoperative abnormalities of the choriocapillaris in exudative age-related macular degeneration. Br J Ophthalmol. 1996; 80: 314–318.
17. Akduman, L., Desai, V., Del Priore, L.V., Olk, R.J., Kaplan, H.J. Visual improvement after subfoveal surgery in POHS depends on perfusion of subfoveal choriocapillaris. Am J Ophthalmol. In press.
18. Korte, G.E., Reppucci, V., Henkind, P. RPE destruction causes choriocapillaris atrophy. Invest Ophthalmol Vis Sci. 1984; 25: 1135–1145.
19. Hsu, J., Thomas, M.A., Ibanez, H., Green, W.R. Clinicopathologic studies of an eye after submacular membranectomy for choroidal neovascularization. Retina. 1995; 15: 43–52.
20. Valentino, T.L., Kaplan, H.J., Del Priore, L.V., Fang, S.F., Berger, A., Silverman, M.S. Retinal pigment epithelial repopulation in monkeys after submacular surgery. Arch Ophthalmol. 1995; 113: 932–938.

21. Del Priore, L.V., Kaplan, H.J., Silverman, M.S., Hornbeck, R., Jones, J., Swinn, M. Debridement of the pig retinal pigment epithelium in vivo. Arch Ophthalmol. 1995; 113: 939–944.
22. Del Priore, L.V., Hornbeck, R., Kaplan, H.J., Jones, Z., Swinn, M. Retinal pigment epithelial debridement as a model for the pathogenesis and treatment of macular degeneration. Am J Ophthalmol. 1996; 122: 629–643.
23. Algvere, P.V., Berglin, L., Gouras, P., Sheng, Y. Transplantation of fetal retinal pigment epithelium in age-related macular degeneration with subfoveal neovascularization. Graefe's Arch Clin Exp Ophthalmol. 1994; 232: 707–716.
24. Jiang, L.Q., Jorquera, M., Streilein, J.W. Immunologic consequences of intraocular implantation of retinal pigment epithelial allografts. Exp Eye Res. 1994; 58: 719–728.
25. Ye, J., Wang, H.M., Ogden, T.E., Ryan, S.J. Allotransplantation of rabbit retinal pigment epithelial cells double-labeled with 5-bromodeoxyuridine (BrdU) and natural pigment. Curr Eye Res. 1993; 12: 629–639.
26. Tezel, T., Del Priore, L.V., Kaplan, H.J. Reattachment of harvested RPE to a substrate prevents apoptosis. Graefe's Arch Clin Exp Ophthalmol. 1996, in press.
27. Chu, P., Grunwald, G.B. Identification of the 2A10 antigen of retinal pigment epithelium as a β1 subunit of integrin. Invest Ophthalmol Vis Sci. 1991; 32: 1757–1762.
28. Chu, P., Grunwald, G.B. Functional inhibition of retinal pigment epithelial cell–substrate adhesion with a monoclonal antibody against the β1 subunit of integrin. Invest Ophthalmol Vis Sci. 1991; 32: 1763–1769.
29. Das, A., Frank, R.N., Zhang, N.L., Turczyn, T.J. Ultrastructural localization of extracellular matrix components in human retinal vessels and Bruch's membrane. Arch Ophthalmol. 1990; 108: 421–429.
30. Avery, R.L., Glaser, B.M. Inhibition of retinal pigment epithelial cell attachment by a synthetic peptide derived from the cell-binding domain of fibronectin. Arch Ophthalmol. 1986; 104: 1220–1222.
31. Ho, T.C., Del Priore, L.V. Reattachment of human RPE to extracellular matrix and human Bruch's membrane. Invest Ophthalmol Vis Sci. Submitted.
32. Ho, T.C., Del Priore, L.V., Kaplan, H.J. En bloc transfer of extracellular matrix in vitro. Curr Eye Res 1996; 15: 991–997.

Box 8096,
Department of Ophthalmology and Visual Sciences
Washington University School of Medicine
660 South Euclid Avenue
Saint Louis
MO 63110, USA

18. Experimental transplantation of human retinal pigment epithelial cells on collagen substrates

N.S. BHATT, D.A. NEWSOME and J.G. DIAMOND

(Bombay, India and New Orleans, LA, USA)

Introduction

Retinal pigment epithelial (RPE) cells play a vital role in providing anatomic, mechanical, and metabolic support for the photoreceptors and outer retina[1]. RPE dysfunction, atrophy and degeneration have been implicated as the cause of many retinal diseases, including age-related macular degeneration[2-4].

Retinal pigment epithelial transplantation has been shown to rescue photoreceptor cells in Royal College of Surgeons dystrophic rats[5-7]. Various types of retinal pigment epithelial grafts[8,9] and surgical techniques[10,11] have been tried with varying degrees of success. In most previous experiments, RPE cells were transplanted in suspension form by the bolus injection technique. This injection of suspended RPE cells can result in various complications, including multiple layer stacking of RPE cells, subretinal fibrosis, invasion of the retina by wandering pigmented cells, the formation of retinal rosettes, and RPE cells in the vitreous causing proliferative vitreoretinopathy[12].

We transplanted human fetal RPE cells cultured on a collagen support into rabbit subretinal space by the transvitreal approach to have a precise and controlled implantation of RPE cells and to avoid these complications. We also performed sham surgery by transplanting the collagen support alone to evaluate its effect on the retina.

Materials and methods

Retinal pigment epithelium isolation and culture

Eyes from fetuses of 16–20 weeks' gestation were procured from the International Institute for Advancement of Medicine, Washington, DC. The RPE was removed mechanically with fine forceps and placed in tissue culture for 5–7 days in Coon's modified Hams F-12 medium (CMF-12) supplemented with L-glutamine (292 mg/l), ascorbic acid (49 mg/l), streptomycin (100 mg/l), penicillin G (100 000 units/l), fetal bovine serum (5%), and epidermal growth factor (10 ng/ml). Sheets of RPE were removed from tissue culture in trypsin/ ethylenediamine tetraacetic acid, and the cells were plated onto collagen supports for an additional 5–7 days of culture.

G. Coscas and F. Cardillo Piccolino (eds.), Retinal Pigment Epithelium and Macular Diseases, pp. 135–141.
© *1998 Kluwer Academic Publishers.*

Preparation of collagen supports

Type I rat tail tendon collagen (Collaborative Research, Bedford, Massachusetts) was used to prepare two types of support. A non-crosslinked support was prepared by placing 150 μl of collagen into 10 mm culture plate inserts (Anocell 10, Whitman, Maidstone, UK) followed by treatment with ammonium hydroxide vapours (5 min) to form a gel support. The support was then rinsed several times in phosphate-buffered saline and used directly. To crosslink the collagen, the insert containing collagen was dried under ultraviolet light in a laminar flow hood overnight. The dried collagen sheet was rehydrated with cell culture medium before use.

Surgical technique

The right eyes of 20 albino New Zealand rabbits, weighing 2–3 g, were used in our study. All procedures involving animals and their handling were conducted in accordance with the applicable Association for Research in Vision and Ophthalmology resolutions and National Institutes of Health guidelines, and approved by the institutional animal care and use committee of Tulane University School of Medicine.

The animals were anaesthetized by IM injection of a mixture of ketamine hydrochloride (10 mg/kg) and xylazine hydrochloride (10 mg/kg). The pupil of the eye to be treated was dilated with topical 1% tropicamide and 2.5% phenylephrine hydrochloride. Proparacaine hydrochloride 0.5% was instilled into the conjunctival sac as a topical anaesthetic. The hair was shaved around the eye, and the area cleaned with povidone-iodine.

A partial perilimbal conjunctival peritomy was made in the temporal 180°. Two sclerotomies were made, one each in the superotemporal and inferotemporal quadrant, 1 mm behind the corneoscleral limbus using a standard microvitreoretinal blade. Through the inferotemporal quadrant sclerotomy, a 2.5 mm infusion cannula was introduced in the vitreous cavity, and intraocular instruments were introduced through the superotemporal sclerotomy. Intraocular infusion consisted of plain balanced salt solution. A traction suture of 5.0 Dacron was placed nasally at the corneoscleral limbus to maneuver the eye. Microscope illumination and corneal contact lens were used to visualize the posterior segment and retina.

Using a vitreous cutter through the superotemporal sclerotomy, a partial vitrectomy was carried out superior to the nerve and the medullary rays. An intraocular cautery was introduced, and the retina was cauterized to reduce the bleeding and to enhance chorioretinal scar formation postoperatively. A 50 μm glass micropipette with its tip tapered by flame and connected to a tuberculin syringe filled with balanced salt solution was then introduced into the eye, and a small retinotomy was made at the site of the cauterized retina. A retinal detachment was produced by injecting balanced saline solution slowly through the micropipette into the subretinal space. A detachment of approximately 2–3 disc diameters was produced. A soft-tipped cannula was then introduced through the retinotomy, and thr rabbit's retinal pigment epithelial cells were carefully scraped off. Care was taken to avoid rupturing Bruch's membrane.

To facilitate visualization of the collagen support during and after transplantation, the support was placed briefly in a culture dish to adsorb HCl-washed charcoal. The collagen support with attached retinal pigment epihtelial cells or a collagen support alone for control experiments was then loaded in a Teflon cannula attached to a 100 μl Hamilton glass syringe containing a 10% sucrose solution in balanced salt solution with calcium and magnesium. The loaded cannula was introduced through the sclerotomy into the eye and the collagen support injected slowly into the subretinal space through the retinotomy.

A total of 20 rabbits received transplants as follows: seven received retinal pigment epithelial transplants on non-crosslinked collagen; seven received retinal pigment epithelial transplants on crosslinked collagen; three received non-crosslinked collagen alone; and three received crosslinked collagen alone. In all cases, we tried to preserve the lens during the surgical procedure and were successful in 19 of 20 eyes (95%). One eye required a lensectomy due to a lens opacity secondary to instrument touch.

After completing the implantation, an air–fluid exchange was performed to facilitate reattachment of the retina. Sclerotomies were closed with the preexisting 6.0 Vicryl sutures and the conjunctiva closed with 7.0 chromic catgut. Tobramycin (1 ml) was injected subconjunctivally, and gentamicin and atropine ointment were instilled in the eye. We did not use corticosteroids or other immunosuppressive medications postoperatively. The eyes were examined on day 1 and then at weekly intervals with the indirect ophthalmoscope.

Harvesting eyes, microscopy

After 6 weeks, the animals were killled and the eyes enucleated for histologic studies. The eyes were fixed in paraformaldehyde (4%, 18 h), dehydrated, embedded in paraffin, and stained with haematoxylin and eosin. Sections were examined by a stereoscopic light microscope and photographed.

Results

In 19 of 20 eyes (95%), the lens remained clear throughout the 6-week examination. Three of 20 eyes (15%) had a retinal detachment from day 1 after the surgery, which persisted throughout. In the one eye with a lensectomy severe intraocular inflammation was seen. In the remaining 16 eyes (80%), examination at the end of one week with an indirect ophthalmoscope showed that the retinas appeared flat at the site of retinal detachment from the surgical procedure. Pigmented areas presumed to be subretinal transplanted pigment epithelial cells were seen superior to the disc and the medullary rays in the eyes with the cell-bearing collagen grafts.

Light microscopy

In nine of the 10 eyes that received a non-crosslinked collagen sheet, little or no evidence existed of the collagen remaining, and presumably it was absorbed. This was true in both control and experimental eyes. In the one case where the non-crosslinked collagen support had not been absorbed at the end of 6 weeks, the support did not appear to be densely packed. It had conformed to the shape of Bruch's membrane and the choroid, there by allowing attachment with the denuded Bruch's membrane.

The transplanted human fetal retinal pigment epithelial cells were identified readily by their pigmentation in contrast to the non-pigmented RPE cells of the rabbit host. The transplanted RPE cells retained their monolayer configuration on the collagen support and appeared to be in continuation with cells attached to the adjacent Bruch's membrane, which had been presumably denuded at the time of the operation. The pigmentation of transplanted RPE cells diminished toward the edge of the collagen support. Since proliferating cells in culture tend to lose pigmentation, the lack of pigmentation at the site of the implant does not rule out the possibility that some of the non-pigmented cells were donor cells that had migrated onto the Bruch's membrane.

In all cases, the morphological appearance of the retina was disrupted at the site of cauterization and retinotomy. Distal to this site, however, the retinas appeared normal with respect to the presence of photoreceptor outer segments and an outer nuclear layer, even over the areas where donor retinal pigment epithelial cells were evident. In 16 of 20 eyes (80%), no evidence was present of retinal pigment epithelial cells migrating into the vitreous, and no epiretinal membranes were noted. No inflammatory or immune cells were seen around the transplanted retinal pigment epithelial cells.

At 6 weeks, the crosslinked, stiffer collagen support appeared more dense than the non-crosslinked counterpart. The crosslinked supports did not conform to the shape of the choroid, nor did they appear to form readily an attachment with the area of denuded Bruch's membrane. The retinal pigment epithelial cells also appeared less likely to remain attached to the crosslinked collagen and were dispersed, forming multiple layers. Eyes receiving crosslinked supports had retinas with abnormal morphologic characteristics, including less attachment, loss of photoreceptor outer segments, and reduced outer nuclear layer density. No evidence was seen of any mononuclear inflammatory cells or epiretinal membrane formation.

Eyes that had received only the crosslinked collagen support without retinal pigment epithelial cells invariably showed degeneration of the outer segments of the retina photoreceptors and attenuation of the outer nuclear layer.

Discussion

Subretinal neovascularization and its complications are a major cause of severe vision loss in patients with age-related macular degeneration[13,14]. Many patients with neovascularization secondary to age-related macular degeneration do not meet laser treatment criteria because of either subfoveal location, extensive neovascularization, poor membrane definition, or scar formation[15,16]. Therefore, attempts have been made to drain surgically submacular haemorrhages and to excise subfoveal nets in patients with exudative age-related macular degeneration[17–21]. Anatomically, surgical procedures have been successful in evacuating the submacular haemorrhage and removing the scar and the subfoveal membrane, but visual improvement in these cases has been limited. This may be caused in part by loss of RPE cells evident after scar removal[18,19], and transplantation of RPE cells may be useful in this situation.

We transplanted human fetal RPE cells cultured on a collagen support into rabbit subretinal space. By transplanting these cells on a support, we had a controlled and precise implantation of the cells at the desired site and also avoided their dispersion of the cells within the subretinal space, the retina and the vitreous cavity. We used two types of collagen supports, including a non-crosslinked collagen support, which was soft and flexible. The non-crosslinked collagen appeared to dissolve or conform to the shape of the Bruch's membrane. In the one case where the collagen was visible, the collagen layer was reduced in thickness but did not totally disappear by 6 weeks. The presence of collagen between the choroid and RPE did not appear to affect the retina as seen on histological slides.

To make the collagen support rigid and more amenable to manipulation during surgical implantation, we crosslinked it with ultraviolet light. The hard crosslinked collagen did not show any sign of resorption, and it did not conform to the shape of Bruch's membrane. The retina overlying this hard crosslinked collagen appeared damaged and disarrayed, which may have been caused, at least in part, by the nature of the collagen support itself. In eyes with the collagen support alone, the photoreceptors overlying the support degenerated, and no beneficial effect resulted. It is likely that the crosslinked condensed collagen acted as a physical barrier to diffusion between the retinal pigment epithelium/choroid and the retina.

During the period of our study, no apparent immune or inflammatory reactions were seen around the transplanted xenograft of RPE cells in eyes with intact Bruch's membrane, even though we did not use any corticosteroids or immunosuppressive drugs. The intraocular transplant site may be immunologically privileged, similar to the phenomenon described as an anterior chamber associated immune deviation[22] Longer periods should be considered for future studies to determine whether an immune reaction may eventually occur.

The histological evidence of photoreceptor integrity in the area of transplanted RPE cells suggests that this technique may supply growth factors or other humoral factors required to prevent or restore retinal deterioration and vision loss[23]. Because of the large number of conditions involving RPE dysfunction, this procedure may have wide application.

Further studies are needed to assess graft rejection and resorption rates of the collagen substrate. In addition, the functional capacity of the transplanted cells requires further scrutiny (for example, ultrastructural examination to assess their association with the interphotoreceptor matrix and phagocytosis of photoreceptor outer segments).

In conclusion, we believe that transplantation of RPE on a collagen support is a precise and controlled method of transplantation and avoids the complications associated with the imprecise transplantation of a cell suspension.

References

1. Zinn, K.M., Benjamin-Henkind, J.V. Anatomy of human retinal pigment epithelium. In Zinn, K.M., Marmor, M.F. (eds.) The Retinal Pigment Epithlium. Cambridge: Harvard University Press, 1979: 3–31.
2. Hogan, M.J. Role of the retinal pigment epithelium in macular disease. Trans Am Acad Ophthalmol Otolaryngol. 1972; 76: 64–67.
3. Sarks, S.H. Aging and degeneration in the macular region. A clinicipathological study. Br J Ophthalmol. 1976; 60: 324–341.
4. Green, W.R., Key, S.N. III. Senile macular degeneration. A histologic study. Trans Am Ophthalmol Soc. 1977; 75: 180–254.
5. Li, L., Turner, J.E. Inherited retinal dystrophy in the RCS rats. Prevention of photoreceptor degeneration by pigment epithelial cell transplantation. Exp Eye Res. 1988; 47: 911–917.
6. Lopez, R., Gouras, P., Kjeldbye, H. *et al.* Transplanted retinal pigment epithelium modifies the retinal degeneration in the RCS rat. Invest Ophthalmol Vis Sci. 1989; 30: 586–588.
7. Sheedlo, H.J., Li, L., Turner, J.E. Functional and structural characteristics of photoreceptor cells rescued in RPE cell-grafted retinas of RCS dystrophic rats. Exp Eye Res. 1989; 48: 841–854.
8. Lopez, R., Gouras, P., Brittis, M., Kjeldbye, H. Transplantation of cultured rabbit retinal epithelium to rabbit retina using a closed-eye method. Invest Ophthalmol Vis Sci. 1987; 28: 1131–1137.
9. Aramant, R., Seiler, M., Ehinger, B. *et al.* Xenografting human fetal to adult rat retina. ARVO abstracts. Invest Ophthalmol Vis Sci (Suppl.) 1990; 31: 594.
10. Yamaguchi, K., Yamaguchi, K., Young, R.W. *et al.* Vitreoretinal surgical technique for transplanting retinal pigment epithelium in rabbit retina. Jpn J Ophthalmol. 1992; 36: 142–150.
11. Wongpicchedchai, S., Weber, P., Dorey, C.K., Weiter, J.J. Comparison of external and internal approaches for RPE transplantation. ARVO abstracts. Invest Ophthalmol Vis Sci. (Suppl.) 1990; 31: 593.
12. Liu, Y., Silverman, M.S., Berger, A.S., Kaplan, H.J. Transplantation of confluent sheets of adult human RPE. Invest Ophthalmol Vis Sci. 1992; 33: 2180–2184.
13. Young, R.W. Pathophysiology of age-related macular degeneration. Surv Ophthalmol. 1987; 31: 291–306.
14. Ferris, F.L. III, Fine, S.L., Hyman, L. Age-related macular degeneration and blindness due to neovascular maculopathy. Arch Ophthalmol. 1984; 102: 1640–1642.
15. Bressler, N.M., Bressler, S.B., Gragoudas, E.S. Clinical characteristics of choroidal neovascular membranes. Arch Ophthalmol. 1987; 105: 209–213.

16. Bressler, N.M., Frost, L.A., Bressler, S.B., Murphy, R.P., Fine, S. L. Natural course of poorly defined choroidal neovascularization associated with macular degeneration. Arch Ophthalmol. 1988; 106: 1537–1542.

17. Lambert, H.M., Capone, A. Jr., Aaberg, T.M., Stenberg, P. Jr., Mandell, B. A., Lopez, P. F. Surgical excision of subfoveal neovascular membranes in age-related macular degeneration. Am J Ophthalmol. 1992; 113: 257–262.

18. Thomas, M.A., Grand, M.G., Williams, D.F., Lee, C.M., Pesin, S.R., Lowe, M.A. Surgical management of subfoveal choroidal neovascularization. Ophthalmology. 1992; 99: 952–968.

19. Berger, A.S., Kaplan, H.J. Clinical experience with the surgical removal of subfoveal neovascular membranes. Ophthalmology. 1992; 99: 969–976.

20. DeJuan, E. Jr., Machemer., R. Vitreous surgery for hemorrhagic and fibrous complicatons of age-related macular degeneration. Am J Ophthalmol. 1988; 105: 25–29.

21. Blinder, K.J., Peyman, G.A., Paris, C.L., Gremillion, C.M. Jr. Submacular scar excision in age-related macular degeneration. Int Ophthalmol. 1991; 15: 215–222.

22. Streilien, J.W. Immune regulation and the eye. A dangerous compromise. FASEB J. 1987; 1: 199–203.

23. Faktorovich, E.G., steinberg, R.H., Yasumura, D., Matthes, M.T., La Vail, M.M. Photoreceptor degeneration in inherited retinal dystrophy delayed by basic fibroblast growth factor. Nature. 1990; 347: 83–87.

Bombay Hospital
Taparia Institute of Ophthalmology
Bombay, India

19. Preinjection fluorescence in indocyanine green angiography

F. CARDILLO PICCOLINO, L. BORGIA, E. ZINICOLA,
S. TORRIELLI and M. ZINGIRIAN

(Genoa, Italy)

Introduction

Preinjection fluorescence of ocular structures, including pseudofluorescence and autofluorescence, has been well documented in fluorescein angiography[1]. The purpose of this study was to verify whether preinjection fluorescence can be also observed in indocyanine green (ICG) angiography. The present digital systems for ICG angiography are highly sensitive to near infrared emissions. They could be also capable of detecting autofluorescent emissions of chorioretinal structures in the near infrared range.

Materials and methods

Infrared fundus photographs were taken prior to dye injection for 450 patients undergoing ICG angiography for different chorioretinal disorders. We used the Topcon IMAGEnet H1024 Digital Imaging System (Ijssel, The Netherlands). Preinjection photographs were taken by inserting the standard ICG filters and using the highest flash energy. The infrared filters in the Topcon system have an overlap of less than 0.5%. Images were stored on optical discs and were evaluated by enhancing the contrast when necessary with the software provided.

When preinjection fluorescence was detected its intensity was arbitrarily graded as 'faint' or 'strong'. For lesions with faint fluorescence, contrast had to be enhanced to obtain a good image definition on the monitor. Lesions having strong fluorescence did not require contrast enhancement.

Results

Preinjection fluorescence was detected in 184 patients (40.8%). Old haemorrhages, lipofuscin-like deposits, some choroidal neovascular membranes and chronic serous retinal detachments resulted in preinjection fluorescence. Table 1 shows the intensity of fluorescence registered for each kind of lesion.

G. Coscas and F. Cardillo Piccolino (eds.), Retinal Pigment Epithelium and Macular Diseases, pp. 143–147.
© 1998 Kluwer Academic Publishers.

Table 1. Preinjection Fluorescent Lesions and Intensity of Fluorescence.

Lesion	Faint fluorescence	Strong fluorescence	Total
Old haemorrhages	0	35	35
Lipofuscin-like deposits	37	28	65
Choroidal neovascular membranes	60	12	72
Chronic serous retinal detachments	12	0	12
Total	109	75	184

Normal structures of the ocular fundus and white atrophic-cicatricial lesions were not fluorescent on the preinjection photographs.

Old haemorrhages

Old greyish coloured haemorrhages dating from several weeks or months had a strong preinjection fluorescence (Fig. 1). Recent haemorrhages of red colour did not appear fluorescent. Fluorescence of old haemorrhages was still discernable in the early photographs of the ICG angiograms which were taken with high flash energy. When the flash energy was reduced due to the intense fluorescence of the choroid, the spontaneous fluorescence of the haemorrhagic material was no longer detectable. During the late phase, when low choroidal fluorescence once again required high flash energy, the same lesions reappeared fluorescent.

Lipofuscin-like deposits

The orange-yellow pigment above choroidal naevi or melanomas had a strong preinjection fluorescence (Fig. 2). This fluorescence was also evident on early

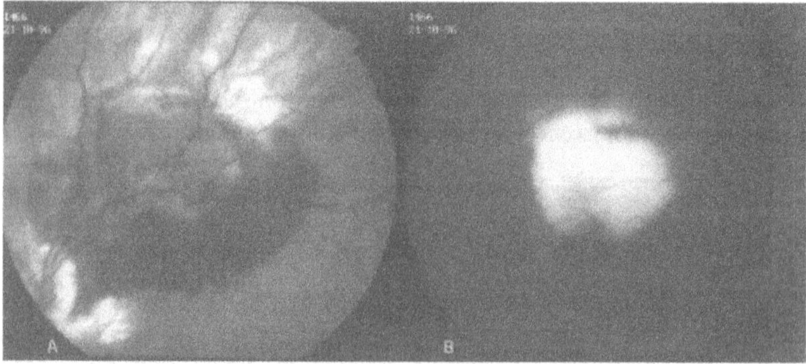

Fig. 1. (a) Subretinal haemorrhage caused by choroidal neovascularization. (b) Preinjection fluorescence of the greyish portion of the haemorrhage.

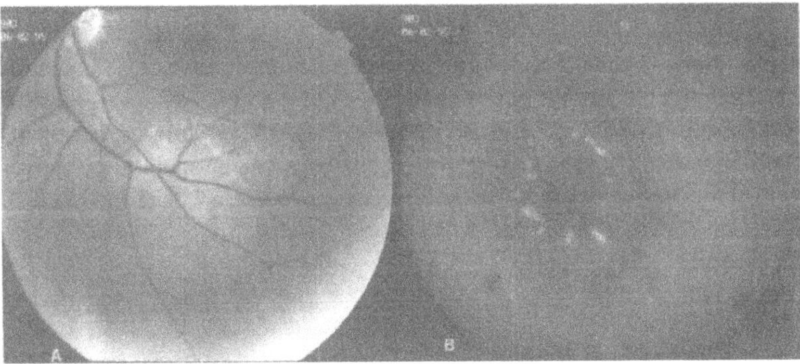

Fig. 2. (a) Suspected choroidal melanoma. (b) Preinjection fluorescence of the subretinal orange-yellow deposits.

and late ICG photographs. A series of other lesions, which could be also interpreted as lipofuscin deposits, resulted in a less intense preinjection fluorescence.

Choroidal neovascular membranes

Choroidal neovascular membranes surrounded by evident or supposed hyper-pigmentation showed preinjection fluorescence in the pigmented border of the lesion (Fig. 3). Fluorescence could be strong or faint. A strong spontaneous fluorescence of choroidal neovascular membranes simulated vascular filling on the early phase of the ICG angiogram.

Hyperpigmentations of scars and inactive Fuchs spots were not fluorescent on the preinjection photographs.

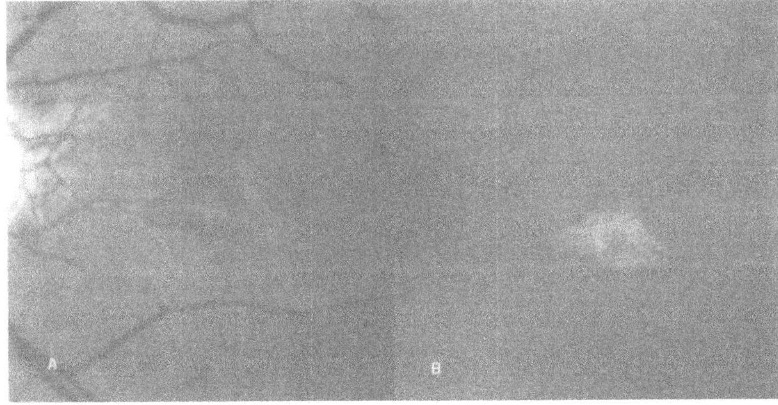

Fig. 3. (a) Pigmented choroidal neovascularization in an eye with angioid streaks. (b) Preinjection fluorescence of the lesion.

Chronic serous retinal detachments

Serous retinal detachments lasting from several months to years demonstrated faint fluorescence on the infrared preinjection photographs (Fig. 4). These chronic serous detachments were associated with a choroidal nevus or were found in eyes with chronic central serous chorioretinopathy. In cases of choroidal nevi, a granular hyperfluorescence corresponding to yellowish subretinal dots was observed within the diffuse fluorescence of the serous detachment.

Conclusions

This study demonstrates that preinjection fluorescence can be observed during ICG examinations, analogous to what has already been observed in fluorescein angiography. Preinjection fluorescence is frequently detectable in patients having diseases requiring ICG examinations. This spontaneous fluorescence of the lesions may result in a misinterpretation of the angiogram.

The preinjection fluorescence found in this study could be interpreted either as pseudofluorescence or as autofluorescence. The overlap between the filter curves in our system was minimal. Furthermore, preinjection fluorescence in our patients did not appear to be related to the reflecting properties of the chorioretinal structures. We can, therefore, hypothezise the possibility of autofluorescence, at least in the cases of strong preinjection fluorescence. All the lesions exhibiting preinjection fluorescence in this study contain biological pigments which have already been shown to have properties of autofluorescence in the long wavelength region of the visible spectrum[2–10]. They might also have near infrared emissions. Table 2 shows the possible sources of infrared autofluorescence in the lesions which presented preinjection fluorescence.

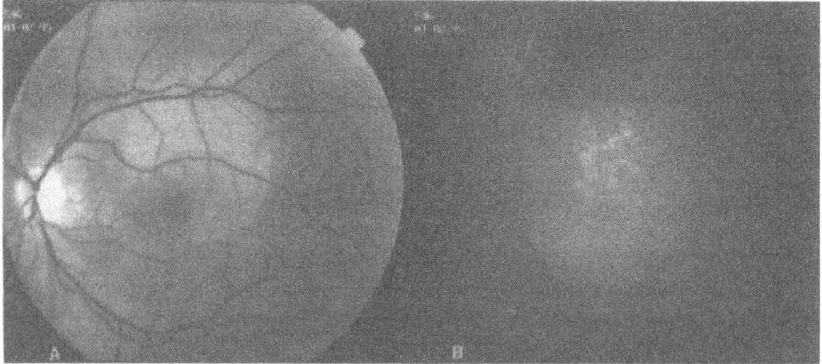

Fig. 4.   (a) Chronic serous retinal detachment associated with a choroidal nevus. (b) Preinjection fluorescence of retinal detachment and subretinal yellowish deposits.

Table 2. Possible sources of infrared autofluorescence.

Lesion	Fluorophores
Old haemorrhages	Degradation products of hemoglobin (porphyrins)
Lipofuscin-like deposits	Lipofuscin components
Choroidal neovascular membranes	Degradation products of hemoglobin, melanin products
Chronic serous retinal detachments	Outer segments products, lipofuscin components

Aside from any interpretations however, the possibility of fluorescence not being related to the presence of dye cannot be disregarded in ICG angiography. This possibility must be considered both during future studies involving ICG angiography and during the clinical utilization of this methodology.

References

1. Schatz, H., Burton, C.T., Yannuzzi, A.L., Rabb, F.M. (eds.). Interpretation of Fundus Fluorescein Angiography. St. Louis, MO: CV Mosby, 1978: 251–268.
2. Schulman, S.G. Molecular luminescence spectroscopy. Methods and applications. New York: Wiley & Sons, 1985: 240–266.
3. Feeney-Burns, L. Lipofuscin and melanin of human retinal pigment epithelium: fluorescence, enzyme cytochemical, and ultrastructural studies. Invest Ophthalmol Vis Sci 1978; 17: 583–600.
4. Eldred, G.E., Miller, G.V., Stark, W.S., Feeney-Burns, L. Lipofuscin: resolution of discrepant fluorescence data. Science. 1982; 216: 757–759.
5. Weiter, J.J., Decori, F.C., Wing, G.L., Fitch, K.A. Retinal pigment epithelial lipofuscin and melanin and choroidal melanin in human eyes. Invest Ophthalmol Vis Sci. 1986; 27: 145–152.
6. Eldred, G.E., Katz, M.L. Fluorophores of the human retinal pigment epithelium: separation and spectral characterization. Exp Eye Res. 1988; 47: 71–86.
7. Katz, M.L., Christianson, J.S., Gao, C.L., Handelman, G.J. Iron-induced fluorescence in the retina: dependence on vitamin A. Invest Ophthalmol Vis Sci. 1994; 35: 3613–3624.
8. Olivecrona, H., Rorsman, H. The effect of roentgen irradiation on the specific fluorescence of epidermal melanocytes. Acta Derm Venereol. 1966; 46: 403–405.
9. Fellner, M.J., Chen, A.S., Mont, M. et al. Patterns and intensity of autofluorescence and its relation to melanin in human epidermis and hair. Int J Dermatol. 1979; 18: 722–730.
10. Miller, A., Barr, R.J. Fixed-tissue binding of fluorescein-conjugate concevalin A to malignant melanomas versus nevi. J Am Acad Dermatol. 1984; 11: 620–624.

Clinica Oculistica dell'Università di Genova
Ospedale S. Martino, Pad. 9
Piazzale Rosanna Benzi
16136 Genova, Italy

20. Infrared light imaging in retinal diseases. A comparison with fluorescein angiography and ophthalmoscopy

G. STAURENGHI, A. LA CAPRIA, M. ASCHERO, P. GONNELLA and
N. ORZALESI

(Milan, Italy)

Purpose

To determine whether infrared imaging (IR) with scanning laser ophthalmoscope (SLO, Rodenstock GmbH) could be used in the diagnosis of retinal diseases.

Methods

Two hundred and fifty consecutive patients with different retinal conditions (including different stages of age-related macular degeneration, central and branch vein occlusion, branch artery occlusion, diabetes, central serous chorioretinopathy, angioid streaks, myopic retinal changes) were studied with both fluorescein angiography (FA) and IR imaging (780 nm) by means of a SLO. Two trained observers, masked for the corresponding colour picture and fluorescein angiography, made the diagnosis based only on infrared image. Sensitivity and specificity of this procedure were evaluated.

Results

Chorioretinal atrophy, drusen, retinal oedema or fluid, retinal pigment, RPE detachment, retinal new vessel, lacquer cracks and angioid streaks were easily visible and diagnosed. Chorioretinal atrophy appears as a highly reflective surface, soft drusen as round shaped grey dots, and hard drusen are less distinct. In indirect mode deposition of material, probably with Bruch's membrane, appears in association with drusen. This material is not seen with regular FA or colour picture. In the presence of retinal oedema the cysts are very well outlined. Retinal pigment epithelium detachment appears as a round dark area masking the choroidal structure as in ICGA. The visualization of proliferating retinal new vessels is similar to that obtained with red free photography. However, the ability to detect these vessels in the presence of the media opacity often associated with diabetic proliferative retinopathy is

G. Coscas and F. Cardillo Piccolino (eds.), Retinal Pigment Epithelium and Macular Diseases, pp. 149–150.
© 1998 Kluwer Academic Publishers.

an important advantage. Lacquer cracks appear as white, well delineated lines. This is particularly useful in cases of macular involvement when lacquer cracks may be masked by macular pigments. Angioid streaks are also very sharply outlined and their relationship with choroidal neovascularization, when present, is almost uniquely shown by IR imaging. Choroidal neovascular membranes appear as a dark area, often surrounded by a white contour. The boundaries of the membrane indicated by IR imaging correspond fairly well to the limit of the histological limit of the membrane. Thin blood deposits and occluded retinal vessels are barely visible. However, in arterial branch occlusion, also of the partial and/or transient type, the boundaries of the ischaemic retinal areas are outlined in a unique way. SLO scotometry indicates in this case a strict correspondence between the area indicated as ischaemic by IR imaging and that suffering from functional impairment.

An overall sensitivity of 0.95 and a specificity of 0.98 in identifying correctly the disease was calculated.

Conclusions

Infrared light imaging is a new, rapid and non-invasive technique of fundus examination. It often combines formations supplied separately by colour picture and FA. It may be used even in cases not amenable to conventional dye injection and/or with moderate opacities of media which are so often present in retinal diseases were it may be usefully applied.

University Eye Clinic
Institute of Biomedical Science
San Paolo Hospital
Milan
Italy

21. Infrared imaging of choroidal neovascularization by scanning laser ophthalmoscope

F. GELISKEN, W. INHOFFEN, U. SCHNEIDER, J.H. GONZALES
and I. KREISSIG
(Tubingen, Germany)

Introduction

Infrared (IR) light penetrates deeper into the fundus and provides some information about subretinal structures. Recent advances made IR imaging with a scanning laser ophthalmoscope (SLO) possible. We performed IR ophthalmoscopy using a SLO in classic choroidal neovascularization (CNV) to determine the role of this technique in clinical use.

Patients and methods

We reviewed 61 eyes of 61 consecutive patients with classic CNV documented by fluorescein angiography (FA). All patients underwent a direct IR ophthalmoscopy using a SLO 101 (Rodenstock).

IR imaging was performed using a 780 nm diode laser, a direct mode, an aperture of 2 mm, a maximal laser energy of 95 μW and a He–Ne laser as aiming beam. FA and IR images were digitized (Topcon IMAGEnet 1024). Borders of the suspected CNV on IR image were mapped in four directions (superior, inferior, nasal, temporal) and traced to FA.

IR images of classic CNVs were classified as well defined if their borders overlapped at least in three directions with FA. If borders in one or two directions overlapped with FA they were ill-defined. They were defined as occult based on IR images if none of the borders correlated with FA.

Results

The Atiology of CNV was age-related macular degeneration (ARMD) in 46 eyes, myopia in six eyes, presumed ocular histoplasmosis syndrome in two eyes and idiopathic in seven eyes.

Digital overlay of IR images revealed that borders of CNV were well-defined in 40 of 61 (66%) eyes. In 18 of 61 (29%) eyes CNV were ill-defined. In three of 61 (5%) eyes, CNV were not detected using IR imaging. All eyes with occult IR imaging had CNV secondary to AMD.

G. Coscas and F. Cardillo Piccolino (eds.), Retinal Pigment Epithelium and Macular Diseases, pp. 151–152.
© *1998 Kluwer Academic Publishers.*

Conclusions

FA is the standard method for diagnosis and therapy of classic CNV. However, our study confirmed that direct IR imaging by a SLO can delineate borders of classic CNV in most of patients. Therefore, non-invasive IR imaging with SLO may be helpful in examination of classic CNV in patients with known allergy for fluorescein dye, in presence of opacities of ocular media or in myotic pupil and in follow-up or non-treatable CNV. More knowledge about IR imaging may reduce the application of angiographic dyes in future.

Ophthalmology III
University of Tübingen
Germany

22. Macular syndromes following cataract surgery: intraoperative and serial postoperative fluorescein angiographic findings

J.G.F. DOWLER, K.S. SHEMI and A.M.P. HAMILTON

(London, UK)

Introduction

The visual outcome of cataract surgery in diabetics with retinopathy is poorer than in non-diabetics, and appears to be particularly poor in eyes with maculopathy[1]. Postoperative macular oedema may represent clinically significant macular oedema unrecognized or untreated because of lens opacity, diabetic macular oedema stimulated or exacerbated by cataract surgery[2-5], or a form of the Irvine Gass syndrome[6,7]. The reduction in incidence of postoperative astigmatism and inflammation associated with the adoption of small incision techniques for cataract surgery permits an attempt to redefine these syndromes, which we undertook using intraoperative and serial postoperative fundus fluorescein angiography.

Materials and methods

Patients

Seven non-diabetic patients without intercurrent ocular or systemic disease likely to modify the nature or postoperative course of cataract surgery or to influence fluorescein angiograms (median age 73; range 40–86) were studied as normal controls.

Twenty-seven diabetics diagnosed after the age of 30 with non-proliferative or quiescent proliferative retinopathy at the time of surgery were studied. Patients with intercurrent ocular or systemic disease likely to modify the nature or postoperative course of cataract surgery or to influence fluorescein angiograms, and patients with neovascularization of the iris or traction retinal detachment were excluded. Median age was 65 years (47–90) and median duration of diabetes was 13 years (1–35). Nine patients took insulin and 18 did not, nine were on antihypertensive medication. Focal macular laser therapy had been applied to eight eyes prior to surgery, and panretinal photocoagulation to three.

G. Coscas and F. Cardillo Piccolino (eds.), Retinal Pigment Epithelium and Macular Diseases, pp. 153–156.
© 1998 Kluwer Academic Publishers.

Intervention

All patients fasted for 6 h prior to surgery. Cardiovascular and respiratory monitoring was undertaken throughout all procedures. An intravenous cannula was sited prior to each procedure. Preoperative medication consisted of G Phenylephrine 5% and G Cyclopentolate 1%. No preoperative systemic or topical antiinflammatory agents were used. In 32 eyes surgery was carried out under peribulbar anaesthesia consisting of 7 ml of a 50 : 50 mix of bupivacaine 0.5% and lignocaine 2% without adrenaline with 300 units of hyaluronidase. A mercury compression bag was used for 5 min prior to surgery. Two patients underwent surgery under topical anaesthesia using 3 drops of amethocaine 1%. All patients underwent phakoemulsification surgery through a sutureless 4 mm scleral tunnel. Capsulorrhexis, then hydrodissection with balanced salt solution was followed by phakoemulsification using balanced salt solution containing 1 ml 1 : 1000 adrenaline per litre. Cortical lens matter was aspirated, a folding silicone intraocular lens implanted, and the anterior chamber inflated with viscoelastic agent. Topical chloramphenicol and a second layer of surgical drapes were applied. Fundus fluorescein angiography was performed using a vertically mounted fundus camera (Fig), using forceps to manipulate eye position. Following angiography, the second layer of surgical drapes was removed, viscoelastic agent was aspirated from the eye, and subconjunctival betamethasone 4 mg and cefuroxime 125 mg administered. Surgery lasted 35–75 min (median 45)

Fundus fluorescein angiography, anterior segment examination, ophthalmoscopy, and measurement of logMAR visual acuity was repeated at 3 days, 10 days, 6 weeks and at 6-week intervals to 6 months. Postoperative inflammation requiring additional medication was noted. Fundus fluorescein angiograms were graded in an unmasked fashion for quality, optic disc hyperfluorescence, focal macular hyperfluorescence, macular capillary nonperfusion and incidental findings

Results

Adverse effects of phakoemulsification combined with fluorescein angiography

One patient was sufficiently nauseated to retch and two other patients complained of transient nausea. No patient suffered an allergic reaction, anaphylaxis, endophthalmitis, death, or any other adverse reaction to fluorescein angiography.

Angiographic findings – intraoperative angiograms

One intraoperative angiogram was ungradeable; the remaining 33 were of good resolution. Focal macular hyperfluorescence was more marked in postoperative angiograms at 3 and 10 days than in intraoperative angiograms.

Generalized macular hypofluorescence was apparent in the intraoperative angiograms of all seven normal controls and in 19 of 27 diabetic patients. Areas of extramacular hyperfluorescence which matched the shape of the operating microscope filament and which evolved rapidly, suggesting subclinical operating microscope phototoxicity, were noted in four patients. Transient choroidal folds, ascribed to peribulbar anaesthetic agent, were noted in one patient. Hyperfluorescence associated with laser burns was noted during intraoperative angiography in six diabetics.

Angiographic patterns – normal controls

Focal hyperfluorescence at macula was absent in the intraoperative angiogram of six of seven normal patients, but appeared on subsequent angiograms in six. Relative optic disc hyperfluorescence was present in some postoperative angiogram of six patients. These changes resolved within 9 months in all cases.

Angiographic patterns – diabetics

Focal hyperfluorescence at the macula was present in all intraoperative angiograms of diabetic patients. This deteriorated in subsequent angiograms in 21 patients, and remained unchanged in six. Five showed spontaneous improvement in angiographic macular oedema by 6 months. Relative optic disc hyperfluorescence occurred in some postoperative angiogram in all patients. Spontaneous improvement in angiographic macular oedema could not be statistically correlated with the occurrence of generalized macular hypofluorescence on intraoperative angiography, the subsequent development of optic disc oedema, or preoperative laser therapy.

Visual acuity

Median preoperative best corrected logMAR acuity was no different in normal individuals (0.18–5.0, median 0.52) and diabetics (0.18–5.0 median 0.72, $p = 0.35$). Six month postoperative acuity was significantly better in non-diabetics (0.08–0.1 median 0) than diabetics (0–0.6, median 0.2, $p = 0.0012$).

Discussion

Intraoperative and serial postoperative fundus fluorescein angiography appears to be a practicable and well tolerated technique generating good quality angiograms. It might be used during cataract surgery in patients with retinal dystrophies, posterior uveitis, etc., during vitrectomy surgery, and in examination under anaesthesia. A larger series would help to define the risks more accurately and to characterize changes in the normal population. Intraoperative fluorescein angiography appears effective in identifying diabetic maculopathy present prior to surgery, and serial postoperative angiography allows the evolution of subsequent macular oedema to be traced. Further study may help to identify angiographic features predictive of likely deterioration or spontaneous resolution of macular oedema, and to define the postoperative interval after which resolution becomes unlikely, thereby providing the basis for appropriate therapeutic intervention.

References

1. Dowler, J.G.F., Hykin, P.G., Hamilton, A.M., Lightman, S.L. Visual acuity following diabetic extracapsular cataract extraction. A meta-analysis. Eye. 1995; 9: 313.
2. Pollack, A., Dotan, S., Oliver, M. Course of diabetic retinopathy following cataract surgery. Br J Ophthalmol. 1991; 75: 2–8.
3. Pollack, A., Leiba, H., Bukelman, A., Oliver, M. Cystoid macular oedema following cataract extraction in patients with diabetes. Br J Ophthalmol. 1992; 76: 221–224.
4. Jaffe, G.J., Burton, T.C. Progression of nonproliferative diabetic retinopathy following cataract extraction. Arch Ophthalmol. 1988; 106: 745–749.
5. Jaffe, G.J., Burton, T.C., Kuhn, E. et al. Progression of nonproliferative diabetic retinopathy and visual outcome after extracapsular cataract extraction and intraocular lens implantation. Am J Ophthalmol. 1992; 114: 448–456.
6. Gass, J.D.M., Norton, E.W.D. Cystoid macular edema and papilledema following cataract extraction. A fluorescein funduscopic and angiographic study. Arch Ophthalmol. 1966; 76: 646–661.
7. Irvine, S.R. A newly defined vitreous syndrome following cataract surgery, interpreted according to recent concepts of the structure of the vitreous. Am J Ophthalmol. 1953; 36: 599.

Retinal Diagnostic Department
Moorfields Eye Hospital
London EC1V 2PD, UK

23. Treatment of macular holes with argon laser evaluated by scanning laser tomography

D. WEINBERGER, O. CRISTAL, H. STEIBEL-KALISH,
R. AXER-SIEGAL, E. PRIEL and Y. YASSUR

(Petah-Tikva, Israel)

Introduction

Surgical treatment of idiopathic macular holes is recommended by many authors and found to be effective and beneficial[1-4]. The user of laser treatment for macular holes has been suggested a few times in the ophthalmic literature[5-9] but was not accepted as a routine procedure because of the low successful rate of visual acuity improvement.

This study evaluated the effect of laser treatment on full thickness macular holes and examined the topographical changes of the macular surface using the confocal laser tomograph (Heidelberg Retinal Tomograph, Heidelberg Engineering, HRT, Germany) following laser treatment. The study was conducted to answer whether laser treatment has any beneficial results compared with the natural history of the disease, and whether one can offer laser treatment for idiopathic full thickness macular holes in selected cases when vitreous surgery cannot be performed.

Patients and methods

Twelve eyes with full thickness macular hole and visual acuity of 20/100 or less, inoperable by vitrectomy, were treated by argon green laser photocoagulation, while 15 untreated eyes served as a control. In the treated group, 50 or 100 µm spot size argon green laser burns were placed in one ring around the hole on the elevated cuff 50 µm apart from the foveal avascular zone, allowing 50–100 µm of untreated space between the applications. The power set-up ranged from 100 to 200 mW and the duration was 0.07–0.1 s. The rationale was to induce flattening of the elevated rim, to stimulate the RPE to proliferate and to absorb the sub-retinal fluid. The laser treatment was not aimed to seal the hole.

The topographical changes of the hole and the rim area, depth of the holes and the height of the rim before and after treatment were evaluated by a confocal scanning laser tomography. The method of confocal scanning laser tomography to evaluate macular holes has been described previously by Bartch *et al.*[10] and Weinberger *et al.*[11]. These authors concluded that the

G. Coscas and F. Cardillo Piccolino (eds.), Retinal Pigment Epithelium and Macular Diseases, pp. 157–159.
© *1998 Kluwer Academic Publishers.*

HRT obtained good reproducibility for height measurements of retinal lesions and can be used to quantify small changes in the retinal surface surrounding the macula.

The results were compared with a control group of untreated macular holes. The anatomical results were also compared to the functional results of visual acuity and threshold sensitivity. In three patients one eye was included in the treated group and the fellow eye, with macular hole as well, was included in the control group.

Examinations of visual acuity, fundus biomicroscopy, fluorescein angiography, macular threshold sensitivity by Humphry perimeter and HRT were taken at the beginning of the study and at 1, 3, 6, and 12 months during the follow-up period.

Results

A reduction in the size of the hole was noted in five treated patients (41.7%) and in none of the untreated patients. A reduction in the size of the rim was observed in 41.7% of the treated eyes compared with 20% of the untreated eyes. A reduction in the height of the rim was observed only in the treated eyes (41.7%) and not in the untreated eyes. An increase in the height of the rim was observed in both groups, but only in 33.3% of the treated eyes as compared to 66% of the untreated eyes. The treatment had no significant effect on the depth of the hole, with no difference between the two groups. Improvement of visual acuity (VA) and threshold sensitivity was observed only in the treated eyes. During the follow-up period visual acuity improved in five eyes, deteriorated in five eyes and was unchanged in two eyes. These results were in comparison to the untreated group in which the visual acuity did not improve but on the other hand decreased only in three eyes and unchanged in 12 eyes. The threshold sensitivity improved only in three treated patients (25%). In all patients where there was an improvement in VA and threshold sensitivity, a reduction in the size and the height of the rim was also noted. There was a direct correlation between decrease in the size of the hole and the rim, flattening of the rim height and improvement of the visual acuity.

In order to evaluate changes in the VA following the laser treatment we compared our results to the published VA results of three groups of macular hole patients; changes of the VA during the natural course of the disease, patients who underwent vitrectomy and patients who underwent laser treatment (including our results). The average improvement of the VA in the natural history series was 7% compared with 63.7% in the vitrectomy series and 33% in the laser-treated series. A decrease in the visual acuity was found in 27.5% of the natural course group, in 17.2% of the vitrectomy group and in 20.7% of the laser-treated group.

The topographical measurements demonstrate a beneficial effect of the laser treatment on the morphological characteristics of the hole and its surrounding rim. Improvement of VA and in threshold sensitivity was found only in the treated eyes and in none of the untreated eyes.

Conclusions

Laser photocoagulation can cause flattening of the elevated rim and improvement of the visual acuity and threshold sensitivity in selected cases of idiopathic full thickness macular holes when compared to the natural history of the disease. There is no doubt that the treatment of choice for full thickness macular hole is vitrectomy, with removal of the posterior vitreous cortex and the release of tangential traction forces. Laser treatment can have a beneficial effect and may be an appropriate alternative in cases where vitreous surgery is not possible.

References

1. Kelly, N.E., Wendel, R.T. Vitreous surgery for idiopathic macular hole: results of a pilot study. Arch Ophthalmol. 1991; 109: 654–659.
2. Glaser, B.M., Michels, R.G., Kuppermann, B.D., Sjaarda, R.N., Pena, R.A. Transforming growth factor β_2 for the treatment of full thickness macular hole. Ophthalmology. 1992; 99: 1162–1173.
3. Lansing, M.B., Glaser, B.M., Liss, H. et al. The effect of pars plana vitrectomy and transforming growth factor-β_2 without epiretinal membrane peeling on full thickness macular holes. Ophthalmology. 1993; 100: 868–872.
4. Tyan, E.H., Gilbert, H.D. Results of surgical treatment of recent onset full thickness idiopathic macular hole. Arch Ophthalmol. 1994; 112: 1545–1553.
5. Schocket, S.S., Lakhanpal, V., Xiaoping, M., Kelman, S., Billings, E. Laser treatment of macular hole. Ophthalmology. 1988; 95: 574–582.
6. L'Esperance, F.A. Jr. Ophthalmic Lasers: Photocoagulation, Photoradiation and Surgery, 2nd edn. St. Louis: C.V. Mosby, 1983: 421–423, 437.
7. Gass, J.D.M. Stereoscopic Atlas of Macular Diseases: Diagnosis and Treatment, 3rd edn. St. Louis: C.V. Mosby, 1987: 676–693, 696–705.
8. Schocket, S.S., Lakhanpal, V., Xiaoping, M. Treatment of macular hole with Argon laser. Trans Am Ophthalmol Soc. 1987; LXXXV: 159–175.
9. Makabe, R. Krypton laser coagulation in idiopathic macular holes. Klin Monatsbl. Augenheilkd. 1990; 196: 202–204.
10. Bartch, D.U., Intellietta, M., Bill, J.F. Confocal laser tomographic analysis of the retina in eyes with macular hole formation and other focal macular diseases. Am J Ophthalmol. 1989; 108: 277–287.
11. Weinberger, D., Steibel-Kalish, H., Gaton, D., Priel, E., Yassur, Y. Three dimensional measurement of idopathic macular holes using a scanning laser tomograph. Ophthalmology. 1995; 102: 1445–1449.

Ophthalmology Department
Rabin Medical Center-Beilinson Campus
Petah-Tikva 49100
Israel

24. Three-dimensional ultrasonography in the evaluation of pathological myopia

J.S. SLAKTER, A.P. CIARDELLA, Y.L. FISHER, L.A. YANNUZZI,
A. FENSTER and R. GERSON

(New York, USA and London, Canada)

Introduction

Pathological myopia remains one of the leading causes of blindness in the world[1]. In spite of the fact that over 2% of the population is estimated to suffer from this condition[2], little is known about its pathogenesis and virtually nothing is known about its treatment[3]. In addition, very little fundamental information on risk factors for severe vision loss have been identified. In the clinical evaluation of pathological myopia, fluorescein angiography has proved to be useful for identifying choroidal neovascularization[4]. More recently, ICG angiography has delineated lacquer crack formation and its association with choroidal neovascularization with increased clarity[5].

The hallmark finding of pathological myopia, however, sometimes independent of axial length, is posterior staphyloma[6-8]. Angiography is not particularly useful in documenting the morphological features of these lesions. Until now, the evaluation of a posterior staphyloma has been limited to the use of A-scan axial length measurement and standard two-dimensional B-scan ultrasound evaluation. With these modalities, a key element of the staphyloma cannot easily been identified: that is, its overall volume. We have recently begun investigating the use of three-diminensional contact B-scan ultrasonography in the evaluation of posterior staphylomas in patients with pathological myopia.

Materials and methods

The three-diminensional ultrasound system consists of a conventional, commonly used B-mode ultrasound device (which is adapted and coupled to a microcomputer). A motorized hand-held transducer rotation assembly unit is used to obtain the three-diminensional images. For the purpose of examination, a standard 'through the lid' approach is used with the transducer and rotation assembly unit placed on the patient's closed lid and coupled with methylcellulose gel. After a two-dimensional image of good quality and appropriate orientation is obtained on the ultrasound screen, the computer system

G. Coscas and F. Cardillo Piccolino (eds.), Retinal Pigment Epithelium and Macular Diseases, pp. 161–164.
© 1998 Kluwer Academic Publishers.

is activated resulting in rotation of the ultrasound transducer through an arc of 200° on the patient's lid. Two hundred slices are obtained at each degree point throughout the rotation. Approximately 10 s are required to obtain the images. After the examination is complete, the computer software program reconstructs the individual 200 slices to create a three-dimensional image of the patient's globe[9-11] (Figs 1, 2).

In order to evaluate the accuracy of this system, a phantom eye was created within an agar gel matrix. A small extension or staphyloma was created in the posterior portion of this phantom eye with a known volume. Serial scans were taken of this phantom eye in a masked fashion to determine the volume of the 'staphyloma'. This was performed on multiple occasions by a single examiner as well as by multiple examiners with multiple scans.

Clinical evaluation of 10 patients with pathological myopia was also performed. The patients ranged in age from 39 to 74 years (mean 56 years) with a refractive error of −9 to −20 diopters. All had an axial length of greater than 26 mm. Volumetric assessment of the staphylomas was performed in these individuals using the ultrasound system.

Results

In evaluating the staphyloma 'phantom eye', the measurements were found to be highly accurate and reproducible. With a single examiner, a mean

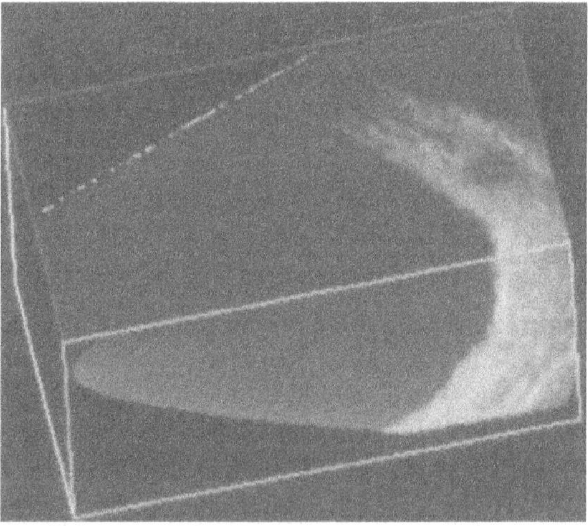

Fig. 1. A three-dimensional reconstruction of an eye with a localized posterior staphyloma. The portion of the image outlined with the lower box is a typical saggital slice of the globe. Above this image (upper box) is the posterior view of this region of the staphyloma.

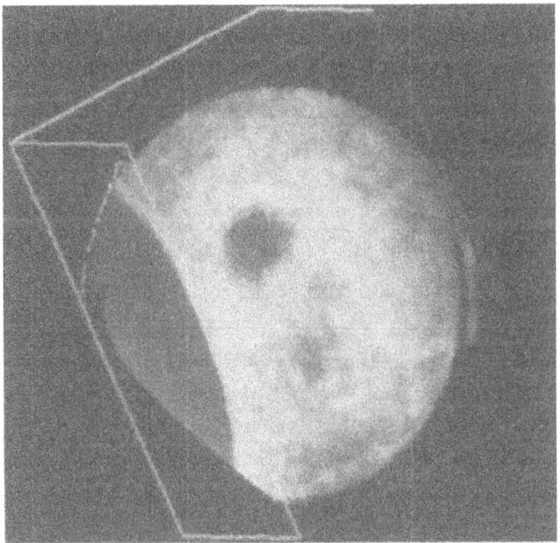

Fig. 2. Further rotation of the image allows for examination of the globe from a posterior approach. In this view, the relationship of the staphyloma (seen superiorly) with respect to the optic nerve (the smaller gray shadow noted inferiorly) can be appreciated.

volume of 40.74 mm^3 was obtained, while the actual volume was 40.80 mm^3. The standard deviation was 0.06. With multiple examiners, a mean volume of 40.92 mm^3 was obtained with a standard deviation of 0.57.

In performing the clinical evaluation of myopic individuals, we found staphyloma volumes ranging from 54.98 to 336.72 mm^3.

Discussion

Previous investigators have clearly identified and correlated increasing axial length with the onset and progression of chorioretinal atrophic changes[6]. No such direct correlation between axial length and the development of lacquer crack formation or choroidal neovascularization has been identified, however. The exact role of the posterior staphyloma itself has not yet been explored. Given the prevalence and severity of this condition, we have begun a prospective case-controlled study of pathologic myopia utilizing three-dimensional ultrasound imaging of the posterior pole in addition to conventional techniques to identify potential risk factors as well as mechanical changes that may relate to vision loss in this condition. We believe that this three-dimensional ultrasound technique is the best means to evaluate the volume of the staphyloma as well as its relationship to other ocular structures. Our initial study demonstrates that this system can produce accurate and reproductive volumetric measurements of these lesions.

There is no question that a study of risk factors for poor vision and pathological myopia must encompass a wide range of demographic, clinical and acquired factors. It is not likely that a single entity, such as the structure of a staphyloma, will represent an overwhelming causative factor. A multifactorial scheme for this complex eye disease is likely. However, it is important to first determine risk factors for poor vision before considering new and sometimes invasive treatment strategies.

References

1. Ghafour, I.M., Allan, D., Foulds, W.S. Common causes of blindness and visual handicap in the West of Scotland. Br J Ophthalmol. 1983; 67: 209–213.
2. National Society for Prevention of Blindness. Fact Book Estimated Statistics on Blindness and Vision Problems. New York: National Society for Prevention of Blindness, 1966: 44.
3. Whitmore, W.G., Harrison, W., Curtin, B.J. Scleral reinforcement in rabbits using synthetic graft materials. Ophthalmic Surg. 1990; 21: 327–330.
4. Hotchkiss, M.L., Fine, S.L. Pathological myopia and choroidal neovascularization. Am J Ophthalmol 1981; 91: 177–183.
5. Quaranta, M., Arnold, J., Coscas, G. *et al.* Indocyanine green angiographic features of pathologic myopia. Am J Ophthalmol. 1996; 122: 663–671.
6. Curtin, B.J., Karlin, D.B. Axial length measurements and fundus changes of the myopic eye. Am J Ophthalmol. 1971; 71: 41–53.
7. Curtin, J.B. Ocular findings and complications: the posterior (central) fundus. In: Curtin, J.B. (ed.) The Myopias. Philadelphia: Harper & Row, 1985: 301–333.
8. Curtin, B.J., Iwamoto, T., Renaldo, D.P. Normal and staphylomatous sclera in high myopia: an electron microscopic study. Arch Ophthalmol. 1979; 97: 912–915.
9. Rankin, R.N., Fenster, A., Downey, D.B., Munk, P.L., Levin, M.F., Vellet, A.D. Three-dimensional sonographic reconstruction. Techniques and diagnostic application. Am J Roentgenol. 1993; 161: 695–702.
10. Fenster, A., Miller, J.M., Tong, S. Three Dimensional Ultrasound Imaging System. U.S. Patent Application. 1993; No. 08/158,267.
11. Fenster, A., Dunne, S., Chan, T. Method and System for Constructing and Displaying Three-Dimensional Ultrasound Images. U.S. Patent Application. 1994; No.08/264,800.

Retinal Research Laboratory
Manhattan Eye, Ear and Throat Hospital
New York, USA

25. The macular choroid and its developments at the embryological stage

P.M. AMALRIC

(Albi, France)

The macula can be considered as the supreme element of differentiation of the eye. Everything is conditioned to increase its efficiency, as it is through this morphoscopic vision that man achieves the plenitude of his action, in coordination with the hand. The eye and the hand are intimately related. Human balance is conditioned by the symmetry of organs, especially of the eyes. Consequently, the development of the latter leads to a geometrical systematization around the horizontal, vertical or oblique axis (Fig. 1). The precision of vision is due to a specialization of both maculas.

During fetal life, numerous circulatory networks disappear in the eye: vascularization disappears in the cornea, the anterior chamber, the lens and

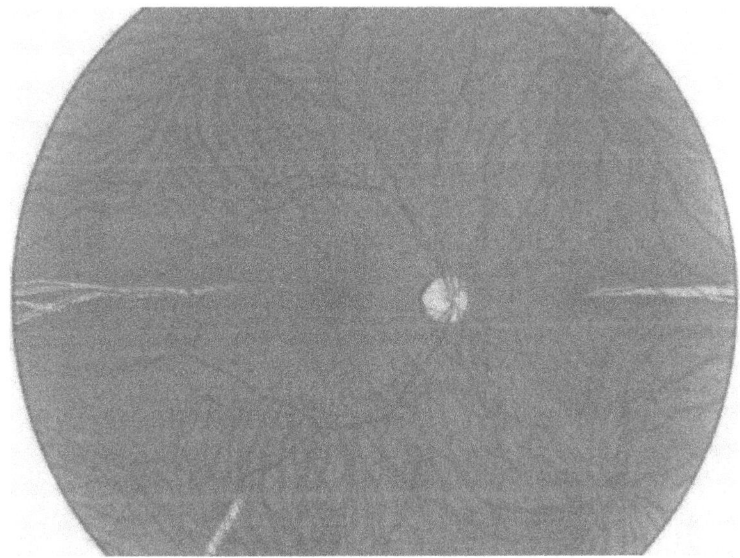

Fig. 1. Choroidal scheme showing the geometrical disposition in relation to the macula and the vertical axis.

G. Coscas and F. Cardillo Piccolino (eds.), Retinal Pigment Epithelium and Macular Diseases, pp. 165–170.
© 1998 Kluwer Academic Publishers.

the vitreous. A new retinal system develops and the macular foveal area remains avascular. At birth, the whole optical system is essentially elaborated and light enables the functions to develop.

Hidden by the pigmentary epithelium, the choroid has long been ignored in this systematization. We know that there is a similar programme of development with, as in the retina, the organization of privileged quadrants. The long posterior ciliary arteries divide the fundus into two parts, superior and inferior, and each quadrant, temporal and nasal, superior and inferior, corresponds to the emergence of four vortex veins.

The macula

The difficulty in obtaining accurate histological examination, and the lack of observations by vascular impregnation with dyes, has prevented the precise definition of the development of the macular choroid during the last months of fetal life. However, as described by Heimann, a ciliary artery which seems to irrigate solely this area can be observed (Fig. 2). Vascular impregnation of the choroid does not show the existence of this artery in the child or adult, however[1-4]. We may conclude that Heimann's artery atrophies or disappears in order to enable a better circulatory balance in an essential area: the fovea. This choriocapillaris corresponds to the avascular area in the retina, as confirmed by angiograms.

Angiograms show the embryological modifications. Heimann's artery is no

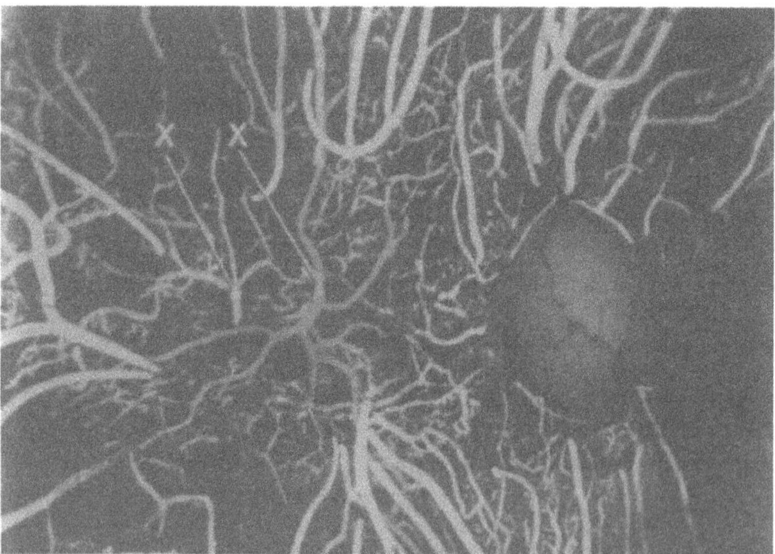

Fig. 2. Heimann's artery.

longer visible and, when visible, the choriocapillaris is only impregnated in the macular area after the first arterial filling. Moreover, the ciliary arteries never originate under the macula; the choroidal triangle originates above and not under the macular oval border, as described on Hayreh's schemes.

At birth, in normal patients, the scheme is particularly precise and in many cases, fluorescein angiography enables the definition of networks. The classical arrangement of ciliary arteries with a spiral direction towards the periphery and the choriocapillaris irrigated by several arteriolar branches originating from the ciliary arteries, can be observed in myopic, partial albinoid or even slightly pigmented patients. The highest vascular density is localized on the macular temporal border, from vessels arranged in triangle and directed to the periphery. The long posterior ciliary artery emerges from the central part of this temporal triangle, its retrograde branches may contribute to the arterial vascularization of the macula. The vortex network of the macular area, directed towards the superior and inferior temporal borders, originates all around the fovea (Fig. 3).

As was observed by Heakel, Darwin's friend, embryogenesis is a short recapitulation of the theory of evolution. At the beginning all the cells are omnipotent, but from the first week, choices are made: organizer genes prevail over development. Most metazooans include a segmented axis, whose genes coding the segmentation, exist in all superimposable species. The DNA sequencies are similar for flie, worms, rodents or humans.

In the field of molecular genetics, it is interesting to note that the modification first observed by Morgan[5] was the difference of colour in the *Drosophilia* eyes he studied.

Our knowledge of the ocular transformation of *Drosophilia* has evolved, since we know that the mutation of a gene can result in the absence of development of the inferior half of the eyes. Moreover, it is amazing to realize that the same result is obtained by including some mammalian HOX proteins in the genetic constitution of the fly.

The DNA sequence implied in this process, was named 'homeobox', the black box of the genetic programme. It forms the family: HOX, HOX 1, HOX 2, HOX 3, etc. The HOX genes, equivalent to the complex of the *Drosophilia*, prevail over the development of similar areas. Today we know all the genes prevailing over the development of *Drosophilia*, and everyday a series of similar organizor genes is discovered.

Homeotical selector genes enable the establishment of organs: the antennapedia ANT-C complex for the organization of the anterior area of the head; bithorax BX-C, for the posterior appendix of the animal.

"The evolution is the result of successive release of the whole body in relation with the liquid element: – the head in relation with the ground, – the hand in relation with the motion, – the brain in relation with the face; allo this enables to take up the conquest of space and time" (André Leroi-Gourhan).

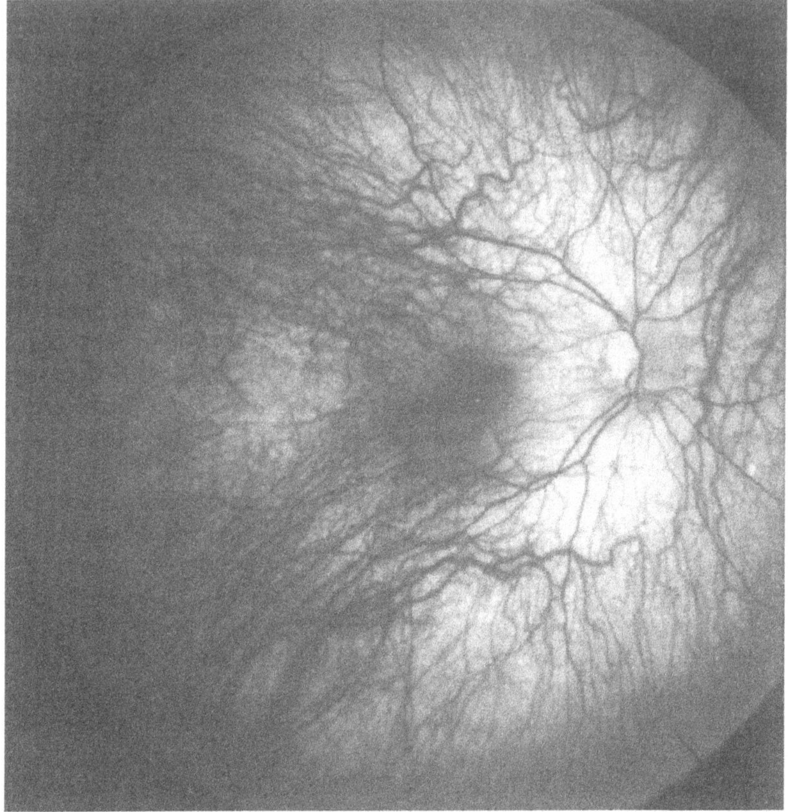

Fig. 3. Vortex network originating in the macula.

What about architect genes for the eye?

From the fly to mouse and man, there is a supergene for the eye. The study of these mechanisms is still in the early stages but the organization of an ocular and cerebral development is fantastic.

Two distinct phenomena occur in the eye: during fetal life, the formation of the organ under the control of homeotic genes; at the end of fetal life, transformation under the influence of a hormone controlling the anatomical remodelling, which results in a real metamorphosis of the eye.

Recently, Gehring's experiments[6] have demonstrated that a single gene is able to entail the formation of such a complex organ as the eye. According to recent studies, a unique gene, located at the top of a series of transformations required 2000–3000 genes, determines the formation of the eye. This master gene has been observed in many species.

The Eyeless gene is the master gene for the formation of the eye. By itself, it is able to originate the development of the organ in areas where it does not usually develop. Mouse DNA, transfected into *Drosophilia*, can generate the formation of eyes in the fly. Darwin asserted that it seemed impossible to him to explain the origin of such a perfect organ as the eye, by simple random variations but Gehring's experiment confirm this possibility. Gehring demonstrate that the eye of the animal has evolved from a single prototype which probably existed in vertebrate as primitive as a flatworm.

Conclusions

The concordance between the choroidal and the retinal vascular networks is absolutely essential in the development of vision to achieve the optical perfection of the eye. Numerous organizing genes must participate in this process, including elective genes for the organization of the macular vision and genes prevailing over the development of the binocular vision. From a phylogenic standpoint, the man, as all quadruped mammals, presents a higher density of visual elements in the superior quadrants, his look being more easily turned downwards than upwards.

Many pathological patterns of the inferior quadrants can be explained by this evolutive law (Figs 4–6)

Today, we must go beyond the strict notion of geometrical lesions caused by arterial or venous vascular occlusion, to think, in some cases, of a genetically transmitted pathology related more to the function than the structure. For a long time, we wondered about some symmetrical or dystrophic bilateral ocular lesions, which did not correspond to the scheme of the choroidal or retinal vascular arrangement. Today, this is clarified, as genetics demonstrates that everything is centred, in a preferential way, on the achievement of a perfect neurovisual function.

Macular vision is primordial and essential. Paracentral peripheral vision extends up to 30°, with a visual preference given to the superior retinal hemifield to get the best vision downwards. Beyond the superior retinal vascular arch, the peripheral vision becomes less and less clear. This is only useful for panoramic vision.

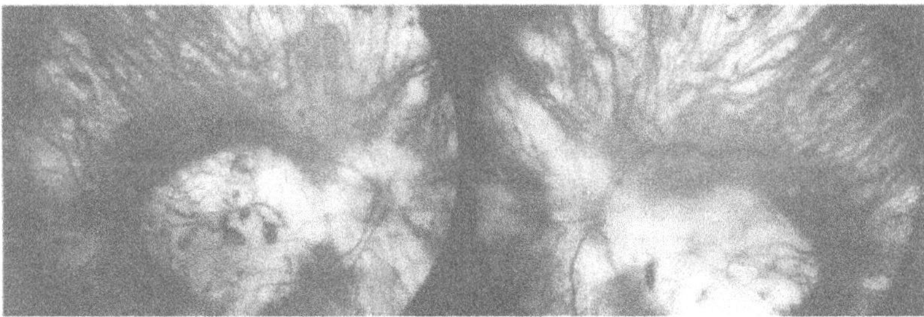

Fig. 4. Congenital symmetrical aplasia of the macular area.

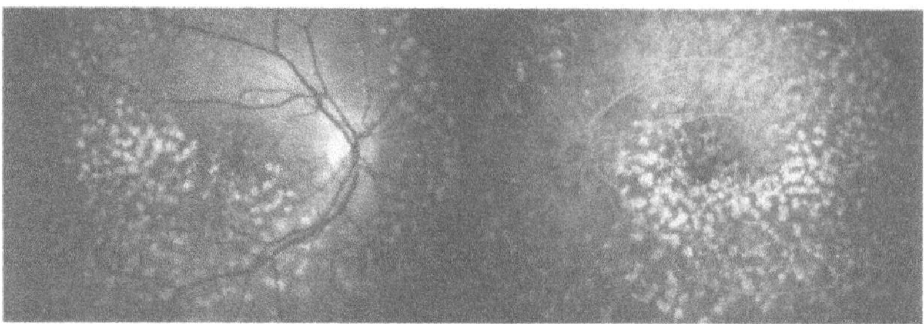

Fig. 5. Paramacular spiroidal symmetrical arrangement of drusen, unexplained by anatomy, but explainable by physiology.

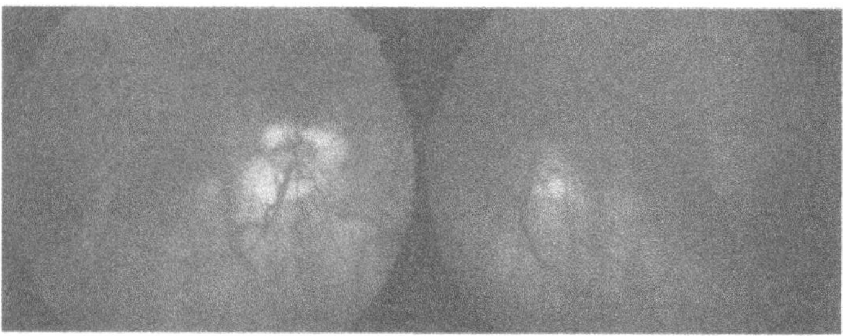

Fig. 6. Symmetrical choroidal and papillary anomaly corresponding to a congenital haemiatrophy.

In embryology, the development of the eye represents a wonderful illustration of all complex phenomena which prevail over the morphogenesis of living beings. For centuries, anatomists, scientists and philosophers have been enthused by its perfect achievement. In the eye, everything works towards the luminous function. Functionality is success in the achievement of an aim.

References

1. Shimizu, K., Ujiie, K. Structure of Ocular Vessels. Tokyo: Igakin Shoin, 1978.
2. Olver, J.M. Functional anatomy of the choroidal circulation – methyl methacrylate casting of human choroid. Eye. 1990; 4: 262–272.
3. Fryczkcowski, A.W. Angioarchitecture of the human submacular choroid. Acta Anat. 1988; 132: 165–169.
4. Fryczkowski, A.W. Diabetic choroidal and iris vasculature: scanning electron microscopic findings. Int Ophthalmol. 1989; 13: 269–279.
5. Morgan, T.H. The physical basis of heredity. Philadelphia, 1919.
6. Gehring, W.J. The master control gene for morphogenesis and evolution of the eye. Genes Cells. 1996; 1: 11–15.

Centre Médical Ophtalmologique
6, rue Saint-Clair
81000-Albi, France

26. The indocyanine green videoangiography in hypertensive choroidopathy

G. LODATO, M. VADALA, G. CARDELLA and M.G. INTORRE

(Palermo, Italy)

Hypertensive fundus changes are most frequently caused by chronic hypertension, mainly affect the retina and are well observed with fluorescein angiography. If hypertensive onset is acute, as in malignant hypertension, choroidal and optic nerve changes are predominant. Choroidal lesions can be actually studied by indocyanine green (ICG) angiography.

We examined seven patients with severe hypertension. Two of these patients suffered from chronic hypertension following pre-eclampsia some years earlier. The features observed by ICG angiography are caused by progressive ischaemia that affects the choriocapillary bed in malignant hypertension[1]. The following angiographic aspects are those which we suggest are related to duration and seriousness of the hypertensive ischaemia:

1. Polygonal and/or triangular perfusion defects of choriocapillary bed, evident on ICG angiography but not by fluorescein angiography (FA). These ischaemic changes are hypofluorescent, regular and well delimited; they are polygonal in the posterior pole and larger and triangular in the periphery, according to the lobule distribution of choriocapillary net[2].
2. Hypofluorescent lesions on ICG angiography that appeared hyperfluorescent in FA, variously sized and shaped. Larger arteries were, however, perfused. When ischaemia was persistent the most sensitive ICG studies showed hypofluorescence due to the absence of a choroidal flush, but fluorescein lesions were still hyperfluorescent because of fluorescein leakage and focal necrosis of retinal pigment epithelium (Elshnig's spots)[1,3]
3. Hypofluorescent lesions on both ICG and FA, circular or multilobed, well defined, usually in the posterior pole or near main vascular arcades. This is an expression of definitive lack of perfusion caused by capillary necrosis.
4. Choroidal hypofluorescent lines, on both ICG and FA, delimited by hyperfluorescent edges assuming the aspect of track; they are mostly radial and in the posterior pole, moving from the optic nerve. They were more clearly visualized and apparently more numerous on ICG than in FA studies. We explain these lesions as choroidal folds: the top part of the fold is hypofluorescent because of narrowing of capillaries due to stretching of choroidal layers, while the sloping edges appear hyperfluorescent.

G. Coscas and F. Cardillo Piccolino (eds.), Retinal Pigment Epithelium and Macular Diseases, pp. 171–172.
© 1998 Kluwer Academic Publishers.

We observed these choroidal folds only in the two cases that were affected by chronic hypertension persisted after pre-eclampsia occurred some years before. We postulate that they could be late-onset degenerative fibrotic alterations in the choriocapillaris layer as a result of ischaemic necrosis.

References

1. Hayreh, S.S., Servais, G.E., Virdi, P.S. Fundus lesion in malignant hypertension. VI. Hypertensive choroidopathy. Ophthalmology. 1986; 93: 1383–1400.
2. Hayreh, S.S. Segmental nature of the choroidal vasculature. Br J Ophthalmol. 1975; 59: 631–648.
3. Kishi, S., Tso, M.O.M., Hayreh, S.S. Fundus lesion in malignant hypertension. I. A pathologic study of experimental hypertensive choroidopathy. Arch Ophthalmol. 1985; 103: 1189–1197.

University Eye Clinic of Palermo
Italy

27. The expanding clinical spectrum of idiopathic polypoidal choroidal vasculopathy (IPCV)

L.A. YANNUZZI, A.P. CIARDELLA, R.F. SPAIDE, M. RABB,
K. FREUND and D.A. ORLOCK

(New York, USA)

Introduction

A peculiar hemorrhagic disorder of the macula, idiopathic polypoidal choroidal vasculopathy (IPCV) was first described, more than a decade ago[1]. The maculopathy was classified and designated by Kleiner *et al.* as posterior uveal bleeding syndrome[2,3] and by Stern *et al.* as multiple recurrent retinal pigment epithelial detachments in black women[4,5]. Yannuzzi *et al.* had suggested the term IPCV because the pathogenesis was unknown, the primary abnormality involved the choroidal circulation and the characteristic lesion was an inner choroidal vascular network of vessels ending in an aneurysmal bulge or outward projection, visible clinically as a reddish-orange, spheroidal, polypoid-like structure[1,6,7]. The disorder was characterized as a distinct clinical entity which was associated with multiple, recurrent, serosanguineous detachments of the retinal pigment epithelium and neurosensory retina, secondary to leakage and bleeding from the peculiar choroidal vascular abnormality. Vitreous haemorrhage, relatively minimal fibrous scarring and the absence of drusen, retinal vascular disease, and signs of intraocular inflammation were also features of the maculopathy.

Indocyanine green (ICG) angiography has been used to detect and characterize the IPCV abnormality with enhanced sensitivity and specificity[7,8]. While some reports exclusively associated IPCV with Black females[4,5,8], it has also been identified in other races[1–3,6,7]. The exact pathogenesis and clinical nature of IPCV is still unclear, but additional case experience based on historical cases and newly recognized observations has provided further information on IPCV.

Patients and methods

An additional 20 cases have been retrospectively reviewed to examine the clinical nature and course of IPCV. Twelve new cases have been examined by the authors and eight other cases have been evaluated by one author through mail consultation from other retinal specialists. A review of the

G. Coscas and F. Cardillo Piccolino (eds.), Retinal Pigment Epithelium and Macular Diseases, pp. 173–183.
© *1998 Kluwer Academic Publishers.*

previously reported 45 cases was also carried out in the overall study of the disorder[1-8]. The new patients seen by the authors were given a complete vitreous-retina-macula examination, including indirect ophthalmoscopy, slit-lamp biomicroscopy with the contact lens, and fluorescein angiography. Most of these new cases were also studied with indocyanine green (ICG) angiography. Although a medical and previous ocular history was obtained in each patient, laboratory testing for systemic disease was not performed within a standard format.

Results

New observations on the clinical spectrum of IPCV were noted with regard to its demographic features, the nature and course of the vascular lesion the possible association with intraocular inflammation, and a newly recognized ICG angiographic characteristic which helps to differentiate the IPCV vascular lesion from typical choroidal neovascularization (CNV).

Demographic features

The diagnosis of IPCV was generally first evident between the ages of 50 and 65 years. The average age of the patients in this report was 60 years. One patient was noted to have clinical manifestations as early as the age of 20; a few patients were first diagnosed in their early 70s, and two patients were first diagnosed at the age of 82 years. The average age of onset of all patients (from the literature and this new series combined) was 60.1 years.

The new patients in this series were mostly females (17 of 20). The disorder predominantly, but not exclusively, involved females by a ratio of approximately 4.7 : 1 (53–12) of all reported patients.

In this series there were 10 Black, 4 White, and 6 Asian patients. There is a definite predilection for the disorder to occur in pigmented individuals. Blacks are at greatest risk in the USA; Asians seem to be at a relative risk compared to Whites with a risk profile of pigmented to White race of approximately 4.2 : 1 (52 : 13).

The vascular lesion

The IPCV lesion is a singular choroidal vascular abnormality. However, there is a marked variability in the nature of the vascular lesion with respect to size, location and course. Sixteen of the 20 newly described patients had bilateral disease.

The width of vascular lesions varied in size from vessels which were smaller than the middle choroid to grossly dilated channels which were larger than the outer choroid (Fig. 1). The lesions with larger calibre vessels were often recognized clinically, whereas angiography was needed to detect vascular

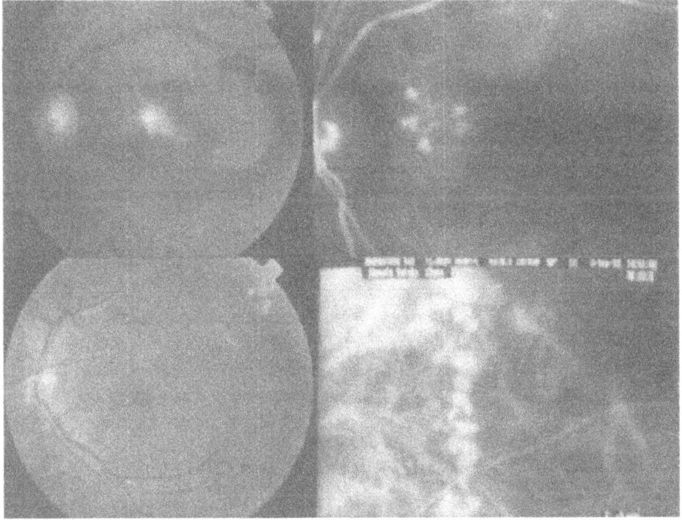

Fig. 1. IPCV. Width of vascular lesions. (A) Clinical photograph of a patient with a haemorrhagic pigment epithelium detachment in the left eye. The polypoidal dilatations of the choroidal
vasculature are barely visible in the papillomacular area. (B) Early phase ICG angiogram of the
same patient. Polypoidal aneurysmal-like dilatations of the choroidal vasculature are evident as
hyperfluorescent lesions temporal to the disc. (C) Clinical photograph of an Asian patient with
IPCV. Large dilatations of the choroidal vessels are clearly visible at the posterior pole. (D) ICG
study of the same patient confirms the presence of large choroidal channels associated with large
polypoidal components

lesions of small dimension. The tubular and polypoidal components of the
vascular lesion correlated in size. In essence, larger channels were associated
with larger polypoidal components.

The vascular lesion was predominantly seen in the peripapillary area. A
few cases presented as a solitary island in the central macula (Figs 2,3).

While IPCV tends to be bilateral, several patients have been followed for
more than a dozen years without evidence of involvement in the other eye[6].
Progression of the vascular lesion within a given eye appears to be based on
enlargement of a focal process rather than confluency of multicentric lesions.
The abnormal vascular lesion may progress in size in at least three different
ways (Fig. 4): by simple proliferation and hypertrophy of the vascular components, by conversion of the polypoidal lesion into the advancing edge of a
vascular channel, or by unfolding of a cluster of aneurysmal elements and
subsequent transformation into enlarging, vascular, tubular components.
When a cluster of aneurysmal, polypoidal elements in the vascular lesion
occurred, it resembled a large, reddish-orange subretinal mass on clinical
examination. With ICG imaging, the vascular mass-like lesion was noted to
be composed of multiple, polypoidal elements which projected anteriorly from

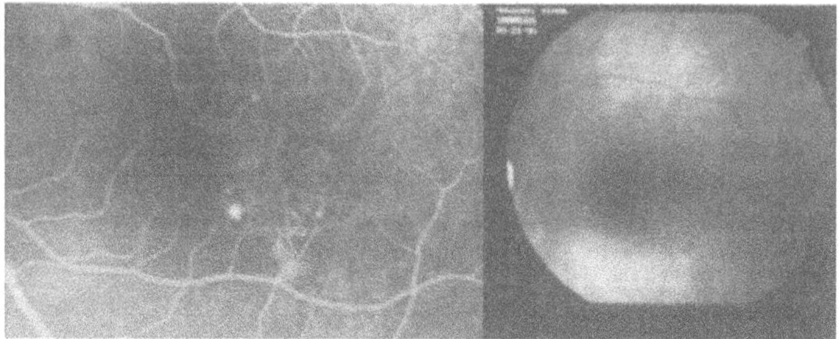

Fig. 2. IPCV. Isolated macular lesion. A) High magnification fluorescein angiography of the left eye of a 41 year-old woman with a positive history for multifocal choroidatis. Temporal to the macula a fine pattern of dilatations of the choroidal vessels is visible. (B) ICG angiogram of the same patient, that shows a vascular pattern corresponding to the lesion in the temporal macula of the left eye. Two nodular areas of staining are evident at the margins of the vascular complex.

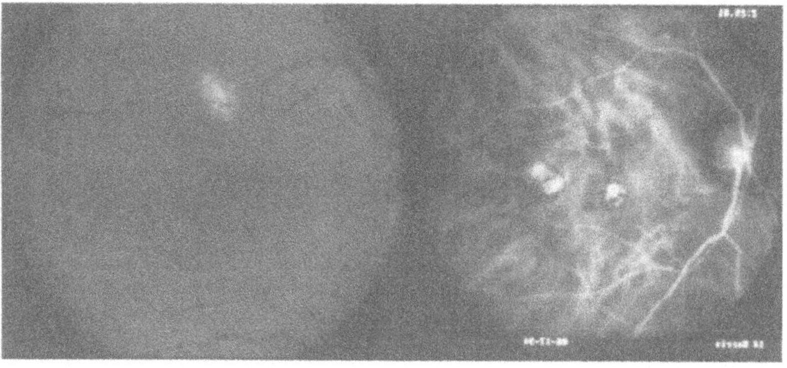

Fig. 3. IPCV. Isolated macular lesion. (A) Clinical photograph of the right fundus of a patient with IPCV. Two isolated large reddish-orange subretinal lesions are evident in the macular area. A fibrotic regressed lesion is evident along the superotemporal arcade. (B) ICG study enhances the recognition of the polypoidal vascular lesions

the inner choroid toward the outer retina. In time, there was eventual flattening of this mass-like vascular lesion and tangential extension of the tubular components in the plane of the inner choroid. When this occurred, the reddish-orange, mass-lesion was no longer evident clinically, leaving a legacy of variable retinal pigment epithelial atrophy overlying the vascular channels of the progressing lesion.

Inflammation

In one patient there was evidence of posterior intraocular inflammation (Fig. 2). Multifocal choroiditis with secondary choroidal neovascularization

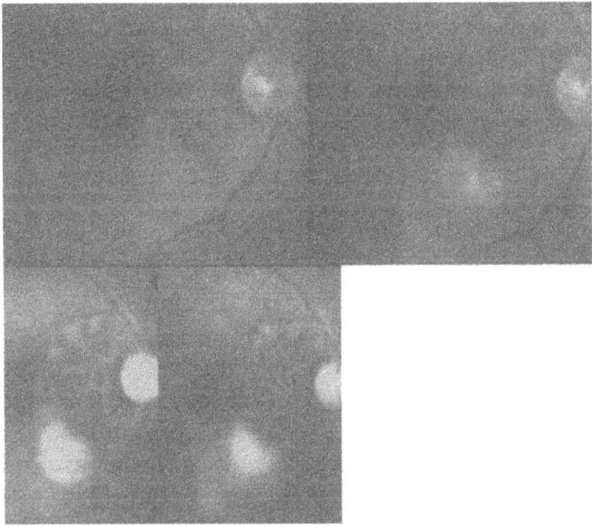

Fig. 4. Progression in size of the vascular lesions in IPCV. (A) Clinical photograph of the right eye of a 61-year-old black male. A reddish-orange elevation is evident in the infero-nasal macula, which communicates with subretinal vascular channels at the level of the inner choroid. (B) Clinical photograph of the same patient two years later. The polypoidal lesion has increased in size and a new component is evident inferiorly. (C) ICG study of the same patient shows dilated choroidal channels partially beneath a serous component of a pigment epithelium detachment (left side). Two years later (right side), the polypoidal lesions are extended inferiorly.

(CNV) had been diagnosed and treated with laser photocoagulation in one eye.

The patient developed a disturbance in the vision of the other eye without real decline in the visual acuity (20/20). The clinical examination did not reveal any discernible exudative abnormality. There were a few inflammatory cells in the posterior vitreous of each eye. The fluorescein angiogram demonstrated an area of subretinal lacy hyperfluorescence suspicious of CNV, but without evidence of late staining. A corresponding ICG study did indicate the presence of polypoidal changes at the margin of the vascular complex, consistent with the IPCV lesion.

In two other patients there were pigment changes within and contiguous with the IPCV vascular abnormality. In the absence of acute clinical signs of inflammation, it could not be determined unequivocally whether these lesions were due to previous inflammatory disease or degenerative manifestation, secondary to antecedent serosanguineous detachments of the macula.

ICG angiography

ICG angiography was useful in this series of patients to image the IPCV choroidal abnormality and described previously[7]. ICG angiography demonstrated an early, choroidal vascular hyperfluorescence as the dye traversed the abnormal vascular components. However, there was a uniform disappearance of the dye (wash out) in the very late stages of the study (Fig. 4) except when polypoidal lesions were actively leaking. The late ICG staining characteristic of classic or occult-CNV was not seen in the IPCV vascular abnormality[8].

Discussion

IPCV appears to be a distinct clinical entity involving the choroidal circulation. The vascular abnormality is in the inner choroid, composed of two fundamental elements, a dilated network of vessels terminating in multiple areas of aneurysmal swelling in a polypoidal configuration (Fig. 4). The polypoidal lesion itself accounts for the episodic leakage and bleeding seen in these patients. Laser photocoagulation treatment has been associated with reversal of leaking polypoidal lesions and resolution of associated serosanguineous detachments in some patients[1,6,7].

The natural course of the disorder is not understood, but numerous patients have demonstrated chronic, multiple, recurrent serosanguineous detachments of the retinal pigment epithelium (RPE) and neurosensory retina with long-term preservation of good vision. Some eyes develop chronic atrophy and cystic degeneration of the fovea with severe vision loss. Other patients have experienced vitreous haemorrhage or even secondary CNV with disciform scarring and profound loss of central vision[1-6]. Most patients have bilateral disease, but a few have only unilateral involvement with more than 10 years of follow-up[7]. No underlying systemic factor has ever been associated with this disorder, except for a recent association in two elderly black females with systemic hypertension and acquired retinal macroaneurysms[8]; nor has there been noted to be any clinical signs of retinal vascular ischaemia or chorioretinal inflammation.

New information is now available to assist in our understanding of the clinical nature of the disorder and its possible causative factors. First, IPCV is not exclusively seen in Black females, as was previously suggested[4,5]. There is, however, a distinct predilection for the disorder to occur in pigmented individuals. Asian patients are also at risk for developing IPCV, but White patients can also develop the disorder. This predisposition for pigmented races contrasts with the relative immunity to age-related macular degeneration (AMD) and disciform scarring in these individuals[10,11]. In spite of multiple, recurrent serosanguineous macular detachments, significant fibrous proliferation typical of end-stage neovascularized AMD is unusual in IPCV.

Although there is no available clinical pathological confirmation, in essence, the vascular abnormality in IPCV appears to be a singular lesion with tubular and polypoidal components which vary in size. The vascular lesion itself appears to be singular and progressive. It does not occur solely in the peripapillary region as originally believed, but it may also present as an isolated island within the central macula (Figs 2,3).

This study also provides a better understanding of the reddish-orange, subretinal mass-like lesion that is seen in IPCV (Fig. 4). It is composed of multiple, polypoidal elements which extend from the IPCV vascular lesion in the plane of the inner choroid, beneath the detached pigment epithelium toward the outer retina. The differential diagnosis of a such a reddish-orange lesion under the retina includes choroidal hemangioma, metastasis from carcinoid syndrome or, more rarely, renal cell carcinoma, posterior scleritis, choroidal osteoma and even CNV. ICG angiography is useful in differentiating the reddish-orange mass as it demonstrates an incomplete ring of polypoidal lesions emanating from the IPCV vascular lesion. The cluster of polypoidal elements may be seen stereoscopically to extend toward the overlying retina. The other mimicking orange mass-like entities are not associated with these dilated inner choroidal vessels and polypoidal vascular elements beneath a pigment epithelium detachment (PED).

The natural course of the IPCV vascular abnormality is also now better understood. Progressive enlargement of the vascular elements through growth of the tubular elements, conversion of the polypoidal change to an advancing tubular structure, and unfolding of the subretinal reddish-orange mass of polypoidal elements on to the plane of the inner choroid coincidental with resolution of the PED has now been documented in patients within this new series.

In spite of increasing case experience, the pathogenesis of the IPCV is still unknown. The association with intraocular inflammation in this series of patients is possibly relevant to our understanding of its aetiology. A clinical correlation of a patient who may have actually had IPCV supports this hypothesis[12]. Histopathological examinations revealed inflammatory cells in the choroid in association with dilated choroidal vessels in a patient who experienced multiple, recurrent, serosanguineous macular detachments and vitreous haemorrhage. No aneurysmal or polypoidal orange choroidal lesions were seen. In this case, there was also a history of hypertension and diabetes. Retinal vascular narrowing and sheathing were also evident clinically in the fellow eye where there was no vitreous haemorrhage. An ICG angiogram performed in the fellow eye was reviewed by the authors, courtesy of Drs Chris Seery and Michael Harris. It did reveal dilated and extremely tortuous choroidal vessels. There were also some aneurysmal-like areas of choroidal leakage which were not evident clinically. In addition, there were at least three areas of choroidal non-perfusion, indicative of ischaemia. Although the choroidal vascular changes could relate to the hypertension and possibly even to the diabetes, an inflammatory-induced ischaemic vasculopathy could also be a contributing factor. Thus, our singular case of IPCV in a patient with multifocal choroiditis, our IPCV patients with possible burned-out chorioretinal inflammatory lesions, and the clinicopathological correlation in a patient with multiple, recurrent, serosanguineous RPE detachments and vitreous haemorrhage suggests that inflammation may possibly be one of the causative factors of the IPCV. One possible explanation linking these cases is the stimulation of embryonic rests by inflammation in a susceptible individual within a multifactorial aetiology. A choroidal osteoma is an example of such a choroidal entity[13].

In spite of these observations, the association with IPCV and inflammation remains attractive but inconclusive. Other potential pathogenetic factors include the possibility of a peculiar choroidal tumour, vascular malformation, or systemic hypertension. One possible choroidal vasculopathy that has a retinal counterpart is idiopathic retinal vascular aneurysms and neuroretinitis[14,15]. In this entity there are multiple large aneurysms in association with signs of inflammation, involving the retinal circulation. A choroidal counterpart consisting of multiple aneurysmal or polypoidal vascular elements in combination with intraocular inflammation is an appealing, yet unproven concept for the pathogenesis of IPCV, as alluded to above.

Finally, the most important consideration in the differential diagnosis of IPCV from other abnormalities of the choroid is the possibility of CNV. It is true that some patients with IPCV present with pure exudative changes mimicking a chronic decompensation of the RPE, a variant of serous chorioretinopathy[7,16]. This is particularly true for a patient who presents with chronic serous and lipid deposition in the central macula due to a submacular IPCV vascular lesion. Most patients, however, develop a serosanguineous detachment of the RPE and neurosensory retina. Generally, this implies the presence of new blood vessel formation or CNV as the underlying causative factor[17]. Indeed, the abnormal vascular lesion in IPCV may merely be a peculiar form of CNV, one that is associated with a separate or independent set of demographic risk factors, clinical features, natural course and visual prognosis. However, the vascular network and the polypoidal lesions of IPCV differ from the classic description of CNV, secondary neovascular maculopathies, particularly with AMD[17–19]. AMD is generally seen in White patients with soft or exudative drusen and/or focal hyperpigmentation[10,19], clinical findings which are not notable in IPCV. New vessel formation with active proliferation in AMD tends to be associated with small calibre vessels which are not detectable clinically and which are associated with a greyish discolouration (dirty grey membrane)[17,18]. Patients with IPCV develop a network composed of vessels of variable dimension and ending with reddish-orange aneurysmal structures that are evident with slit lamp biomicroscopy unless they are obscured by exudate or blood[5–7].

There are other histopathological and angiographic factors which serve to differentiate CNV from IPCV. First, the choroid in AMD, according to Arnold and Sarks[20], tends to diminish in thickness and to show signs of stromal fibrosis without significant alteration in the dimensions of the choriocapillaris and without significant inflammatory cell involvement. These factors are inconsistent with the clinical-pathological case report of IPCV. Second, diffuse, late staining of this stromal matrix in CNV is evident with fluorescein and ICG angiography as a so-called plaque[9]. In contrast, ICG angiography of the vascular lesion in patients with IPCV reveals a prominent vascular network in the early stages of the study, but there is clearing or wash out of the dye in the late stages. This is a newly recognized ICG angiographic feature seen in IPCV, distinguishing its vascular abnormality from CNV. In IPCV the late ICG photographs reveal only a silhouette of the large choroidal vessels in the vascular abnormality, except for any polypoidal lesions which are actively leaking. In this case, there is staining of the wall of the aneurysmal lesion and leakage into the surrounding choroid and subretinal space[7].

Some eyes with CNV may reveal late staining with ICG angiography in the form of a plaque in association with a more intense area of hyperfluorescence which is evident in the early and more prominent in the later stages of the study at the margin of the plaque, so-called focal CNV or a 'hot spot'[8,21]. The occult CNV in such eyes does not reveal the phenomenon of wash out seen in the IPCV vascular abnormality; rather, diffuse staining is typical of such a plaque of occult CNV as reported in a clinicopathological correlation of occult CNV secondary to AMD and studied with ICG angiography[22].

Finally, the clinical location and course of IPCV is also different from that of CNV. Occult CNV is usually in the macula and will tend to organize into a fibrotic or disciform scar, leading to severe macular damage and vision loss[17]. The PEDs seen in IPCV do not necessarily involve the central macula, and they virtually never organize into a fibrotic scar[6,7]. Consequently, the visual prognosis is much better in IPCV than in AMD associated with occult CNV and a PED. Thus, the demographic profile, the clinical manifestations, the fluorescein and ICG angiographic characteristics, the natural course, the response to laser photocoagulation treatment and the visual prognosis of patients with IPCV are distinctly different from individuals with CNV secondary to AMD. Treatment of IPCV to date has been presumptive and anecdotal, but rational. If the inflammation is indeed a part of the pathogenesis of IPCV, pharmacotherapeutics might play an important role in its management. Steroid treatment, however, did not appear to have any beneficial effect on the patient reported in the clinicopathological correlation[12]. Laser photocoagulation treatment of leaking polypoidal lesions with serosanguineous exudate threatening or involving the fovea is unproven but rational. Photocoagulation of the leaking polypoidal lesions with ICG angiographic guidance can result in resolution of associated detachments without stimulation or fertilization of the vascular components and with consequent resolution of the exudate and improvement of the vision[1,6,7]. The same empirical treatment approach applies to secondary CNV[6].

In summary, IPCV appears to be a distinct clinical entity that can and should be differentiated from typical CNV and other known choroidal degenerative, inflammatory and ischaemic disorders. The principle abnormality seen in IPCV, notably the branching vascular network and polypoidal structures at the border of the lesion, are unique to the disorder. In patients with serosanguineous detachment of the retinal pigment epithelium, particularly Blacks and other pigmented races, ICG angiography should be performed to evaluate the choroidal vasculature in an attempt to establish a more definitive diagnosis. If the characteristic vascular lesion of IPCV is seen, a conservative approach to management should be entertained unless there is persistent or progressive exudative change that is threatening the central vision. In that event, there may be a rationale for photocoagulation treatment of leaking aneurysmal or polypoidal components within the vascular lesion, but not the entire vascular complex. It is important to keep in mind that definitive clinical trials to establish the efficacy and safety of laser treatment in the management of these patients have not been undertaken, and because of the rarity and variability of the disorder, probably never will be. When in doubt, the relatively favourable natural course seen in IPCV compared with other haemorrhagic detachments of the macula mitigates in favor of a conservative form of management. Finally, a concerted effort should also be made by physicians to obtain other clinicopathological correlations to assist in the identification of pathogenetic factors related to this disorder and in turn to establish more appropriate treatment strategies.

References

1. Yannuzzi, L.A. Idiopathic polypoidal choroidal vasculopathy. Presented at the 1982 Macula Society Meeting.
2. Kleiner, R.C., Brucker, A.J., Johnston, R.L. Posterior uveal bleeding syndrome. Ophthalmology. 1984; 91 (suppl. 9): 110.
3. Kleiner, R.C., Brucker, A.J., Johnston, R.L. The posterior uveal bleeding syndrome. Retina. 1990: 10: 9–17.
4. Stern, R.M., Zakov, N., Zegarra, H., et al. Multiple recurrent serous sanguineous retinal pigment epithelial detachments in black women. Am J Ophthalmol. 1985; 100: 560–569.
5. Perkovich, B.T., Zakov, Z.N., Berlin, L.A., Weidenthal, D., Avins, L.R. An update on multiple recurrent serosanguineous retinal pigment epithelial detachments in Black women. Retina. 1990; 10: 18–26.
6. Yannuzzi, L.A., Sorenson, J., Spaide, R.F., Lipson, B. Idiopathic Polypoidal choroidal vasculopathy. 1990; Retina. 10: 1–8.
7. Spaide, R.F., Yannuzzi, L.A., Slakter, J.S., Sorenson, J.A., Orlock, D.A. Indocyanine green videoangiography of idiopathic choroidal vasculopathy. Retina. 1995; 15: 100–110.
8. Ross, R.D., Gitter, K.A., Cohen, G., Shomaker, K.S. Idiopathic polypoidal choroidal vasculopathy associated with retinal arterial macro aneurysm and hypertensive retinopathy. Retina. 1996; 16: 105: 111.
9. Yannuzzi, L.A., Slakter, J.S., Sorenson, J.A. et al. Digital indocyanine green videoangiography and choroidal neovascularization. Retina. 1992; 12: 191–223.
10. Ferris, F.L. III. Senile macular degeneration: review of epidemiologic features. Am J Epidemiol. 1983; 118: 213–221.
11. Capone, A. Jr, Wallace, R.T., Meredith, T.A. Symptomatic choroidal neovascularization in blacks. Arch Ophthalmol. 1994; 112: 1091–1097.
12. MacCumber, M.W., Dastgheib, K., Bressler, N.M. et al. Clinicopathological correlation of the multiple recurrent serosanguineous retinal pigment epithelial detachments syndrome. Retina. 1995; 15: 100–110.
13. Trimble, S.N., Schatz, H., Schneider, G.B. Spontaneous decalcification of a choroidal osteoma. Ophthalmology. 1988; 95: 631–635.

14. Kinkaid, J., Schatz, H. Bilateral retinal arteritis with multiple aneurysmal dilations. Retina. 1983; 3: 171–175.
15. Chang, T., Aylward, W., Davis, J.L., et al. Idiopathic retinal vasculitis, aneurysms, and neuro-retinitis. Ophthalmology. 1995; 102: 1089–1097.
16. Yannuzzi, L., Slakter, J.S., Kaufman, S.R., Gupta, K. Laser Treatment of diffuse retinal pigment epitheliopathy. Eur J Ophthalmol. 1992; 2: 103–114.
17. Green, W.R., McDonnel, P.J., Yeo, J.H. Pathological features of senile macular degeneration. Ophthalmology. 1985; 92: 615–627
18. Gass, J.D.M. Stereoscopic Atlas of Macular Diseases. St. Louis, MO: CV Mosby, 1987.
19. Hyman, L.G., Lilienfeld, A.M., Ferris, F.L., III. Senile macular degeneration: a case control study. Am J Epidemiol. 1983; 118: 213–221.
20. Arnold, J.J., Sarks, S.H., Killingworth, M.C., Sarks, J.P. Reticular pseudodrusen. Retina. 1995; 15: 183–191.
21. Guyer, D.R., Yannuzzi, L.A., Ladas, I., Slakter, J.S., Sorenson, J.A., Orlock, D.A. Indocyanine-green guided laser photocoagulation of focal spots at the edge of plaques of choroidal neovascularization. Arch Ophthalmol. (In press.)
22. Chang, T.S., Freund, K.B., de la Cruz, Z., Yannuzzi, L.A., Green, W.R. Clinico-pathological correlation of choroidal neovascularization demonstrated by indocyanine green angiography in a patient with retention of good vision for almost 4 years. Retina. 1994; 14: 114–124.

Manhattan Eye, Ear and Throat Hospital
Retinal Research Department
210 East 64th Street
New York
NY 10021, USA

28. ICG angiographic evaluation of choroidal abnormalities associated with multifocal choroidopathies

A. GIOVANNINI, B. SCASSELLATI-SFORZOLINI,
E. D'ALTOBRANDO and C. MARIOTTI

(Ancona, Italy)

Introduction

Fluorescein angiography (FA) has not been helpful in the study of the pathogenesis of choroidal diseases because of its limits in exploring the choroid. The introduction of indocyanine green angiography (ICGA) in the clinical practice has opened new frontiers in the field of chorioretinal diseases, and this technique has several advantages over FA. Indocyanine green shows 98% binding to plasma proteins, which accounts for the very slow leak through the fenestrated choriocapillaris. Moreover the absorption and fluorescence of the dye is in the near infrared, thus overcoming the screen formed by retinal pigment epithelium, exudates, haemorrhages and opaque ocular media. These characteristics of ICG, together with the recent development of digital high resolution videoangiography, have led to great improvements in the imaging of the choroid[1]. Multifocal choroidopathies (MC) have benefited to a great degree from this new technique[2-4]. The purpose of our study is to report the ICG angiographic findings in MC.

Materials and methods

Using high definition videoangiography (TOPCON IMAGEnet H1024), 74 patients affected by MC, comprising 59 inner punctate choroidopathies without pigment epithelium detachment (PED), two inner punctate choroidopathy with PED, one acute idiopathic blind spot enlargement syndrome (AIBSES)[5], five multifocal choroiditis associated with panuveitis, one presumed ocular histoplasmosis syndrome (POHS), two macular punctate epitheliopathies and four idiopathic choroidal neovascularizations[3] (112 eyes with ophthalmoscopic or ICG angiographic evidence) were studied. There were 51 females and 23 males, age 16–73 years (mean age 36.8) with a follow-up period of 3–44 months (mean 21). All patients underwent a complete ophthalmic examination, colour and red-free fundus photography, and FA and ICGA of both eyes.

G. Coscas and F. Cardillo Piccolino (eds.), Retinal Pigment Epithelium and Macular Diseases, pp. 185–191.
© 1998 Kluwer Academic Publishers.

Results

In the majority of patients ICGA added no further information to that obtained by FA (Fig. 1): the number of choroidal spots was the same on ICGA and FA. On FA the spots were always hyperfluorescent; on ICGA the spots were hypofluorescent in 69 patients (107 eyes), hyperfluorescent in five patients (five eyes). In one case hypo- and hyperfluorescent spots were observed in the same eye. In the other patients, however, ICGA showed choroidal alterations undetectable with FA. In 16 patients (23 eyes) the ICG revealed hypofluorescent spots (Figs. 2–4); in 3 patients (three eyes) the ICGA showed a dark halo around the optic disk or in the macular area (Fig. 4); in two cases these were associated with hypofluorescent spots, alone in the case of AIBSES). In five patients (five eyes) hyperfluorescent spots were seen (Fig. 5); in one patient these were associated with hypofluorescent spots, and in 15 patients (19 eyes) choroidal hyperpermeability was a further ICG finding. This was present even in the unaffected fellow eye in three patients (Fig. 2).

The spots were round or oval, with a diameter of 400–500 µm (spots up to 1000 µm can be observed as secondary enlargement of the scar in the atrophic phase in myopic patients). The number of spots ranged from a few to tens (those visible only by ICGA were usually numerous, diffuse and sometimes confluent). In order to evaluate the number and seat of the spots visualized on ICGA, we divided the fundus into zones: the macula, pericentral area and periphery; for every zone we evaluated the number of the choroidal hypo- and hyperfluorescent spots as < 10 or > 10 (Table 1).

A systemic steroid therapy (1 g intravenous metilprednisolone for 5 consecutive days) induced the complete regression or the reduction of the ICG hypofluorescent spots in three patients (Figs. 3, 4) and of the dark halo in three patients (Fig. 4), in two cases the hyperfluorescent spots disappeared on ICGA after antibiotic therapy. In three cases a reduction of the spots visible in ophthalmoscopy was observed after steroids and antibiotic therapy (Fig. 2).

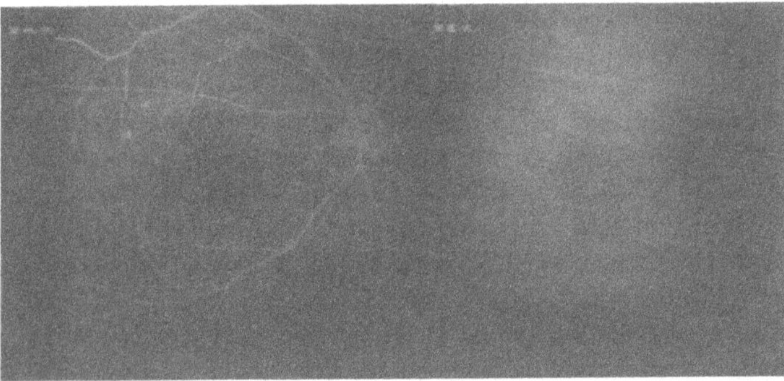

Fig. 1. Typical case of MC in a 23-year-old female. (a, b) Choroidal spots visible on FA correspond to those visualized on ICGA.

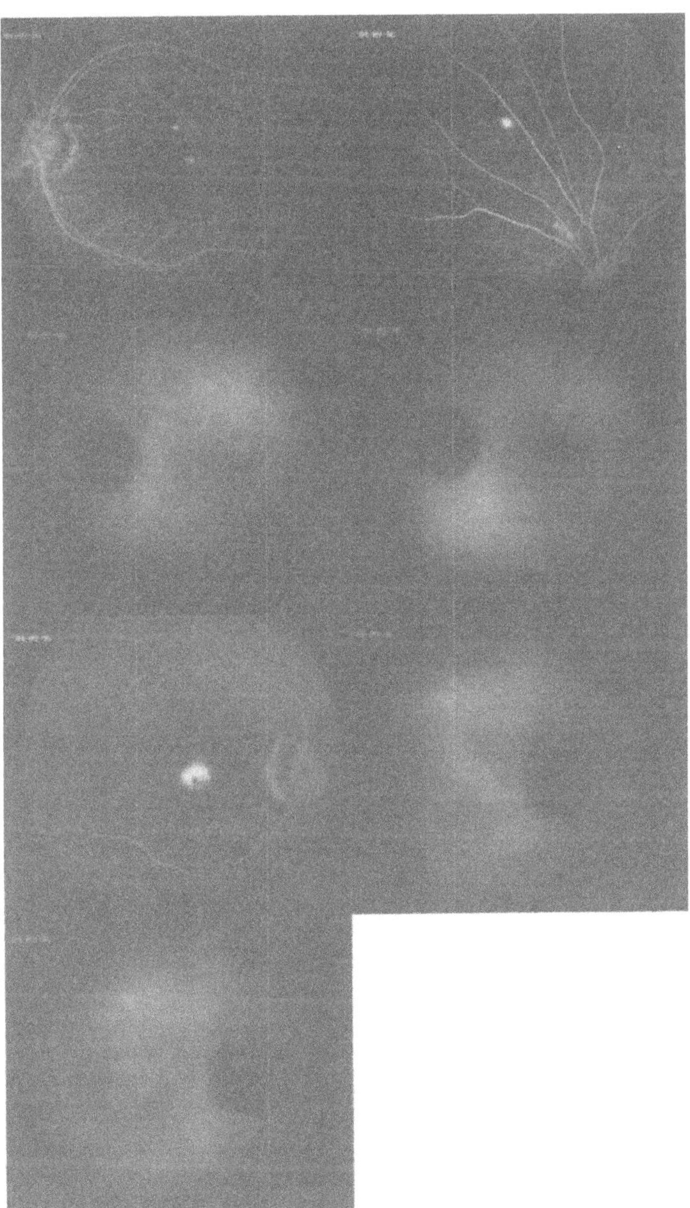

Fig. 2. MC in a 43-year-old man. (a, b) The FA shows choroidal spots in the macular area and in the nasal periphery. (c) ICGA at 20–25 min. Areas of choroidal permeability, hypofluorescent spots and a hyperfluorescent spot are visible. (d) ICGA at 44:49: the choroidal spots are more evident. (e) The FA of the fellow eye shows a subfoveal CNV. (f, g) Choroidal hyperpermeability and peripapillary hyperfluorescent spots are visible in the late phases of ICGA.

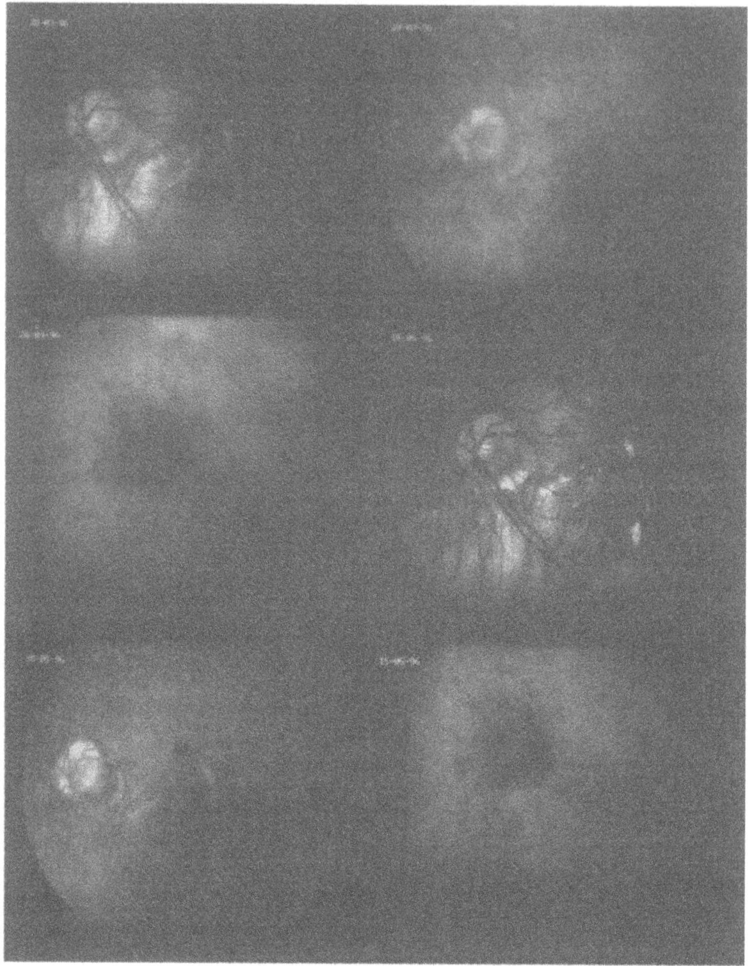

Fig. 3. MC with panuveitis and subretinal fibrosis in a 35-year-old female. The onset of the disease was preceded by an episode of retrobulbar optical neuritis. (a) Red-free photograph. (b) FA. (c) ICGA late phase: hypofluorescent spots are evident at the posterior pole, in the peripapillary area and nasally to the papilla. (d, e) Red-free and FA after steroids: the vitreous opacity is no longer present. (f) ICGA late phase: the hypofluorescent spots regressed after steroid therapy.

Discussion

The MC are a composite group of disease characterized by choroidal spots, peripapillary atrophy and choroidal neovascularization (CNV). Subretinal fibrosis and uveitis can be observed in these group of diseases, except uveitis in POHS.

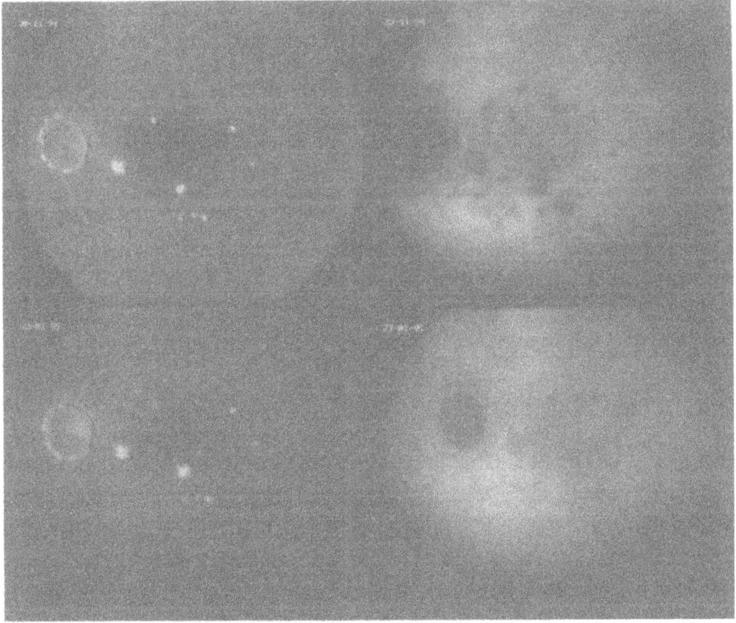

Fig. 4. MC in a 30-year-old female. Few cells in the vitreous were observed. The ICGA (b) shows more spots than FA (a) and a dark halo in the peripapillary area, not visible on FA. (c) Steroids caused the regression of the dark halo and of the spots detectable only on ICGA.

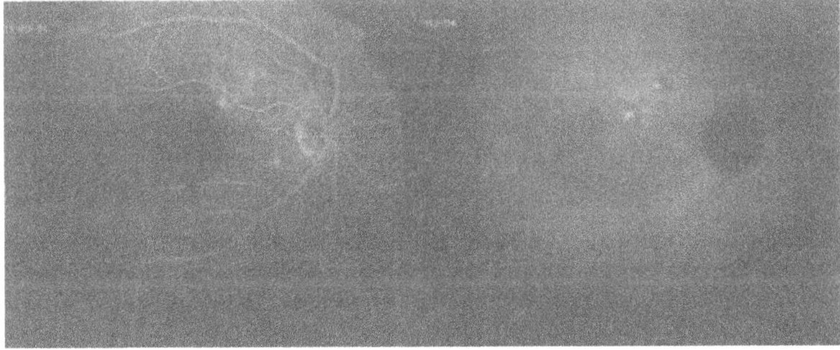

Fig. 5. MC in a 21-year-old male. (a) The FA shows three spots in the macular area. (b) On ICGA the spots are hyperfluorescent.

Table 1. Number of spots in the three zones of the fundus (112 eyes).

	< 10 Spots	> 10 Spots	Total
Zone 1	25	28	53
Zone 2	14	14	28
Zone 3	12	19	31
Total	51	61	112

If the hypopigmented spot is the ophthalmoscopic hallmark of MC, hypofluorescent and hyperfluorescent spots are the key signs of the disease on ICG. In the light of the evidence provided by ophthalmoscopy, FA and ICG we propose the following classification of MC in three stages.

Stage 1 of ICG choroidal activity (11 eyes)

In this group we included those patients who complained of visual changes due to CNV, cells in the vitreous or to acute symptomatic blind spot enlargement. At this stage no spot could be detected with ophthalmoscopy and/or FA. Hypofluorescent spots (nine eyes in eight patients) and hyperfluorescent spots (two eyes in two patients), were visualized only in the late phases of ICGA. These spots were frequently grouped, and sometimes many confluent spots gave the image of a halo in the peripapillary or macular area.

Stage 2 of clinically evident choroidal activity (75 eyes)

One or more of the classic signs of activity were evident. The choroidal spots could be visualized on ophthalmoscopy, being hypofluorescent in the early phases and hyperfluorescent with a slight diffusion in the late phases of FA. On ICGA we observed either hypofluorescent spots, sometimes more numerous than on FA (15 eyes) or, less frequently, hyperfluorescent spots (three eyes) and choroidal permeability alterations (17 eyes).

Stage 3 or healed stage (26 eyes)

No sign of activity was evident. In FA the spots were hyperfluorescent without late leakage, whereas in ICGA they were hypofluorescent during all angiographic phases.

The absence, in the early phases, of choroidal dynamic alterations corresponding to the hypofluorescent spots, the anatomo-pathological findings observed in POHS[6,7] and their regression after steroid treatment suggest that the black spots could be choroidal inflammatory structures and not caused by choroidal ischaemia. ICG, dut to its ability to detect deep choroidal infiltration, allows us to confirm the hypothesis of Nüssenblatt and Palestine about POHS[8]. They suggested the presence of 'invisible' choroidal lesions that become visible and cause the spot if immunologically activated.

Hyperfluorescent spots and choroidal hyperpermeability are signs of choroidal activity which cannot be detected by FA or ophthalmoscopy, and can be usually observed associated with other signs of activity of the disease such as cells in the vitreous or sometimes the onset of a CNV. The hyperfluorescent spots are similar in shape and slightly smaller than hypofluorescent spots, always multiple, and diffuse in wide areas of the fundus. They seem to be more typical of POHS (in this disease they have been found in 40% of cases)[2]. POHS, in contrast to MC commonly observed in Europe, is characterized by hyperfluorescent spots usually smaller than the hypofluorescent spots of the other MC.

Choroidal permeability alterations could be explained by choroidal inflammation, in particular of the choroidal vessels. From the hyperfluorescent spots, if we consider that hyperfluorescence means an alteration of choroidal permeability and absence of signs of delayed choroidal filling, we hypothesize that we are dealing with subclinical inflammation of the choriocapillaris (non-occlusive subclinical choriocapillaritis).

In our study ICG angiography revealed choroidal alterations not seen on FA. This allowed better evaluation of the stage of the disease and therapeutic monitoring; ICG angiography seems, therefore, to represent an important tool in the diagnosis and management of these diseases.

References

1. Yannuzzi, L.A., Slakter, J.S., Sorenson, J.A., Guyer, D.R., Orlock, D.A. Digital indocyanine green videoangiography and choroidal neovascularization. Retina. 1992; 12: 191–223.
2. Slakter, J.S., Giovannini, A., Yannuzzi, L.A., Scassellati Sforzolini, B., Guyer, D.R., Orlock, D.A. Indocyanine green videoangiography of multifocal choroiditis and the presumed ocular histoplasmosis syndrome. Abstr Macula Soc., Rancho Mirage 1994, 110.
3. Giovannini, A., Scassellati Sforzolini, B., D'Altobrando, E., Mariotti, C. Indocyanine green angiographic findings in idiopathic choroidal neovascularization. Int Ophthalmol. In press.
4. Giovannini, A., Scassellati Sforzolini, B., D'Altobrando, E., Mariotti, C. Indocyanine green angiographic findings in multifocal. Bull Soc Belge Ophtalmol. In press.
5 Callanan, D., Gass, J.D.M. Multifocal choroiditis and choroidal neovascularization associated with the multiple evanescent white dot and acute idiopathic blind spot enlargement syndrome. Ophthalmology. 1992; 99: 1678–1685.
6 Ryan, S.J. Histopathological correlates of presumed ocular histoplasmosis. Int Ophthalmol Clin. 1975; 15: 125.
7 Gass, J.D. Pathogenesis of disciform detachment of the neuroepithelium. Am J Ophthalmol. 1967; 63: 678.
8 Nüssenblatt, R.B., Palestine, A.G. Uveitis. Year Book Medical Publisher Inc, Chicago 1989; 382–383.

Clinica Oculistica dell'Università di Ancona
Nuovo Ospedale Regionale di Torrette
60020 Ancona, Italy

29. Vogt–Koyanagi–Harada-type disease: a case report

G. BOLOGNESI, A. PECE, U. INTROINI, C. SANNACE, G. PACELLI,
F. CARDILLO PICCOLINO and R. BRANCATO

(Milan, Italy)

Introduction

The Vogt–Koyanagi–Harada syndrome (VKH) is characterized by bilateral uveitis with serous detachments and signs of systemic disease, including skin disorders (alopecia, poliosis), hearing problems (loss of hearing, dizziness) and signs of meningeal irritation[1,2]. The aetiology of the disease is still not known although recent findings point to an autoimmune reaction against melanocytes[3].

The patient described here had fluorescein angiographic findings characteristic of Harada disease, but no signs of meningeal irritation or systemic disease. This fits the definition of Harada-type syndrome. ICGA[4] brought to light the diffuse inflammatory alteration of the choroid in this disease[5].

Case report

A 33-year-old man presented at this Department on 19 April 1994 complaining of sudden visual loss in both eyes the day before. The history was negative for current or past pathology. Blood samples were taken for routine tests and to check for any immune or inflammatory abnormalities. The findings were unremarkable. Cerebrospinal fluid was not tested for pleiocytosis. Visual acuity was 20/100 in both eyes, not improving with correction. The anterior segment was quiet, but there was slight Tyndall flare in the vitreous in both eyes. Intraocular pressure was 16 mmHg in both eyes. Biomicroscopy showed retinal serous lifting at the posterior pole and multiple detachment of the RPE and folds in the limiting membrane. Multiple greyish areas were visible in the RPE. The optic nerve was hyperaemic.

The patient was examined by retinal FA and ICGA (Fig. 1). In the early FA phases both eyes showed numerous rounded subretinal hypofluorescent areas at the posterior pole, extending to the vascular arcades. In the macular region there were numerous RPE detachments, the largest occupying the central region. In the late FA phases the optic disc became hyperfluorescent and the hypofluorescent areas visible in the earlier phases were no longer visible. The retinal periphery appeared undamaged.

In the early ICGA phases both eyes presented numerous hypofluorescent

G. Coscas and F. Cardillo Piccolino (eds.), Retinal Pigment Epithelium and Macular Diseases, pp. 193–197.
© 1998 Kluwer Academic Publishers.

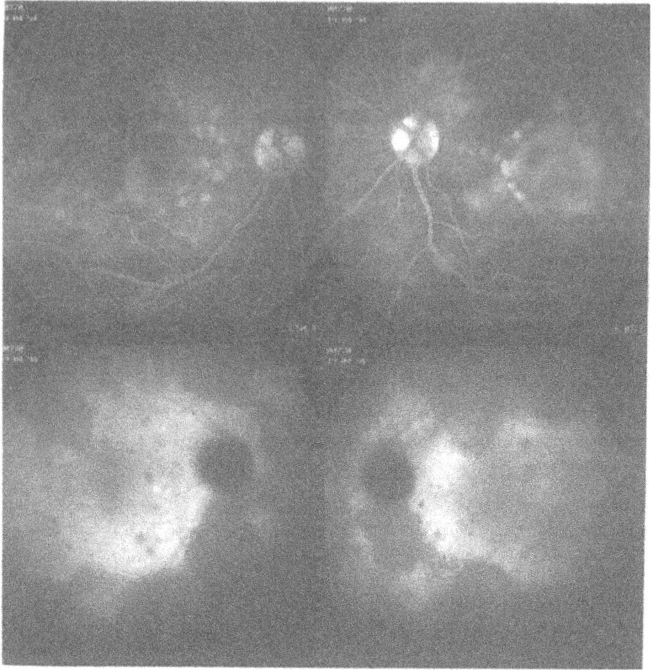

Fig. 1. Fluorescein angiography and indocyanine green angiography of both eyes at the first examination (April, 1994).

dots at the posterior pole, corresponding to the hypofluorescent areas seen with FA. From the middle phases of the examination (10–15 min) a large, clearly outlined map-like hyperfluorescent plaque gradually appeared in the macular region, lying at the posterior pole, but extending beyond the vascular arcades and the optic nerve. In the later phases of the examination (after 30 min) the hyperfluorescent area became more clearly defined, and finely granular. Some hypofluorescent dots were still visible within it. The periphery appeared uninvolved.

The patient was given 200 mg methylprednisolone i.v. for 3 days, followed by 50 mg orally on alternate days for a month. Eight days and 1 month after the start of this therapy the patient returned for biomicroscopy, FA and ICGA.

At 8 days visual acuity was 20/50 in the OD and 20/40 in the OS. FA showed multiple detachments of the RPE and neuroepithelium; hyperfluorescence persisted at the optic disc and some of the hypofluorescent dots seen before in the early phases of the examination were still visible, though fewer and weaker. ICGA confirmed that the hypofluorescent dots had regressed, as had the macular region hyperfluorescent plaque. In the late phases the optic nerve was weakly hyperfluorescent.

The examination repeated at 30 days gave virtually the same results. Natural vision at this time was 20/20 in both eyes. The patient was seen again on 5 June 1996 and visual acuity was still 20/20 in both eyes. FA and ICGA gave normal findings (Fig. 2).

Discussion

The clinical course of VKH usually moves through several stages, starting with a prodromic phase marked by flu-like syndrome, and acute uveitis lasting several weeks. Systemic symptoms appear later during the chronic phase, and relapses may subsequently occur, with ocular complications such as cataract, glaucoma and subretinal neovascularization developing[6].

In the acute phase FA gives a typical picture with diffuse areas of staining

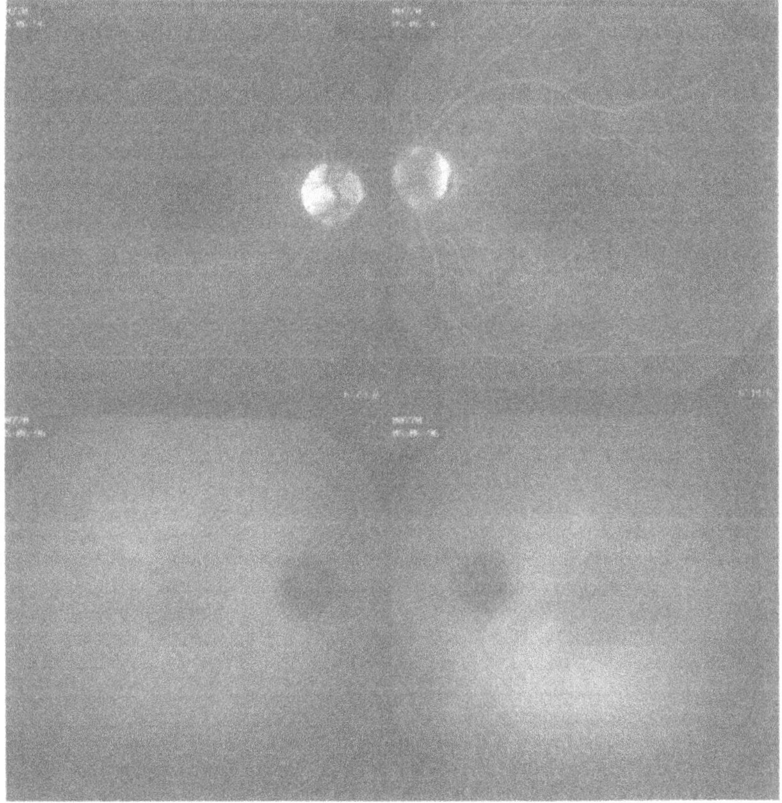

Fig. 2. Fluorescein angiography and indocyanine green angiography of both eyes at the last examination (June, 1996), showing complete regression of the alterations previously described.

in the RPE. Histological examination shows diffuse granulomatous inflammation of the uvea and Dalen-Fuchs nodules consisting of lymphocytes, macrophages and epithelioid cells, with loss of choroidal melanocytes in the chronic stage of the disease[7].

The case reported here presented a typical FA picture of VKH with no systemic disorders, and can thus be classified as Harada-type disease. No notewortly alterations to choroid vessels were seen in the arterio-venous phase of the ICGA which did, however, show up two types of alteration: diffuse hypofluorescent dots and a large hyperfluorescent plaque visible mainly in the late phases of the examination.

The small hypofluorescent areas seen in the initial ICGA phases have two possible causes: either choriocapillaris filling defects, or a block in dye uptake caused by abnormal RPE cells, damaged photoreceptors and; above all, inflammatory cells in the choroidal interstitial tissue.

The late phase hyperfluorescent plaque had clear-cut edges and involved the whole posterior pole, extending beyond the vascular arcades and optic nerve. It may be related to the high affinity of the dye for the proteins found widely throughout the choroidal structure, damaged by the inflammatory disease[8,9]. ICGA showed that these alterations definitely regressing after only 8 days treatment. However, one month ICGA follow-up still showed some choriocapillary damage, despite full functional recovery.

This case of Harada-type disease, presenting no systemic alterations, showed diffuse choroidal damage, clearly detected by ICGA. It is not clear why these alterations arise. ICGA not only showed up the choroidal lesions, which were not visible with FA, but proved particularly useful in assessing the response to therapy.

References

1. Beniz, J., Forster, D.J., Lean, J.S. et al. Variations in clinical features of the Vogt–Koyanagi–Harada syndrome. Retina. 1991; 11: 275–280.
2. Moorthy, R.S., Inomata, H., Rao, N.A. Vogt–Koyanagi–Harada syndrome. Surv Ophthalmol. 1995; 39: 265–292.
3. Broekhuyse, R.M., Kuhlmann, E.D., Winkens, H.J. Experimental autoimmune anterior uveitis (EAAU). Induction by immunization with purified uveal and skin melanins, Exp Eye Res. 1993; 56: 575–583.
4. Yannuzzi, L.A., Slakter, J.S., Sorenson, J.A. et al. Digital indocyanine green videoangiography and choroidal neovascularization. Retina. 1992; 12: 191–223.
5. Yannuzzi, L.A., Sorenson, J.A., Guyer, D.R., Slakter, J.S., Chang, B., Orlock, D. Indocyanine green videoangiography: current status. Eur J Ophthalmol. 1994; 4: 69–81.
6. Chang, T., Freund, B., Green, W.R., Yannuzzi, L.A. Clinicopathologic correlation of indocyanine green angiography of occult choroidal neovascularization. Retina. 1994; 14: 114–124.
7. Lubin, J.R., Ni, C., Albert, D.M. A clinicalpathological study of the Vogt–Koyanagi–Harada syndrome. Int Ophthalmol Clin. 1982; 22: 141–156.
8. Cherrick, G.R., Stein, S.W., Leevy, C.M. et al. Indocyanine green: observations on its physical properties, plasma decay and hepatic extraction. J Clin Invest. 1960; 39: 592–600.

9. Ho, A.C., Yannuzzi, L.A., Guyer, D.R., Slakter, J.S. et al. Intraretinal leakage of indocyanine green dye. Ophthalmology. 1994; 101: 534–541.

Department of Ophthalmology and Visual Sciences
Scientific Institute H S. Raffaele
University of Milano
Via Olgettina, 60
20132 Milano
Italy

30. Indocyanine green angiographic findings in a case of Harada's disease

A.U. MAGNASCO, F. CARDILLO PICCOLINO, L. RAVAZZONI and
E. ZINICOLA

(Genoa, Italy)

Introduction

Vogt-Koyanagi-Harada (VKH) syndrome is a multisystemic disease involving melanocytic organs such as eyes, ears, skin and meninges. The ocular involvement is a bilateral panuveitis associated with exudative retinal detachments that occurs most often in darkly pigmented individuals and is probably the result of an autoimmune process directed primarily aganist choroidal melanocytes[1,2]. The diagnostic criteria for VKH syndrome, established by the American Uveitis Society, include at least three of the following features: (a) bilateral iridocyclitis; (b) posterior uveitis, including exudative retinal detachment or 'sunset glow' fundus; (c) central nervous system findings, including headache, meningismus, tinnitus, dysacousis, neck stifness, or cerebrospinal fluid pleocytosis; (d) cutaneous findings, including alopecia, poliosis, or vitiligo[3]. There ahve been few reported studies concerning indocyanin green (ICG) angiography in VKH syndrome[4,5] We report a case of VKH syndrome studied with ICG angiography before and after resolution of the subretinal exudation.

Case report

A 21-year-old Peruvian woman presented in May 1994, complaining of blurred vision in both eyes associated with headache, slight deafness and hair-aching. Visual acuity was 20/70 in both eyes. Slit-lamp examination of both eyes revealed a normal anterior segment. Ophthalmoscopic and biomicroscopic fundus examinations showed a large serous neuroepithelial detachment at the posterior pole in both eyes, peripherical yellowish spots of pigment epithelium and mild optic disk swelling. Fluorescein angiography and indocyanin green angiography were performed with the Topcon IMAGEnet H1024 Digital Imaging System (Paramus, NJ). Fluorescein angiography showed punctate hyperfluorescence within the serous neuroepithelial detachments, which became diffusely fluorescent in the late phase. Late staining of the disc was also observed. ICG angiography revealed a number reduction of large

G. Coscas and F. Cardillo Piccolino (eds.), Retinal Pigment Epithelium and Macular Diseases, pp. 199–202.
© *1998 Kluwer Academic Publishers.*

choroidal vessels. In the midphase multiple small hypofluorescent areas could be observed, and choroidal veins showed a segmental fluorescence. The serous neuroepithelial detachments were hypofluorescent in the late ICG angiographic phase with some pinpoint hyperfluorescent leaks on the borders. A diffuse background hyperfluorescence, attributable to choroidal staining, surrounded the hypofluorescent area of serous retinal detachment in the very late ICG photographs (Fig. 1).

The neurological signs of neck stifness, marked CSF pleocytosis and reduction of blood lymphocyte subpopulations confirmed the diagnosis of Vogt-Koyanagi-Harada syndrome. The patient was treated with a 12-day course of intravenous corticosteroids followed by oral prednisone for 3 months, with complete regression of the retinal exudative phenomena and improvement of visual acuity to 20/25 in both eyes. The neurological signs and the slight deafness disappeared. After 2 months of therapy, fluorescein angiography showed only a slight mottled pigmentation temporally to the macular region.

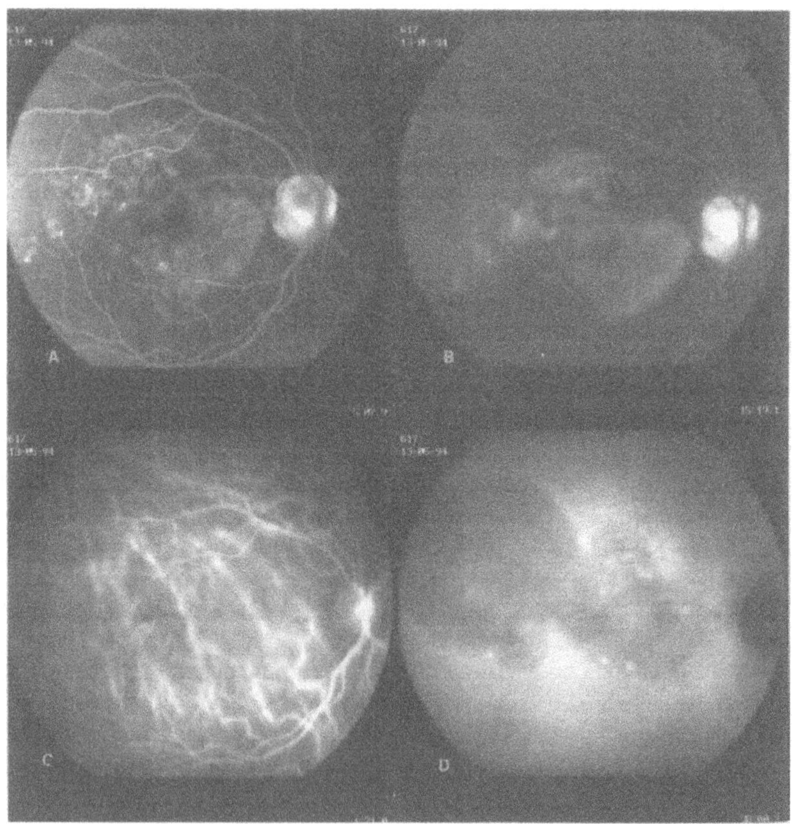

Fig. 1.   Fluorescein (A,B) and ICG (C,D) photographs at the first observation.

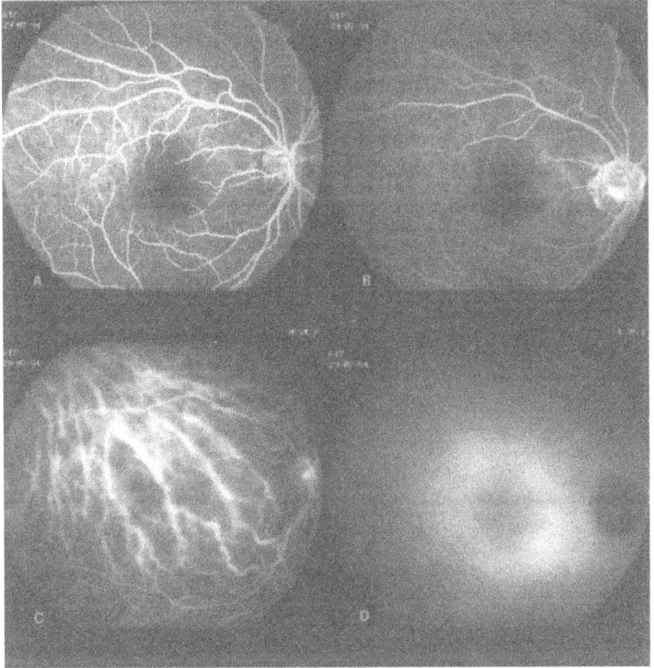

Fig. 2.   Fluorescein (A,B) and ICG (C,D) photographs after systemic corticosteroid treatment.

ICG angiography revealed an increased number of large choroidal vessels with choroidal veins better delineated with respect to the pretreatment examination (Fig. 2). Some hypofluorescent lesions were still visible among the large vessels in the midphase ICG angiogram. A slight diffuse perimacular hyperfluorescence due to choroidal leakage was present in the very late phase.

Conclusions

In this typical case of VKH syndrome ICG angiography revealed the existence of choroidal circulation abnormalities attribuitable to the inflammatory process affecting the choroid. Diffuse reduced vascularity at the posterior choroid was the main ICG angiographic finding. The ICG study was able to demonstrate improvement of choroidal circulation after systemic administration of corticosteroids.

References

1. Sakamoto, T., Murata, T., Inomata, H. Class II major histocompatibility complex on melano-cytes of Vogt-Koyanagi-Harada disease. Arch Ophthalmol. 1991; 109: 1270 1274.

2. Rubsamen, P.E., Gass, J.D. Vogt-Koyanagi-Harada syndrome. Arch Ophthalmol. 1991; 109: 682–687.
3. Moorthy, R.S., Inomata, H., Rao, N.A. Vogt-Koyanagy-Harada syndrome. Surv Ophthalmol. 1995; 39: 265–292.
4. Yuzawa, M., Kawamura, A., Matsui, M. Indocyanine green video-angiographic findings in Harada's disease. Jpn J Ophthalmol. 1993; 37: 456–466.
5. Oshima, Y., Harino, S., Hara, Y., Tano, Y. Indocyanine green angiographic findings in Harada's disease. Am J Ophthalmol. 1996; 122: 58–66.

University Eye Clinic
S. Martino Hospital, Pad. 9
Largo R. Benzi, 10
16132 Genoa
Italy

31. Indocyanine green angiography in choroidal osteoma

B.A. LAFAUT, T. KOHNO, J.D. DE LAEY, C. MESTDAGH
and A. GAUDRIC

(Ghent, Belgium)

A choroidal osteoma appears ophthalmoscopically as a yellow to orange choroidal mass which is irregular and slightly elevated and usually situated adjacent to the optic disc. Its diagnosis is essentially based on ophthalmoscopy, ultrasonography and computer tomodensitometry of the orbit, which shows a plaque-like lesion in the posterior pole with the density of normal bone. The osteoma is most commonly found in young women and is of unknown cause. The tumour is considered to be a choristoma, although it has not been fully established whether it is congenital. An osteoma consists of compact bone lying in the choroid. The intratrabecular spaces are filled with loose connective tissue containing blood vessels. Some vascular tufts may extend outside the tumour mass and lie external to Bruch's membrane. These tufts must be differentiated from choroidal new vessels, a possible sight threatening complication of choroidal osteomas.

On infrared angiography an early hypofluorescence, corresponding to the osteoma is observed. In the middle phase the hypofluorescent zone is smaller than in the early phase and rather corresponds to the yellow-white zone of the tumour. Abnormal choroidal vessels may be seen, which leak ICG dye. On late phases variable areas of hypo- and hyperfluorescence are observed. The areas of late hypofluorescence may be larger than that of early hypofluorescence, suggesting either absent or hypoperfused choriocapillaris as a secondary effect of the osteoma. Infrared angiography highlights the superficial vascular structure of the tumour. Hyperfluorescent dots can sometimes be seen most probably corresponding to vessels in compact bone. They are present in the yellow-white portion of the lesion and not in the yellow-orange part. Although one of the three cases studied here, presented subretinal haemorrhages, suggestive of subretinal new vessels, a clear network of choroidal neovascularization could not be identified with fluorescein angiography or with ICG angiography.

Infrared angiography is of limited value in determining the extent of the

G. Coscas and F. Cardillo Piccolino (eds.), Retinal Pigment Epithelium and Macular Diseases, pp. 203–204.
© *1998 Kluwer Academic Publishers.*

osteoma but provides some more information on the vascular component of the tumour.

A full report of this presentation has been submitted to *von Graefe's Archives for Clinical and Experimental Ophthalmology.*

Department of Ophthalmology
University Hospital
Ghent, Belgium

32. Indocyanine green angiography of choroidal naevi and suspected melanomas

E. ZINICOLA, F. CARDILLO PICCOLINO, L. BORGIA and
S. TORRIELLI

(Genoa, Italy)

Introduction

Current diagnosis of pigmented choroidal tumours is based on ophthalmo-scopic evaluation, on standard fluorescein angiography and standardized A-scan echography[1,2]. Modern indocyanine green (ICG) angiography using high resolution digital imaging procedures, has to a great extent overcome the limits of fluorescein angiography in imaging of the choroidal vasculature[3-7].

The purpose of our study was to evaluate the utility of ICG angiography in the clinical assessment of choroidal naevi and suspected melanomas.

Patients and methods

Twenty-six consecutive patients with choroidal naevi or suspected melanomas underwent ultrasonography, colour fundus photography, fluorescein angiography and indocyanine green angiography. For inclusion in the study lesions had to be larger than 2 disc diameters and less than 2 mm thick. Lesions were classified as suspected melanomas on the basis of the ultrasonographic findings and presence of orange pigment and/or serous retinal detachement.

Each patient underwent digital fluorescein and ICG videoangiography utilizing the Topcon IMAGEnet H1024 Digital Imaging System (Ijssel, The Nederlands).

Eighteen patients were re-examined every 6 months with a follow-up period of 6–26 months (mean 13 months).

Results

Better evidence and delineation of tumours was obtained with ICG angiography than with fluorescein angiography and fundus photography. The lesions appeared very dark and had well defined borders on the ICG angiogram in early, middle and late phases. Intrinsic vascularization of the tumour was not seen in any case.

G. Coscas and F. Cardillo Piccolino (eds.), Retinal Pigment Epithelium and Macular Diseases, pp. 205–207.
© 1998 Kluwer Academic Publishers.

In three cases the middle-late phase of ICG angiography revealed an area of choroidal leakage adjacent to the lesion, attributable to hyperpermeability of the choriocapillaris.

During the follow-up period, ultrasonography showed no significant changes in the thickness of the tumour in any of the cases, while ICG angiography revealed enlargement of the lesion in three patients. Variations of the extension of the tumour were much more evident by comparing the ICG angiograms than evaluating the photographic and fluorescein angiographic records (Fig. 1).

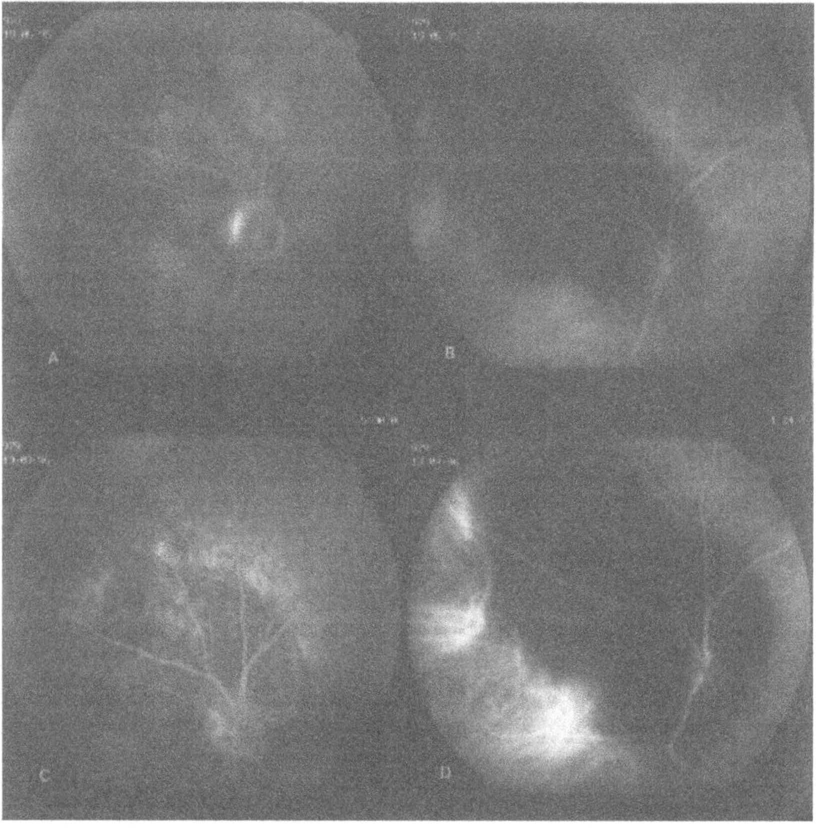

Fig. 1. (a,b) Fluorescein and ICG photographs of a suspected choroidal melanoma. (c,d) The same case 6 months later. The enlargement of the pigmented lesion is well documented by the ICG examination.

Conclusions

ICG angiography appears more reliable and accurate than fundus photography and fluorescein angiography in identifying and delineating choroidal naevi and suspected melanomas. Along with ultrasonography it seems to be useful in the follow-up evaluation of these lesions.

References

1. Mukai, S., Gragoudas, E.S. diagnosis of choroidal melanoma. In: Albert, D.M., Jacobiec, F.A. (eds) Principles and Practice of Ophthalmology. Vol. 5. Philadelphia: W.B. Saunders, 1994: 3209–3217.
2. Ossoing, K.C., Lohmeyer, M. Choroidal nevi: diagnosis with standardized echography. In: Sampaolesi, R. (ed) Ultrasonography in Ophthalmology. Dordrecht: Kluwer Academic Publishers, 1990: 173–180.
3. Scheider, A. Schroedel, C. High resolution indocyanine green angiography with scanning laser ophthalmoscope. Am J Ophthalmol. 1989; 108: 458–459.
4. Yannuzzi, L.A., Slakter, J.S., Sorenson, J.A., Guyer, D.R., Orlock, D.A. Digital indocyanine green videoangiography and choroidal neovascularization. Retina. 1992; 12: 191–223.
5. Cardillo Piccolino, F., Borgia, L., Zingirian, M. Indocyanine green choroidal videoangiography during induced intraocular hypertension. Am J Ophthalmol. 1993; 115: 817–818.
6. Cardillo Piccolino, F., Borgia, L., Zinicola, E., Zingirian, M. Indocyanine green angiographyc findings in central serous chorioretinopathy. Eye. 1995; 9: 324–332.
7. Cardillo Piccolino, F., Borgia, L., Zinicola, E. Indocyanine green angiography of circumscribed choroidal hemangiomas. Retina. 1996; 16: 19–28.

Clinica Oculistica dell'Università di Genova
Ospedale S. Martino, Pad. 9
Piazzale Rosanna Benzi
16136 Genova (Italy)

33. An anomalous case of angioid streaks and multiple and recurrent detachments of retinal pigment epithelium

M. MARULLO, A. SCUPOLA, G. SIMI, V. DE IORIO and
E. BALESTRAZZI

(L'Aquila, Italy)

Introduction

Angioid streaks (AS) are typical lesions of the ocular fundus produced by linear breaks of Bruch's membrane[1]. Generally, patients affected by AS are asymptomatic for many years. A sudden decrease of visual acuity can be caused by choroidal breaks due to mild bulbar contusions[2], retinal haemorrhages due to mild bulbar trauma[3], AS extended to the foveal area[4] or growth of the choroidal neovascular membrane (CNVM)[5] The growth of new subretinal vessels is the most frequent complication[6] and it is usually restricted to the posterior pole, where it may appear as a serous or haemorrhagic detachment of the retinal pigment epithelium (RPE)[7,8]. A clinical case of AS complicated by multiple, recurrent choroidal neovascular membrane (CNVM) and by RPE detachment localized mostly in the peripheral area is reported, as far as we know, similar cases have not been described in literature.

Case report

A 61-year old white man presented with a loss of visual acuity in both eyes in October 1989. Familial clinical history was negative for chorioretinal pathologies. Medical history revealed bronchial asthma, ostheoarthrosis of knees and of proximal interphalangis joints. Systemic arterial pressure was normal. The patient was not taking anticoagulant or antiaggregating drugs. Best visual acuity was 20/32 in both eyes and intraocular pressure was normal.

Ocular fundus examination of the right eye revealed AS extending peripherally and joined in a ring around the optic disc and a fibro-atrophic scar with irregular edges in the posterior pole. In the peripheral zone, a serous-haemorrhagic detachment of the RPE of almost $1\frac{1}{2}$ optic disc diameters, was localized at 4 o'clock (Fig. 1). In the left eye, besides the presence of AS, there was also a large fibro-atrophic scar involving most of the posterior pole and estending nasally to the optic disc. Examination of the retinal peripheral area revealed two serous-haemorrhagic RPE detachments at 1 and 6 o'clock respectively and a large area of RPE dystrophy in the nasal sector (Fig. 2).

G. Coscas and F. Cardillo Piccolino (eds.), Retinal Pigment Epithelium and Macular Diseases, pp. 209–218.
© *1998 Kluwer Academic Publishers.*

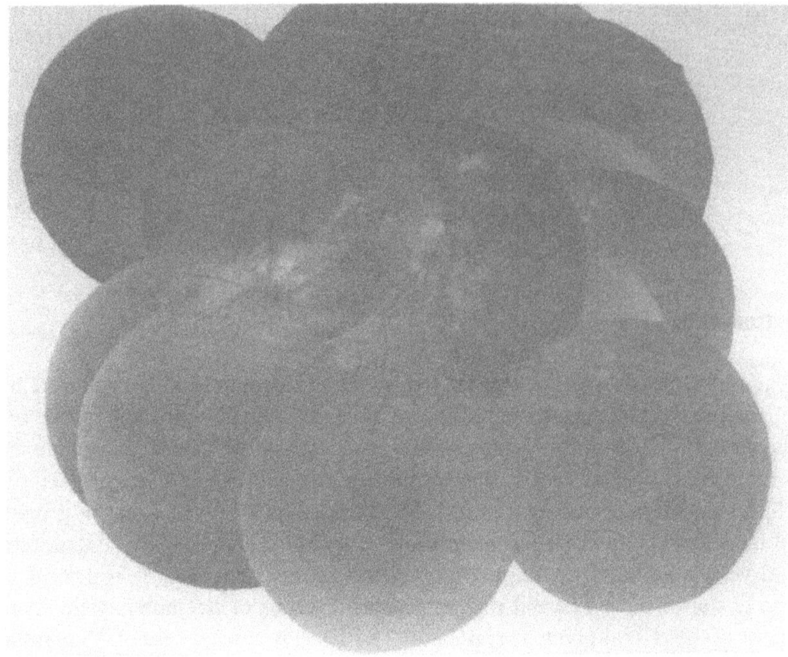

Fig. 1. Ophthalmoscopic findings, right eye. AS extended to the medium periphery. Atrophic scars with irregular edge at the posterior pole. In peripheral area there is a serous haemorrhagic detachment of RPE at 4 o'clock.

Fluorescein angiography confirmed the ophthalmoscopic findings in both eyes. Moreover in the optic disc temporally to the macula, typical 'leopard-like spots' indicated the site of a previous haemorrhage (Fig. 3). In the left eye small hyperfluorescent spots inside the RPE detachments proved the vascular origin of two peripheral RPE detachments localized in the superior and inferior areas (Fig. 4).

The patient refused laser treatment of the CNVM. General physical examination excluded AS-associated diseases such as pseudoxanthoma elasticum, sickle cell anaemia or Paget's disease of bone. Results of laboratory investigations, including blood coagulation, chest X-ray and antibody titers for common microrganisms causing choroiditis were normal.

In June 1991 visual acuity was unchanged. Fluorescein angiography of the right eye disclosed a new neovascular membrane in the peripheral temporal area and a serous RPE dethacment in the nasal area of the retinal periphery (Fig. 5). In the left eye, a round hyperfluorescence indicating atrophy secondary to the RPE detachment in the peripheral nasal area and new CNVM in the inferior and temporal peripheral areas were found (Fig. 6).

In September 1993, although visual acuity was still unchanged, a worsening

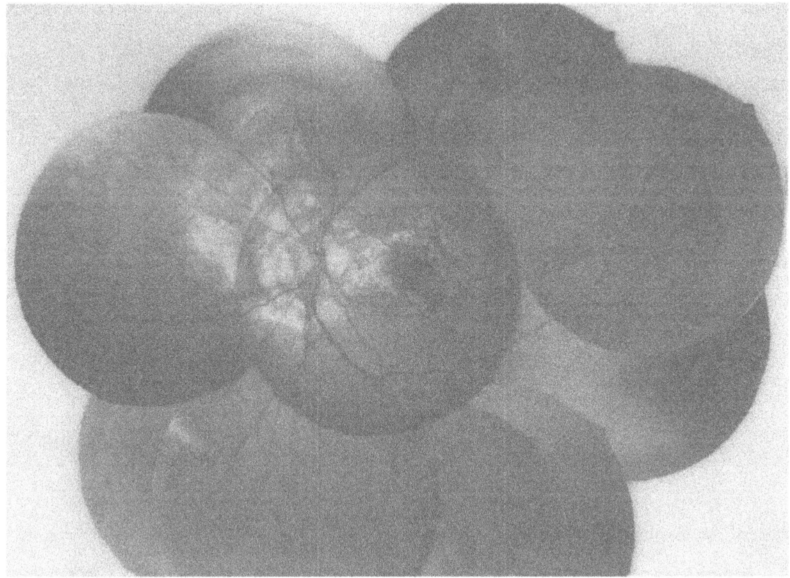

Fig. 2. Ophthalmoscopic findings, left eye. AS joint in a peripapillar ring. Atrophic scar with irregular edge interests a large part of the posterior pole, with juxtamacular pigment accumulation. In the periphery two small serous-haemorrhagic RPE detachments are visible at 1 and 6 o'clock.

of the ophthalmoscopic findings was confirmed in both eyes by fluorescein angiography. While the CNVM in the periphery of the right eye showed complete regression with dystrophic alterations, CNVM increased in the posterior pole (Fig. 7). In the left eye a large hypofluorescent area due to a subretinal haemorrhage could be seen in the temporal area of the posterior pole, probably due to bleeding of a subretinal neovascularization. It was possible to observe a large number of other CNVM not only in the nasal area of the optic disc but also in the periphery (Fig. 8). At the last examination, in August 1995, neither the retroequatorial ophthalmoscopic findings nor visual acuity were unchanged in the right eye (20/32), while in the extreme periphery a large number of small detachments of the RPE and new CNVM were evident (Fig. 9). Visual acuity was reduced to 20/200 in the left eye because of the development of new neovascular membranes at the interpapillo-macular tract. Moreover a large RPE serous detachment in the superior temporal area of the left eye and new numerous CNVM appeared in the peripheral area (Fig. 10).

Discussion

Fibrovascular tissue growth through the breaks of Bruch's membrane is very common in patients affected by AS, with a frequency ranging from 42 to

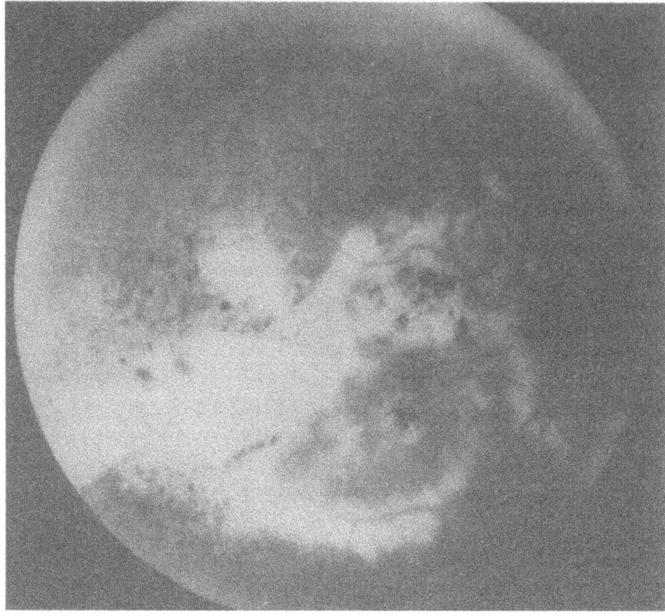

Fig. 3. Fluorangiographic findings, right eye. Typical 'leopard-like spots' in the temporal part of the posterior pole indicating the site of a previous haemorrhage.

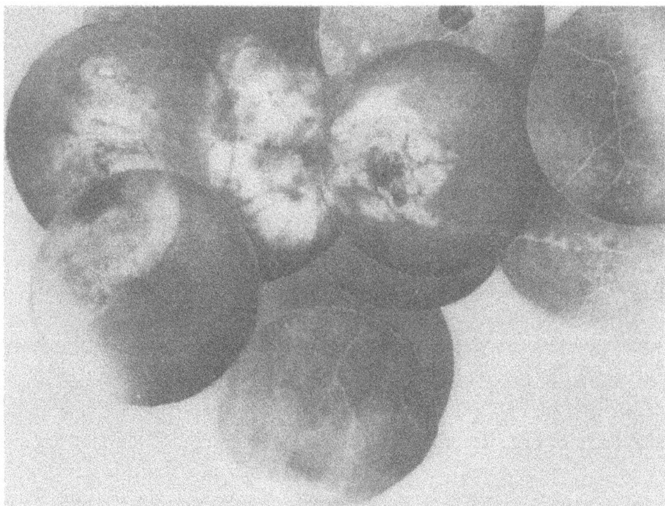

Fig. 4. Fluorangiographic findings, left eye. Small hyperfluorescent spots inside the RPE haemorrhagic detachment, indicating its vascular origin. Multiple phenomena of neovascularization associated with RPE dystrophic effects are evident due to a probable previous detachment.

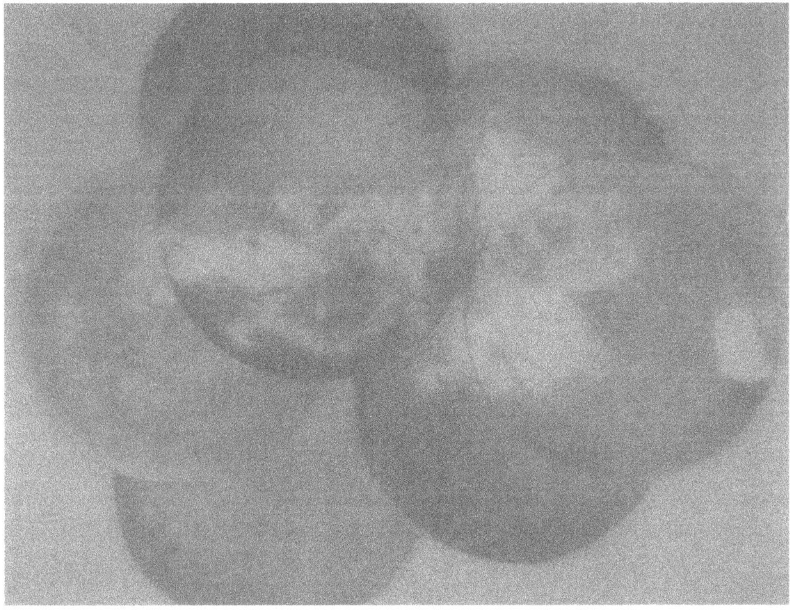

Fig. 5.   Fluorangiographic findings, right eye. Presence of CNVM at 9 o'clock and of a new RPE serous detachment at 4 o'clock.

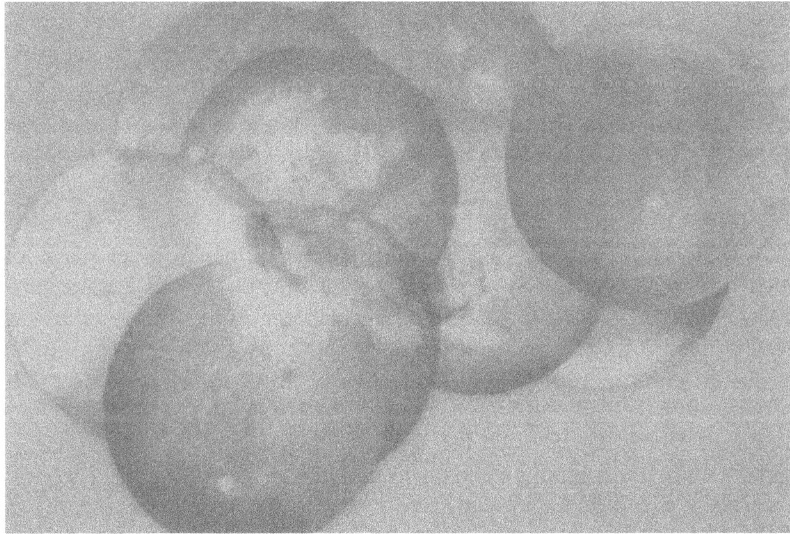

Fig. 6.   Fluorangiographic findings, left eye. The situation indicates no changes compared with the previous control in the peripherical sectors. New CNVM phenomena are evident.

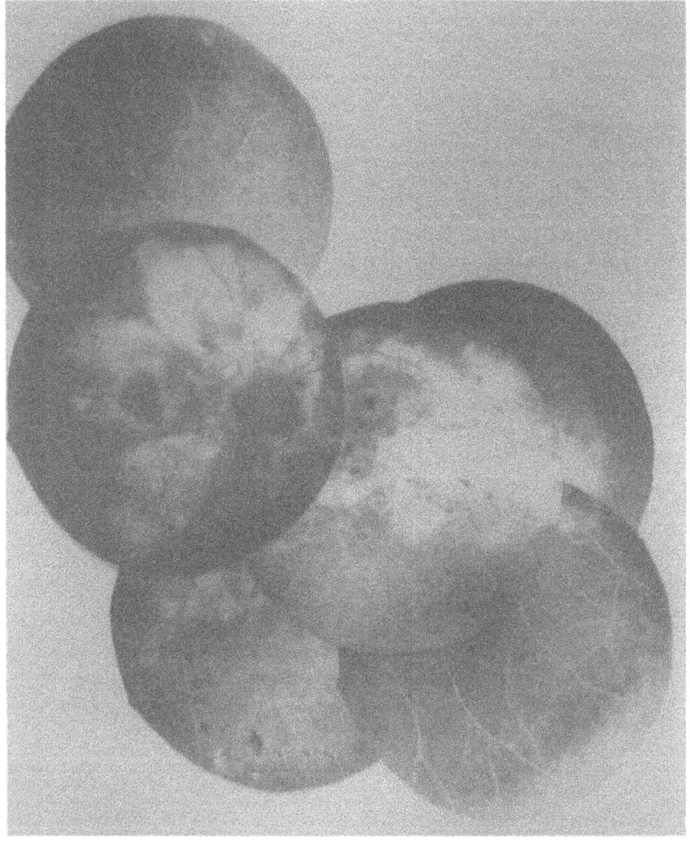

Fig. 7. Fluorangiographic findings, right eye. The previously described neovascularization, after 2 years, shows a total regression with the appearance of dystrophic alteration. At the posterior pole new CNVM are evident.

80%[6,8]. The CNVM are localized at the margins of the AS, especially in the interpapillo-macular tract where they can cause serous/serous-haemorrhagic detachments of the RPE or neuroepithelium, or both. These lesions are responsible for the abrupt reduction in visual acuity and for the appearance of the metamorphopsia[8]. The phenomenon of neovascularization occurs by proliferation, through the fracture lines in Bruch's membrane, of one or more endothelial buds which reach the subepithelial space where they proliferate and mature, transforming themselves into capillaries[9,10]. The progressive increase in blood flow is responsible for the exudation which causes for the RPE detachment, which may be serous or haemorrhagic in case of vessel rupture[11]. These haemorrhages can occur either spontaneously or may follow mild trauma[11].

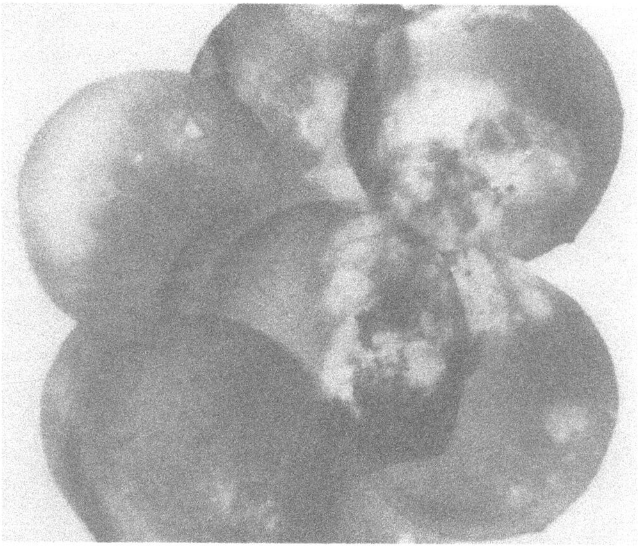

Fig. 8.   Fluorangiographic findings, left eye. Not only nasal to the optic disc, but also in the extreme periphery, a large number of small hyperfluorescence areas with leakage of fluorescein due to neovascularization phenomena are visible.

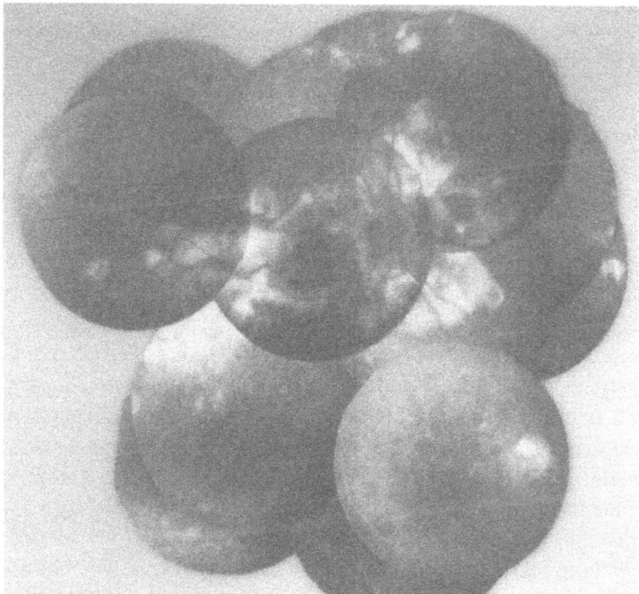

Fig. 9.   Fluorangiographic findings, right eye. In the extreme periphery a large number of small RPE dethachments and CNVM are evident.

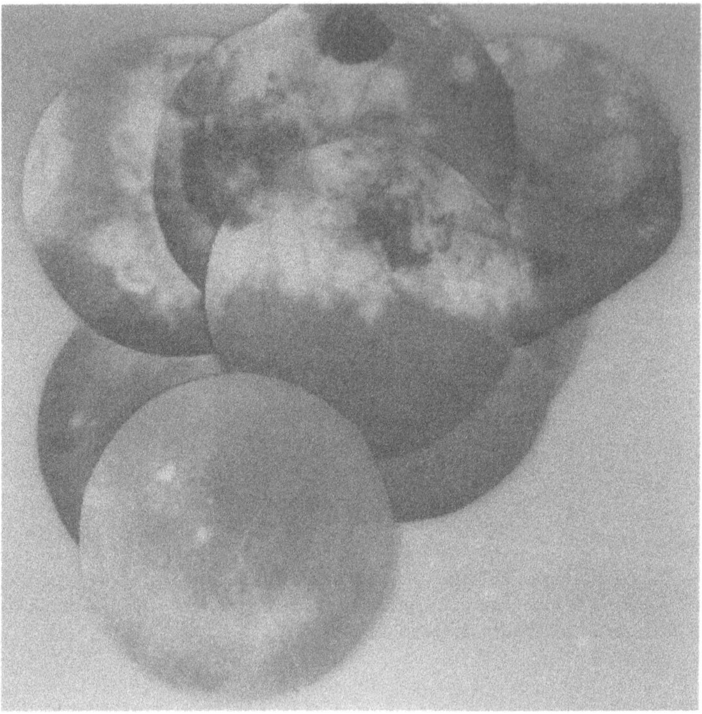

Fig. 10. Fluorangiographic findings, left eye. Development of new neovascular membranes at the posterior pole.In the superior temporal sector a large RPE serous detachment has appeared.

Bruch's membrane is merely a mechanical barrier to the free advancement of newly formed vessels from the choriocapillaris. The interruptions in Bruch's membrane, which are present in AS retinopathy, therefore favour, but do not themselves determine subretinal neovascularization. Histopathological studies have demonstrated that vessel formation can occur even in the absence of break points in Bruch's membrane[12–14]. The endothelial buds are capable of producing certain metalloproteases and collagenases which are responsible for connective tissue degradation[15]. Moreover, Glaser[16] has shown that RPE cells *in vitro* release a factor which inhibits the growth of newly formed vessels; alterations in the RPE reduce the production of this inhibitory growth factor, hence favouring the growth of new vessels. The vasoformative process is a complex and not yet understood phenomenon, and many factors modulate neovascular growth[17].

The clinical case described is undoubtedly an awkward case of AS, the most surprising features being the diffuse proliferation of new vascular membranes along with the multiple and recurrent detachments of the RPE localized for the most part peripherally. In this case it is possible that the CNVM, the RPE detachments and AS may, or may not be, independent phenomena.

Ultrastructural alterations of Bruch's membrane could explain the peripheral CNVM and the RPE detachments in areas where AS are not evident. It is possible that the vasoformative process was favoured by the presence of microruptures not evident at ophthalmoscopic and fluorangiographic examinations. The possible co-existence of AS and age-correlated peripheral degeneration could be suggested as a pathogenetic hypothesis[18,19].

Foos and Trese[13] found vascular diseases, diabetes mellitus and ictus cerebri to be associated to the formation of new peripheral vessels. Dalaney[20] has studied patients affected by peripheral haemorrhagic RPE detachments in whom age-correlated macular degeneration was often also seen.

In conclusion, this case could represent a new clinical entity or an unusual variant of AS. Certainly it is strange that no similar cases have been reported.

References

1. Giuffrè, G. Stries angioides et lèsions associèes: Interpretation ophthalmoscopique et à l'angiographie fluorescèinique. J Fr Ophthalmol. 1986; 9: 811–824.
2. Grand, M.G., Isserman, M.J., Miller, C.W. Angioid streaks associated with pseudoxantoma elasticum in a 13 years old patient. Ophthalmology. 1987; 94: 197–200.
3. Shilling, J.S., Blach, R.K. Prognosis and therapy of angioid streaks. Trans Ophthal Soc UK. 1975; 95: 301–306.
4. Schivo, G., Battaglia Parodi, M., Orione, C. et al. La retinopatia a strie angioidi: complicanze e trattamento. Boll Ocul. 1989; 68: suppl. 4: 425–427.
5. Gass, J.D.M. Stereoscopic Atlas of Macular Disease. Edn. 3a, St. Louis: C.V. Mosby Co., 1987: 102–109.
6. Piro, P.A., Scheraga, D., Fine, S.L. Angioid streaks: natural history and visual prognosis. In Fine, S.L., Owens, S.L.(eds) Management of Retinal Vascular and Macular Disorders. Baltimore: Williams and Wilkins, 1983: 136–139.
7. Zografos, L., Chamero, J. Evolution au cours des ruptures indirectes traumatiques de la choroide. J Fr Ophthalmol. 1990; 13: 269–275.
8. Clarkson, J.G., Altman, R.D. Angioid streaks. Surv Ophthalmol. 1982; 26: 235–246.
9. Gass, J.D.M. Serous retinal pigment epithelial detachment with a noch: a sign of occult choroidal neovascularization. Retina. 1984; 4: 205–220.
10. Green, W.R., McDonnel, P.J., Yeo, J.H. Pathologic features of senile macular degeneration. Ophthalmology. 985; 92: 615–627.
11. MacCumber, M.W., Dastgheib, K., Bressler, N.M. et al. Clinicopathologic correlation of the multiple recurrent serosanguineous retinal pigment epithelial detachments syndrome. Retina. 1994; 14: 143–152.
12. Sarks, S.H. New vessel formation beneath the retinal pigment epithelium in senile eyes. Br J Ophthalmol. 1973; 57: 951–965.
13. Foos, R.Y., Trese, M.T. Chorioretinal juncture; vascularization of Bruch's membrane in peripheral fundus. Arch Ophthalmol. 1982; 100: 1492–1503.
14. Heriot, W.J., Henkind, P., Bellhorn, R.W., Burns, M.S. Choroidal neovascularization can digest Bruch's membrane. Ophthalmology. 1984; 91: 1603–1607.
15. Rifkin, D.B., Gross, J.L., Moscatelli, D. et al. In Nossel, H.L., Vogel, H.J. (eds) Pathology of the Endothelial cell. New York: Academic Press. 1982: 191–197.
16. Glaser, W.R., Campochiaro, P.A., Davis, J.L. et al. Retinal pigment epithelial cells release an inhibitor of neovascularization. Arch Ophthalmol. 1985; 103: 1870–1875.
17. Jampol, L.M., Acheson, R., Eagle, R.C. et al. calcification of Bruch's membrane in angioid streaks with homozygous sickle cell disease. Arch Ophthalmol. 1987; 105: 93–98.

18. Hagedoorn, A. Angioid streaks. Arch Ophthalmol. 1939; 21: 746–774; 935–965.
19. Coleman, K., Ross, M.H., McCabe, M., Coleman, R., Mooney, D. Disk drusen and angioid streaks in pseudoxanthoma elasticum. Am J Ophthalmol. 1991; 112: 166–170.
20. Dalaney, W.V., Torrisi, P.F., Hampton, G.R. Hemorrhagic peripheral pigment epithelial disease. Arch Ophthalmol. 1988; 106: 646–650.

Viale Nizza, 5
67100 L'Aquila
Italy

34. Conservative treatment of choroidal melanomas of the posterior pole

C. MOSCI, A. POLIZZI and L. RAVAZZONI

(Genoa, Italy)

Introduction

Conservative treatment of ocular melanoma is used whenever possible. The Genoa ocular oncology study group (GOOSG) treated small and medium choroidal melanomas (thickness < 5 mm) with ruthenium plaque, except for tumours located near the optic disc. These and medium-large melanomas were treated with proton beam irradiation. We evelueted the results of such conservative treatment for choroidal melanomas of the posterior pole.

Methods

During the period January 1991–January 1996, 75 cases of choroidal melanoma were studied by the Genoa Study Group, of which 25 cases were located at the posterior pole or touching the optic disc. One patient refused treatment and one is under observation. All patients but one underwent conservative therapy. The present study considered cases with a follow-up longer than 6 months.

Results

The study took into consideration 17 patients, three of whom were treated with ruthenium plaque and 14 with proton beam. All but one had a reduction in visual acuity. Tumour thickness reduction (measured by standard ecography) was achieved in all patients. The most relevant complication appeared to be optical atrophy and actinic retinopathy.

Conclusion

Conservative management of choroidal melanomas has become very important in recent years following the encoranging pioneering work of Gragoudas[1] and Lommatzsch[2]. Zografos[3] showed that the mortality rate with cobalt 60

G. Coscas and F. Cardillo Piccolino (eds.), Retinal Pigment Epithelium and Macular Diseases, pp. 219–220.
© *1998 Kluwer Academic Publishers.*

therapy was 7% at 5 years and 12% at 10 years after treatment while with the proton beam it was 11% 5 years after treatment. These findings were similar to those observed by Gragoudas[1]. Therapy using Ru plaques gave a mortality curve equal to that for Co60[2]. The preliminary resuts of the Genoa study group are in accord with these authors[4]. The results obtained in this study are interesting; however, a longer follow-up and more cases are needed. We suggest that for tumours located at the posterior pole conservative treatment is the best choice, unless the tumour is large.

References

1. Gragoudas, E.S., Seddon, J.M., Egan, K.M. et al. Metastasis from uveal melanoma after proton beam irradiation. Ophthalmology. 1988; 95: 992–999.
2. Lommatzsch, P.K., Kirsch, I.H. 106 Ru/106 Rh plaque radioterapy for malignant melanomas of the choroid. Doc Ophthalmol. 1988; 68: 225–238.
3. Zografos, L., Bercher, L., Egger, E., Chamot, L., Uffer, S., Gailloud, C. Surviving rate of patients with choroidal melanomas treated by proton beam irradiation and cobalt 60 applicators. Atti Int Symposium on Intraocular Tumors 1990; 1991: 247–251.
4. Mosci, C., Ravazzoni, L., Polizzi, A. et al. Conservative treatment of uveal melanoma: preliminary reports. In: Frenzzotti, R., Balestrazzi, E., Falco, L., Esente, S. (eds.) International Symposium on Intraocular and Epibulbar Tumors, Florence, Italy, March 3–5, 1994. Bologna: Monduzzi, 1994, 117–120.

35. Assessment of the sympatho-vagal interaction in central serous chorioretinopathy measured by power spectral analysis of heart rate variability

P. BERNASCONI, E. MESSMER, A. BERNASCONI and A. THÖLEN

(Zurich, Switzerland)

Purpose

It has been postulated that patients with central serous chorioretinopathy (CSCR) frequently have Tape A behaviour with increased catecholamine release. Therefore modulation of the central nervous system may be of value in the treatment of CSCR. The purpose of this study was to measure the activity of the sympathetic nervous system in patients with CSCR by a power spectral analysis (PSA) of heart rate (RR interval) variability. PSA is a suitable non-invasive method to reflect the balance of sympatho-vagal interactions and is already used in the assessment of the autonomic nervous system in various diseases, including essential hypertension, diabetic neuropathy and cardiovascular diseases.

Methods

According to history and the results of the fluorescein angiography we divided the patients with CSCR into four groups: group 1 (n = 8) with acute CSCR (Fig. 1), group 2 ($n = 7$) with acute recurrent CSCR (Fig. 2), group 3 ($n = 2$)

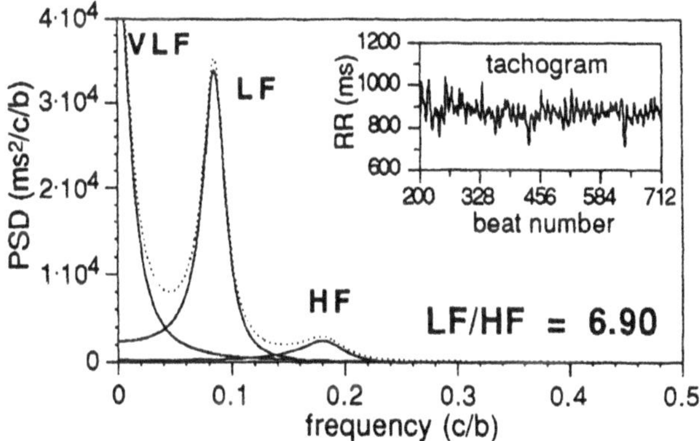

Fig. 1. Acute CSCR.

G. Coscas and F. Cardillo Piccolino (eds.), Retinal Pigment Epithelium and Macular Diseases, pp. 221–224.
© *1998 Kluwer Academic Publishers.*

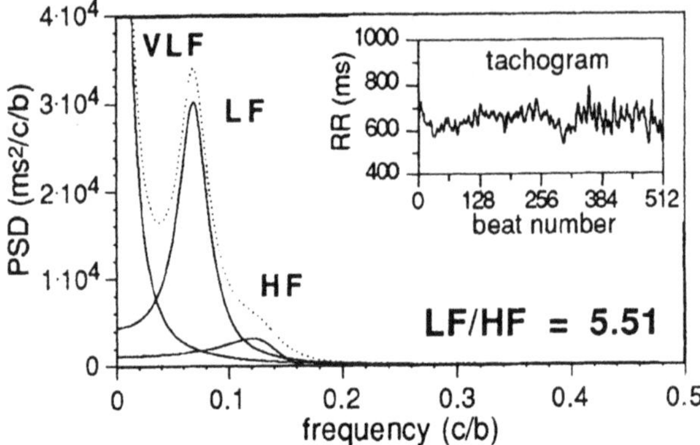

Fig. 2. Acute recurrent CSCR.

with chronic persistent CSCR (Fig. 3) and group 4 ($n = 7$) after CSCR (Fig. 4). Thus we obtained RR interval measurement data for 24 patients (23 men and 1 woman), with an average age of 44 years (range: 32–52). These data were compared with the data of 15 healthy volunteers (Fig. 5) of the same age. Variability of the RR interval can be seen by plotting RR as a function of the beat number, a representation which is usually defined as the tachogram. To obtain more information about heart rate fluctuations the data can be quantified and displayed by using the spectral analysis. Off-line analysis was performed with an autoregressive method (maximum entropy method) with a Macintosh program (proBeat, Switzerland). The resulting ratio of low frequency component (LF) and high frequency component (HF) of the power spectrum serves as a measure of sympathetic-vagal balance with LF representing mainly sympathetic activity and HF representing vagal activity.

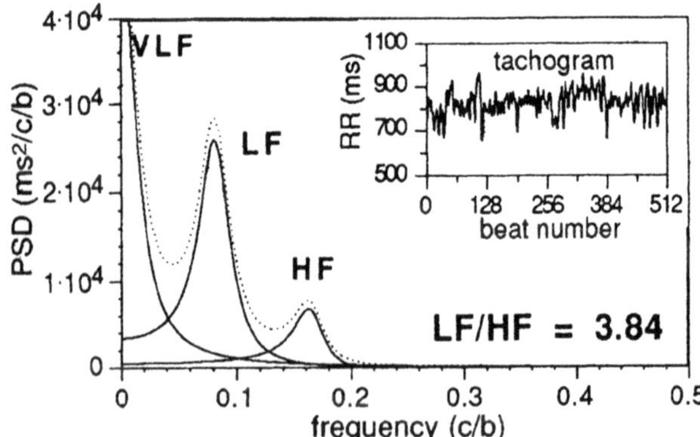

Fig. 3. Chronic persistent CSCR.

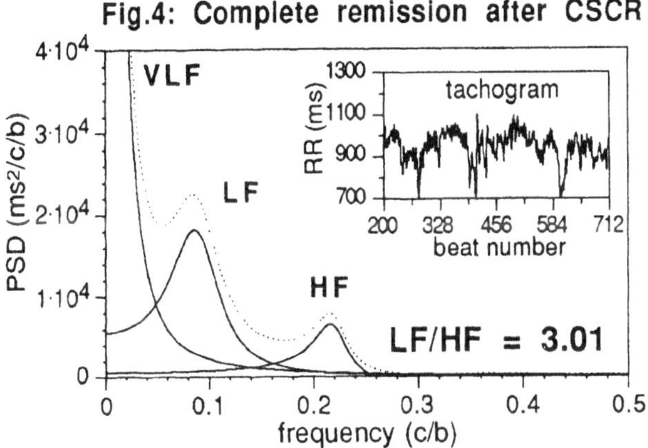

Fig. 4. Complete remission after CSCR.

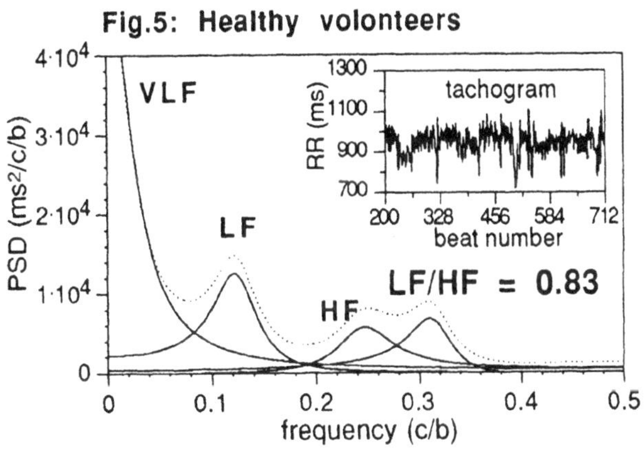

Fig. 5. Healthy volunteers.

Results

When comparing the LF/HF ratios of CSCR patients with normal controls (LF/HF ratio of 1.1) significant differences were found for all but one subgroup (Fig. 6): group 1: LF/HF ratio of 5.5 ($p < 0.01$), group 2: LF/HF ratio of 5.4 ($p < 0.05$), group 3: LF/HF ratio of 4.2 ($p < 0.1$) and group 4: LF/HF ratio of 3.0 ($p < 0.05$). Significant differences ($p < 0.05$) were also found between active CSCR (groups 1 and 2) and inactive CSCR (group 4).

Conclusions

These results support the view that the pathogenesis of CSCR related to an increased sympathetic activity of the autonomic nervous system. Furthermore

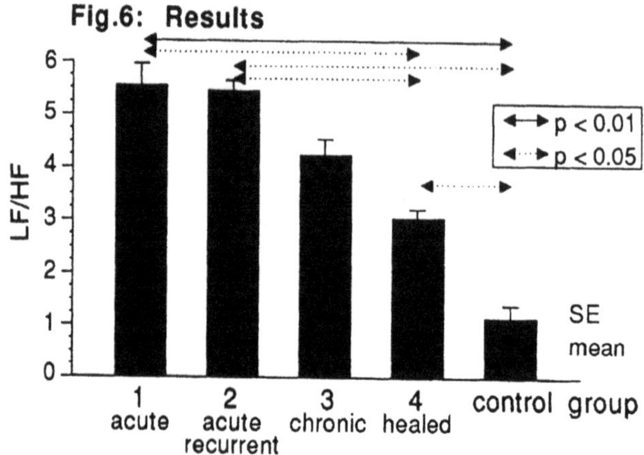

Fig. 6. Results.

the LF/HF ratios correlate well with the activity of the disease. PSA may be useful in assessing the changes of sympathetic activity in acute and chronic CSCR, yielding additional information for a rational therapy, such as β-blockade.

University Eye Clinic
University of Zürich Medical School
Switzerland

36. Central serous chorioretinopathy: an endocrine screening

R. NUZZI, A. CERRUTI and L. VLACHOS

(Turin, Italy)

Introduction

Central serous chorioretinopathy (CSC) is a serous detachment of the retinal neuroepithelium, whose aetiopathogenesis has not yet been completely clarified. In an attempt to identify possible causal factors, we carried out an endocrine screening in 16 patients with clinically and fluoroangiographically demonstrated CSC. The aim of the research was to evaluate links between laboratory parameters of and two peculiar aspects of CSC, widely confirmed in literature: the prevalence in male subjects and the role played by 'stress'. We measured blood concentrations of reproductive hormones and the ACTH-cortisol axis, and plasma and urinary concentrations of catecholamines.

Materials and methods

We studied 16 male patients, aged 27–51 years (mean age 36.1 years), suffering from CSC in its active phase. This was evident both at the ophthalmoscopic examination, as serous oedema at the posterior pole, and at fluoro-angiographic examination, where at least one leakage point was observed. Fourteen cases were unilateral and two bilateral. Eleven patients were in the first episode of illness, three were in their first relapse state, one was in his fourth episode of active CSC and one was in his fifth.

The history included data about their dietary habits (i.e. if they smoked or/and drank beverages like coffee or tea) and the presence of systemic diseases, with particular attention to those in which 'stress' may be a factor. We also sought information regarding whether the subjects had gone through emotional trauma during the previous two months.

We noted the duration of the symptoms from the onset until the moment of the examination.

The laboratory parameters measured are given in Table 1.

The blood samples were collected between 7 and 9 a.m.

The range of analytical sensitivity, the intra-assay and inter-assay variability and reference values (normal range) for normal subjects were validated by a

G. Coscas and F. Cardillo Piccolino (eds.), Retinal Pigment Epithelium and Macular Diseases, pp. 225–232.
© 1998 Kluwer Academic Publishers.

Table 1. Laboratory parameters measured.

---

1. Reproductive hormones (plasma levels)
    Follicle stimulating hormone (FSH; enzyme immunoassay, EIA);
    Luteinizing hormone (LH; EIA);
    Prolactin (immunoradiometric assay; RIA);
    Testosterone (RIA);
    Dehydroepiandrosterone solphate (DHEAS; RIA);
    β-Oestradiol (RIA)
2. ACTH-cortisol axis (plasma levels)
    Andrenocorticotrope hormone (ACTH; RIA);
    Cortisol (RIA);
3. Adrenomedullary-sympathetic system (plasma and urinary levels)
    Plasma catecholamines (including epinephrine, norepinephrine and dopamine;
        high perormance liquid chromatography, HPLC)
    Urinary catecholamines (including epinephrine, norepinephrine and dopamine; HPLC)

---

control group of age- and sex-matched subjects submitted to the same laboratory tests and methodology by our clinic laboratory. The control group was composed of 20 men whose mean age corresponded well (36.3 years, standard deviation 3.10).

Neither local nor systemic therapy was carried out until the samples were collected. All patients were informed of the research aim and methods and each gave their consent.

Results

Table 2 shows the clinical parameters at the time of examination. Twelve patients reported they had always had good health, while two reported systemic hypertension, one gastritis and one both of these diseases. All patients reported emotional trauma during the 2 months before the examination took place and where signs of illness were revealed.

Table 3 shows the results concerning plasmatic and urinary levels of catecholamines. The plasma values were above the normal range in 56.3% of the cases (nine patients; 378–1190 pg/ml, mean 603 pg/ml), and normal in 43.7% (seven patients). No specific link with dietary habits was noted. Both patients with bilateral disease had abnormal catecholamine levels. Urinary catecholamine levels were all in the normal range.

Table 4 shows the plasma levels of prolactin and hormones of the pituitary-gonadal axis: all were in normal range. Table 5 shows the plasma levels of ACTH and cortisol: all values were in the normal range.

Discussion

Plasma catecholamine levels in these patients were interesting, as they were above the highest normal value in 56.3% of the cases. In these patients, the

Table 2. Clinical parameters.

Patient	Age (years)	Episode of illness	Mono or bilaterality	Smoke (cigarettes per day)	Systemic pathological history	Duration of ocular symptoms (weeks)
R.S.	43	I	Monolateral	0	Stress	4
M.M.	35	I	Monolateral	0	Stress	20
B.M.	30	II	Monolateral	> 20	Stress	3
C.G.	31	I	Monolateral	0	Stress	1
B.G.	38	IV	Monolateral	< 5	Stress	4
S.P.	27	II	Monolateral	> 20	Stress, gastritis	2
M.E.	39	I	Monolateral	0	Stress	1
B.A.	40	I	Monolateral	0	Stress	3
I.S.	41	V	Monolateral	10–20	Stress	2
S.A.	31	II	Monolateral	> 20	Stress	8
B.A.	27	I	Monolateral	< 5	Stress	3
Z.R.	37	I	Monolateral	< 5	Stress	1
P.S.	41	I	Monolateral	10–20	Stress	2
S.R.	27	I	Monolateral	0	Stress	3 days
S.L.	51	I	Bilateral	0	Stress, gastritis, hypertension	3 days
S.U.	39	I	Bilateral	0	Stress, hypertension	2

Table 3. Plasma and urinary catecholamine levels.

Patient	Plasma catecholamines (pg/ml)	Urinary catecholamines (μg/24 h)
R.S.	1190	31
M.M.	535	28
B.M.	380	29
C.G.	553	53
B.G.	540	18
S.P.	490	30
M.E.	378	22
B.A.	221	29
I.S.	224	27
S.A.	230	36
B.A.	185	26
Z.R.	157	47
P.S.	167	30
S.R.	175	20
S.L.	714	34
S.U.	650	24

illness began between 3 days and 5 months before our examination, and
plasma values appeared independent from duration of illness and whether it
was the first episode or a relapse. Urinary catecholamine levels were, however,

Table 4. Plasma levels of reproductive hormones.

Patient	Follicle stimulating hormone (mUI/ml)	Luteinizing hormone (mUI/ml)	Prolactin (ng/ml)	Testosterone (ng/ml)	Dehydro-epiandro-sterone sulphate (μg/dl)	17-β-estradiol (pg/ml)
R.S.	6.0	4.0	15.0	5.5	350	24
M.M.	2.1	4.0	4.4	5.5	180	25
B.M.	2.0	2.5	6.2	4.2	180	20
C.G.	4.3	2.1	13.5	4.5	220	20
B.G.	4.5	2.1	8.5	3.6	100	15
S.P.	2.6	2.4	9.0	7.0	180	30
M.E.	4.3	2.0	2.0	5.5	207	21
B.A.	3.4	2.1	9.0	4.5	182	24
I.S.	2.2	2.6	10.2	3.6	100	20
S.A.	2.4	2.2	10.1	3.9	158	20
B.A.	3.2	4.1	9.8	4.3	202	30
Z.R.	4.5	5.1	4.6	5.2	161	16
P.S.	5.3	2.0	9.8	4.5	230	30
S.R.	2.6	2.8	9.2	4.7	325	30
S.L.	5.1	2.4	2.2	5.5	100	15
S.U.	6.3	4.3	4.6	6.8	198	18

Table 5. Plasma levels of ACTH and cortisol.

Patient	ACTH (pg/ml)	Cortisol (μg/dl)
R.S.	61	20.0
M.M.	34	16.8
B.M.	19	10.8
C.G.	59	15.0
B.G.	16	13.3
S.P.	33	20.0
M.E.	35	13.6
B.A.	12	16.2
I.S.	30	16.5
S.A.	25	15.8
B.A.	40	14.2
Z.R.	20	15.0
P.S.	40	19.6
S.R.	30	19.4
S.L.	33	8.0
S.U.	51	10.2

always normal, confirming their correct peripheral metabolism. The elevated plasma levels must, therefore, be due to increased release and not to reduced catabolism.

The episodic increase of plasmatic catecholamines may be considered as the expression of a particular sensitivity of the adrenomedullary-sympathetic system to different stimuli. It has to be stressed that the general adrenergic activity is higher during the morning and this could explain the frequency of the abnormal values we observed. If this hypothesis is true, these subjects may have an extreme adrenergic response to stress, which is known to be an important stimulus in CSC.

Stress causes neurovegetative repercussions mediated by the activity of limbic system and, especially of the locus ceruleus[1]. The limbic system comprises a group of neurological structures situated between diencephalon and telencephalon; it acts as an integration zone between the part of encephalon that is at the head of psychic elaboration (cerebral cortex) and that of emotional and vegetative activity (hypothalamus and thalamus). Thus, the limbic system, which is very complex in mammals and especially in human beings, integrates the instinctive and emotional reactions. The sympathetic system is controlled by these superior centres in order to get a subject in an emergency situation ready for fight or flight, through a high increase of plasmatic catecholamines[2].

Elevated catecholamine plasma levels provide laboratory confirmation of the hypothesis that, in many cases, CSC could be caused by emotional trauma in subjects who are particularly susceptible to it[3]. Indeed, it is likely that the subjects with abnormal values are those with Type A behaviour subjects, which Yannuzzi asserts to be 60% of CSC patients[4]. A funduscopic finding, very similar to CSC, was provoked in experimental animal models by the injection of epinephrine[5-11]. However, 43.7% of our patients with ophthalmoscopically and fluoroangiographically demonstrated CSC had normal plasma catecholamine levels. This group was also heterogeneous for the duration of the symptoms and the number of relapses.

This observation is likely to support a multifactorial hypothesis in the aetiopathogenesis of this disease. Nevertheless, it cannot be excluded that these patients, who reported emotional trauma in their recent past, may have had an adrenergic response. The onset and duration of the disease, which could have escaped our notice, may be attributed to this. Repeated evaluation in the same subject of plasma catecholamine levels would be very interesting, in order to relate them to the spontaneous evolution of the disease.

All other laboratory parameters were within the normal range. In particular, ACTH and cortisol levels are normal. A sample taken in the morning cannot be considered representative of the correct functioning of this axis, but simply gives an indication of gross alterations. For this reason, our data cannot exclude subtle functional modifications: these need to be investigated by dynamic tests, particularly by the evaluation of glucocorticoid release during the evening and the night. Previous publications report that corticosteroid hormones can be involved in the pathogenesis of the illness: cases of CSC have been reported in patients suffering from Cushing's disease or in patients under corticosteroid therapy for another illness[12-16]. Nevertheless, the supporting action of corticosteroid hormones towards the catecholamine action and their production is well known. Thus, in these patients, the situation of stress associated with a previous illness may have caused increased adrenergic production, supported by hypercortisolism. This gives rise to doubts about the use of corticosteroid therapy in this disease, even though we did not find hypercortisolism in our patients.

Pituitary-gonadal hormones were also in the normal range. It remains to be explained why CSC is an illness typical of adult males, a very unusual feature for a disease without any hereditary origin. Thus, screening in female subjects would be very interesting, even if they are extremely uncommon, as widely confirmed in literature[17,18]. A possible involvement of sexual hormones in the pathogenesis is supported by cases of CSC during pregnancy[19-22] and hyperprolactinemia[23].

In conclusion, catecholamines seem to play an important role in the pathogenesis of CSC, which is likely to be multifactorial.

The recent application of indocyanine green angiography has shifted the attention from pigment epithelium[24] to choroid, whose vascular flow seems to be modified during CSC. According to Scheider[25], the typical report is a reduced choroidal blood flow, while, according to Guyer *et al.*[26], it is increased. In both cases, injury to the pigment epithelium would be a consequence, and the neuroepithelial detachment would result from a compromised function of ionic channels of the external blood retinal barrier. The presence of β-receptors was demonstrated both in the choroid and in the pigment epithelium. In the choroid, adrenergic stimulation would provoke vasodilatation[27]; the effect on pigment epithelium is not so clear. According to Browning[28], it would increase its functionality, while, according to Colombati *et al.*[29], the β-adrenergic receptors activation would provoke the release of Ca^{2+}, reducing the pump activity of the pigment epithelium.

Further studies will be necessary to elucidate the role played by pigment epithelium, choroid and its innervation as to onset of CSC. As widely suggested by recent research, the adrenergic response seems to be important. In spite of this, the systemic therapy with β-blockers did not give univocal results: Browning[28] believes they are useless, while Avci *et al.*[30] reported that they are effective in shortening the duration of illness, even if they do not prevent relapses.

Prospective studies, concerning wider casuistry, should be carried out to evaluate the role of catecholamines in CSC and to determine why the eye is a target organ, especially in male adults. We are continuing to carry out a research to assess the efficacy of local α-blockers and β-blockers, free from side effects typical of the systemic ones.

References

1. Angeli, A., Masera, R.G., Orlandi, F., Terzolo, M. Sindromi da Eccesso di Glicocorticoidi. Rome: Luigi Pozzi Ed., 1994.
2. Covelli, I., Frati, L. Patologia Generale. Naples: Florio Ed., 1986: 982–983.

3. Rigal, K., Harrer, S., Titscher, G. Psycosomatic factors in the etiology of central serous retinopathy. Folia Ophth Leipzig. 1987; 12: 173–179.
4. Yannuzzi, L.A. Type A behavior and central serous chorioretinopathy. Trans Am Ophthalmol Soc. 1986; 84: 799–845.
5. Yoshioka, H., Sugita, T., Nagayoski, K. Fluorescein angiographic findings in experimental retinopathy produced by intravenous adrenaline injection. Folia Ophthalmol Jpn. 1970; 21: 648–652.
6. Nagayoski, K. Experimental study of chorioretinopathy by intravenous injection of adrenaline. Acta Soc Ophthalmol Jpn. 1971; 75: 1720–1727.
7. Miki, T., Sunada, I., Higaki, T. Studies on chorioretinitis induced in rabbit by stress (repeated administration of epinephrine). Acta Soc Ophthalmol Jpn. 1972; 76: 1037–1045.
8. Yasuzumi, T., Miki, T., Sugimoto, K. Electron microscopic studies of epinephrine choroiditis in rabbits: I. Pigment epithelium and Bruch's membrane in the healed stage. Acta Soc Ophthalmol Jpn. 1974; 78: 588–598.
9. Yoshioka, H., Katsume, Y., Akuma, H. Experimenta central serous chorioretinopathy in monkey eyes: II. Fluorescein angiographic findings. Ophthalmologica. 1982; 185: 168–178.
10. Yoshioka, H., Katsume, Y. Experimenta central serous chorioretinopathy: III. Ultrastructural findings. Jpn J Ophthalmol. 1982; 26: 397–409.
11. Oshioda, H., Katsume, Y., Akune, H., Nagasaki, H. Experimental central serous chorioretinopathy. Fluorescein angiography and electron microscopy. Kerume Med. 1984; 31: 89–99.
12. Harada, T., Harada, K. Six cases of central serous choroidopathy induced by systemic corticosteroid therapy. Doc Ophthalmol. 1985; 60: 37–44.
13. Wakakura, M. Serous retinal detachment in thrombotic thrombocytopenic purpura and corticosteroid therapy. Arch Ophthalmol. 1986; 104: 177–178.
14. Miura, K., Ueno, M., Miura, Y., Seo, T. Central serous chorioretinopathy induced by systemic corticosteroid therapy. Folia Ophthalmol Jpn. 1989; 40: 59–64.
15. Petracci, M., Nuti, A., Pannini, S. *et al.* Central serous chorioretinopathy: iatrogenic illness during systemic corticosteroid treatment. Ann Ottalmol Clin Ocul. 1990; 116: 13–18.
16. Bouzas, E.A., Scott, M.H., Mastorakos, G. *et al.* Central serous chorioretinopathy in endogenous hypercortisolism. Arch Ophthalmol. 1993; 111: 1229–1233.
17. Knave, B., Tengroth, B., Voss, M. Age and sex distribution of some macular diseases: senile and presenile macular degeneration and central serous retinitis. Acta Ophthalmol. 1984; 161 (Suppl.): 95–103.
18. Mutlak, J.A., Dutton, G.N. Fluorescein angiographic features of acute central serous retinopathy. Acta Ophthalmol. 1989; 67: 467–469.
19. Chumbley, L.C., Frank, R.N. Central serous retinopathy and pregnancy. Am J Ophthalmol. 1974; 77: 158–160.
20. Gass, J.D.M. Unusual ocular complication of pregnancy. In: Franklin, R.M. (ed.), Retina and Vitreous. Amsterdam: Kugler Publication, 1993: 309–310.
21. Gass, J.D.M. Central serous chorioretinopathy and white subretinal exudation during pregnancy. Arch Ophthalmol. 1991; 109: 677–681.
22. Sunness, J.S., Haller, J.A., Fine, S.L. Central serous chorioretinopathy and pregnancy. Arch Ophthalmol. 1993; 11: 360–364.
23. Coppeto, J.R. Central serous retinopathy, the Fransworth-Munsell 100-Hue test and prolactin. Arch Ophthalmol. 1985; 103: 323–325.
24. Spitznas, M. Pathogenesis of central serous retinopathy: a new working hypothesis. Graefe's Arch Clin Exp Ophthalmol. 1986; 224: 321–324.
25. Scheider, A., Nasemann, J.E., Lund, D.E. Fluorescein and indocyanine green angiographies of cental serous choroidopathy by scanning laser ophthalmoscopy. Am J Ophthalmol. 1993; 115: 50–56.
26. Guyer, D.R., Yannuzzi, L.A., Slakter, J.S. *et al.* Digital indocyanine green videoangiography of central serous chorioretinopathy. Arch Ophthalmol. 1994; 112: 1057–1062.
27. Grajewski, A.L., Ferrari-Dileo, G., Feuer, W.J., Anderson, D.R. Beta-adrenergic responsiveness of choroidal vascolature. Ophthalmology. 1991; 98: 989–995.

28. Browning, D.J. Nadolol in the treatment of central serous retinopathy. Am J Ophthalmol. 1993; 116: 770–771.
29. Colombati, S., Clabacchi, F.M., Longhena, P.L. Acute and chronic serous epitheliopathy. Hypothesis of topical treatment with beta-blockers. Ann Ottalmol Clin Ocul. 1991; 117: 1185–1188.
30. Avci, R., Deutman, A.F. The treatment of central serous choroidopathy with a beta-blocker: metoprolol. Klin Monatsbl Augenheilkd. 1993; 202: 199–205.

I Ophthalmologic Clinic
via Juvarra 19
10122 Turin, Italy

37. Digital indocyanine green angiography of central serous chorioretinopathy

S. BALTATZIS, J. LADAS, D. PANAGIOTIDIS, S. KOKOLAKIS,
G. ANAGNOSTAKI and G. THEODOSSIADIS

(Athens, Greece)

Central serous chorioretinopathy (CSC) is a condition usually seen in younger patients in which a neurosensory retinal detachment is noted with or without an associated pigment epithelial detachment. There has been great controversy about the pathogenesis of this condition. Some investigators believe that the primary abnormality is an alteration of the permeability of the choroidal blood vessels, while others have postulated that the permeability alterations are of RPE origin[1-4].

Using indocyanine green (ICG) angiography, we studied 78 consecutive eyes with acute CSC to determine whether this technique could provide information concerning the pathogenesis of this disease.

Patients and methods

Our study included 41 consecutive patients (78 eyes) with acute CSC. All our patients had in one or both eyes, localized idiopathic neurosensory detachments in the macula with or without pigment epithelial detachments (PEDs) secondary to one or more focal fluoroangiographic leaks at the level of the retinal pigment ipithelium (RPE). The patients ages ranged from 20 to 40 years (median 30 years). Thirty were males and 11 females.

The patients had no other signs of ocular disease, including age-related macular degeneration, pathological myopia, intraocular inflammation, previous laser photocoagulation, angioid streaks, presumed ocular histoplasmosis syndrome or choroidal rupture.

Each patient underwent general ophthalmoscopic examination, fundus biomicroscopy with Goldman lens, fundus photography and digital fluorescein and ICG angiography. The angiograms were performed with the TOPCON IMAGEnet H 1024 Imaging System that was connected to an ICG camera (Topcon TRC-501A).

ICG (25 mg) was injected intravenously, and angiograms were then obtained for 45 min. FA and ICG findings were then compared.

G. Coscas and F. Cardillo Piccolino (eds.), Retinal Pigment Epithelium and Macular Diseases, pp. 233–236.
© *1998 Kluwer Academic Publishers.*

Results

In all 78 eyes, all active leakage points observed with FA could also be identified with ICG. ICG angiography did not identify any active leakage that was not noticed with FA, except in one case where we noticed one leaking point on FA and two on ICG (Fig. 1).

During the mid- and late frames of the ICG angiography areas of choroidal

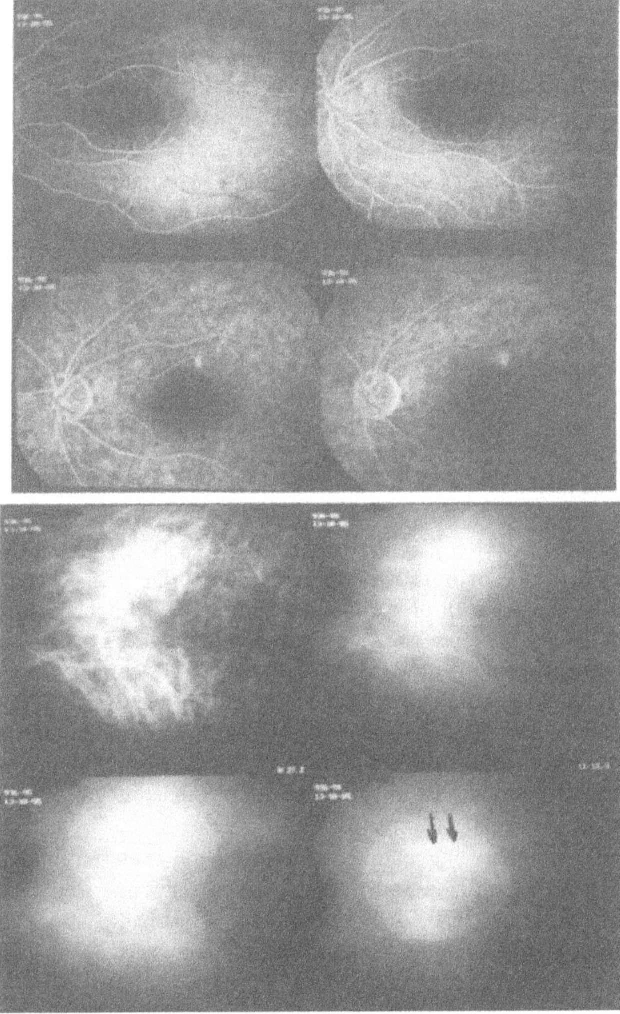

Fig. 1.   One leaking point on fluorescing angiography (above). Two leaking points in indocyanine green angiography (below).

hyperfluorescence were observed in the great majority of patients. Some of these areas surrounded active leakage points or were associated with abnormalities of the RPE that were more or less detectable by the FA.

In 44 eyes (56%) we observed confluent hypofluorescent spots of varying size and of irregular shape. The great majority of these spots coincided with slightly hyperfluorescent areas on FA due to RPE changes. In contrast, Piccolino observed these spots in slightly hypofluorescent areas on FA[3].

Fifty eyes (64%) had pigment epithelial detachments (PEDs) on the FA. The observed PEDs had a unique pattern on the ICG. In the late phases a hyperfluorescent ring surrounded the hypofluorescent central portion. In one patient we noticed a small PED on FA, that was not identified on ICG. In the same eye, we oserved a window defect lesion on FA, which corresponded to hypofluorescent spots on ICG angiography. We also noticed a window defect on FA which corresponds to the typical appearance of PED on ICG angiography. This lesion is probably described as 'presumed' PED on ICG angiography by Guyer *et al*[4].

In one of our patients, we noticed a rather peculiar phenomenon: a large neurosensory retinal detachment (NSRD) in the macula was detected as a round homogeneous diffuse hyperfluorescent area with a well-defined border in the late transit frames of the ICG angiography. This area was identified with typical appearance of NSRD on the FA: (i.e. a slight masking effect because of the fluid under the NSRD). We could not find this strange appearance of NSRD on ICG angiography in any of the other patients (Fig. 2). We need a further explanation as to how the indocyanine dye, in contrast to fluorescein, fills the area of NSRD in this patient.

Conclusions

Our findings are in general agreement with other investigators and support the theory that the primary abnormality of this disease is an alteration of the permeability of the choroidal blood vessels.

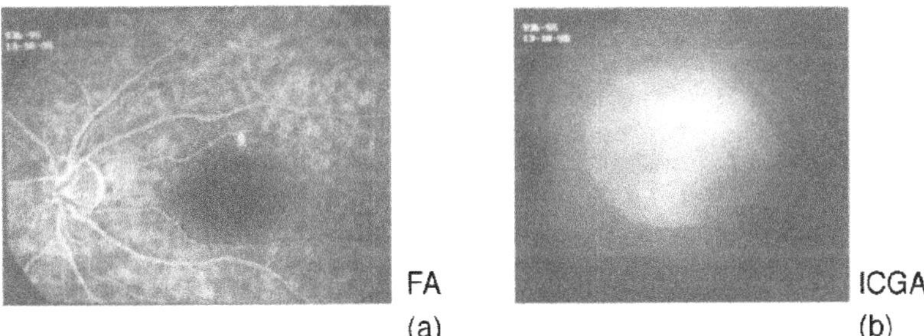

Fig. 2. (a) A neurosensory retinal detachment (NSRD) in the macule was identified as slight masking effect because of the fluid under the NSRD on FA, but (b) in ICGA (late transit frame) this large neurosensory retinal detachment was detected as a round homogeneous diffuse hyperfluorescent area with a well-defined border.

The number of leakage points or PEDs detected by FA was not always the same as that seen on the ICG angiography. All the detected areas of choroidal hyperfluorescence on the ICG angiography surrounded active leakage points or associated with RPE abnormalities on FA. All the hypofluorescent spots on ICG angiography were noticed in hyperfluorescent areas due to RPE changes, and were more or less detectable on the FA, and for the case with the peculiar phenomenon of pooling of the indocyanine green dye under the NSRD, a further explanation can be needed.

References

1. Gass, J.M. Idiopathic central serous chorioretinopathy. Am J Ophthalmol. 1967; 63: 587–615.
2. Marmor, M. New hypothesis on the pathogenesis and treatment of serous retinal detachment. Graefes Arch Clin Exp Ophthalmol. 1988; 226: 548–552.
3. Piccolino, F.C. Borgia, L. Central serous chorioretinopathy and indocyanine green angiography. Retina. 1994; 14: 231–242.
4. Guyer, D.R. Yannuzzi, L.A. et al. Digital indocyanine green angiography of central serous chorioretinopathy. Arch Ophthalmol. 1994; 112: 1057–1062.

Athens University Eye Clinic
Athens
Greece

38. Indocyanine green angiography: utility in chronic central serous chorioretinopathy

A. ROMANI, M. DE LUCA, G. GABBRIELLINI, G. CARDINI,
P. MELANI and M. NARDI

(Pisa, Italy)

Introduction

Chronic central serous chorioretinopathy (C-CSC), also known as diffuse retinal epitheliopathy or gravitational epitheliopathy was first recognized as an independent disease by Zweng and Little in 1977[1]. C-CSC is characterized by a diffuse, frequently bilateral alteration of the retinal pigment epithelium (RPE), prevalently at the posterior pole. It has a chronic and progressive course and the final prognosis for preservation of a good visual acuity is usually unfavourable[1−6].

The alterations of the fundus in C-CSC may be barely visible on ophthalmoscopic examination. Fluorescein angiography, however, may reveal irregular atrophy of the RPE, small pigment epithelium detachments (PED), and areas of active leakage and serous retinal detachment. In some cases atrophic tracks, corresponding to a previous neurosensory detachment and extending towards the inferior periphery of the fundus, are visible.

The similarity of this disease with central serous chorioretinopathy (CSC) yields the idea that C-CSC represents the late evolution of a recurrent CSC[6]. This hypothesis is supported by ICG angiography studies of patients with C-CSC and CSC, which have shown similar alterations of the choroid in these two diseases[3]. A study with indocyanine green videoangiography (V-ICG) was performed in some cases of C-CSC to identify the entity of choroidal involvement in C-CSC. A comparison between fluorangiography (FA) and V-ICG results in the same patients was also performed.

Materials and methods

Thirty patients, 22 with bilateral disease, were studied. The mean age was 49 years (range 36–69 years), and 22 were male. All patients received a complete ophthalmological examination including visual acuity assessment, Amsler grid testing, slit lamp biomicroscopy of the anterior segment, applanation tonometry, posterior segment examination with a Goldman contact lens and/or a non-contact 90 diopters lens, fundus photographs, FA and V-ICG

G. Coscas and F. Cardillo Piccolino (eds.), Retinal Pigment Epithelium and Macular Diseases, pp. 237–241.
© 1998 Kluwer Academic Publishers.

angiography. Each patient was examined again after a month and subsequently every 6 months. The same tests were repeated during each follow-up examination. Both FA and V-ICG angiography were performed with Topcon IMAGEnet H1024 Digital Imaging System.

V-ICG angiography was performed injecting 25 mg of ICG (Cardiogreen) into the antecubital vein, followed by the injection of 5 ml of physiological solution. Photograms of the early, intermediate (15–30 min) and late (40–60 min) phases were recorded. Five eyes were treated with argon laser. The mean duration of follow-up was 12 months (range 4–24 months).

Results

One or more localized areas of early hyperfluorescence were identified with V-ICG angiography (Fig. 1). These hyperfluorescent areas appeared 2–3 min after injection of the dye, were more evident in the intermediate phases, and tended to fade in the late phases. After 30 min they were still present, although with attenuate intensity, in 23 eyes, while they had completely vanished in nine eyes. In 19 eyes the areas of active leakage were more evident with V-ICG angiography than with FA. All the areas of window defect with FA showed a diffuse hyperfluorescence with V-ICG angiography. This hyperfluorescence appeared 10 min after the injection of the dye, and faded completely in the late phase. These hyperfluorescent areas were larger with V-ICG angiography than with FA. In 32 eyes V-ICG angiography was able to identify a diffuse hyperfluorescence in areas where FA failed to show any alteration. Five eyes showed the characteristic gravitational pattern of atrophic areas, located at the base of the most hyperfluorescent choroidal zone (Fig. 2). In four eyes an area of early hyperfluorescence was identified; this area increased in the intermediate phase, and persisted in the late phase. This area probably corresponds to a subretinal neovascularization. In seven of the eight unilateral cases (which showed no alteration of the fellow eye with clinical examination and fluorescein angiography), V-ICG angiography revealed a diffuse choroidal hyperpermeability also in the fellow eye. Such hyperpermeability was more evident in the intermediate phase and faded in the late phase.

Discussion

On the basis of FA two different pathogenetic hypothesis of acute and chronic CSC have been proposed in the past. The first hypothesis identifies the RPE as the principal area of an immunitary or inflammatory damage, causing a breakdown of the external haematoretinal barrier and pooling of fluid under the neurosensory retina[6]. The second hypothesis identifies the initial cause of CSC in an ischemic or inflammatory damage to the choriocapillaris, which provokes secondarily, an alteration of the RPE[7]. V-ICG angiography has

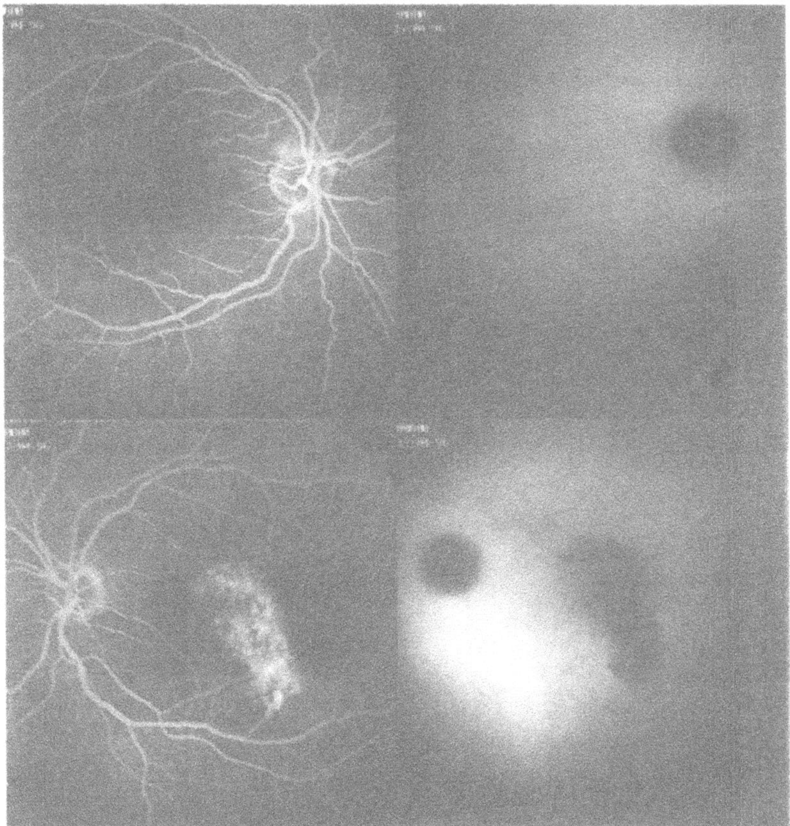

Fig. 1. V-ICG angiography reveals in OD a diffuse choroidal hyperpermeability, that is not seen with FA; in OS V-ICG reveals a more diffuse damage than FA.

recently shown a diffuse alteration of the choriocapillaris as the possible causing factor of CSC[3,8]. In fact, V-ICG angiography of CSC patients has revealed a diffuse choroidal hyperpermeability at the posterior pole, probably related to a damage of the choriocapillaris. This area of hyperpermeability was not limited to the area of neurosensory detachment, but extended to the surrounding choroid. The increased hyperfluorescence in the intermediate phases could be explained by a staining of the damaged RPE. In a significant number of cases, V-ICG angiography shows hyperfluorescence in areas where FA fails to reveal any alteration. These observations may support the hypothesis that diffuse choriocapillaris hyperpermeability may cause leakage of plasma proteins in the interstitial space, and as the ultimate result, damage to the RPE, a breakdown in the external haematoretinal barrier, and eventually a neurosensory detachment[5]. When this situation becomes chronic, the

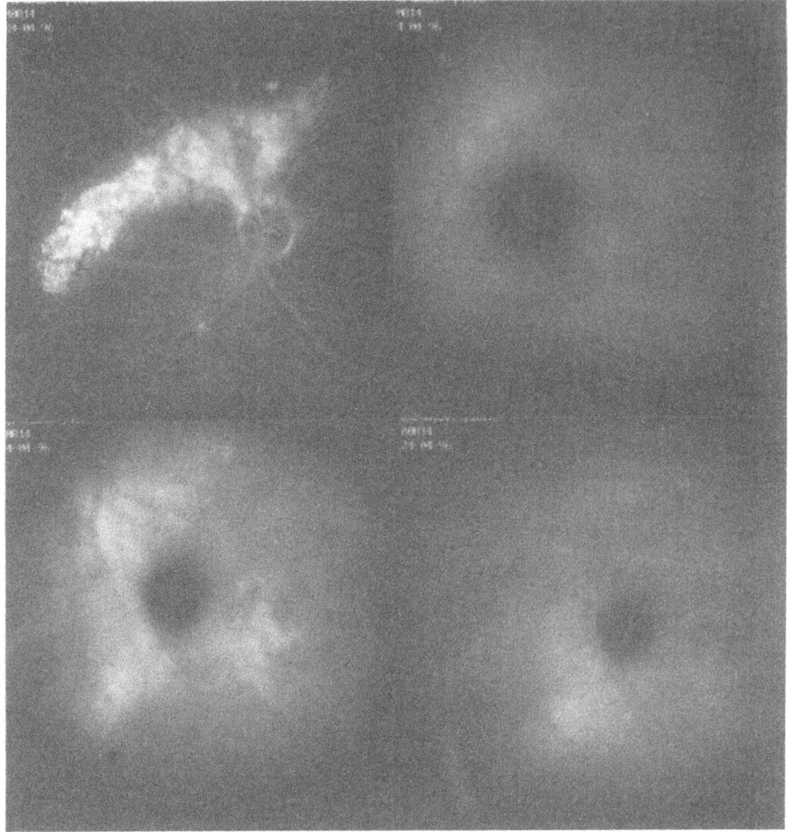

Fig. 2. FA shows a typical RPE track. V-ICG angiography shows hyperfluorescence of the RPE track in the intermediate phase, and a diffuse alteration of the RPE in the late phase.

fluid under the retina gravitates inferiorly causing linear areas of RPE atrophy, which appear as atrophic tracks.

In conclusion, V-ICG, showing a diffuse hyperpermeability of the choroid also in areas that were silent with FA and in apparently normal eyes, may enhance the ability of early diagnosis and prognosis assessment of C-CSC patients. V-ICG is indispensable for identification of occult subretinal neovascularization. However further clinical and pathological studies are necessary to understand fully the aetiology and pathogenesis of CSC.

References

1. Zweng, H.C., Little, H.L. Diffuse retinal pigment epitheliopathy. In: Argon Laser Photocoagulation. St. Louis: CV Mosby Co, 1977: 340–349.

2. Gilbert, C.M., Owens, S.L., Smith, P.D., Fine, S.T. Long-term follow-up of central serous chorioretinopathy. Br J Ophthalmol. 1984; 68: 815–820.
3. Guyer, D.R., Yannuzzi, L.A., Slakter, J.S., Sorenson, J.A., Ho, A., Orlock, D. Digital indocyanine green videoangiography of central serous chorioretinopathy. Arch Ophthalmol. 1994; 112: 1057–1062.
4. Yannuzzi, L.A., Shakin, J., Fischer, Y., Altomonte, M.A. Peripheral retinal detachments and retinal pigment ephithelial atrophic tracks secondary to central serous pigment epitheliopathy. Ophthalmology. 1984; 91: 1554–1572.
5. Marmor, M.F. New hypothesis on the pathogenesis and treatment of serous retinal detachment. Graefes Arch Clin Exp Ophthalmol. 1988; 226: 548–552.
6. Spitznas, M. Pathogenesis of central serous chorioretinopathy: a new working hypothesis. Graefes Arch Exp Ophthalmol. 1986; 224: 321–324.
7. Gass, J.D.M. Pathogenesis of disciform detachment of the neuroepithelium. Am J Ophthalmol. 1967; 63: 587–615.
8. Scheider, A., Nasemann, J.E., Lund, O.E. Fluorescein and indocyanine green angiographies of central serous chorioretinopathy by scanning laser ophthalmoscopy. Am J Ophthalmol. 1993; 115: 50–56.

Neuroscience Department
Eye Clinic
University of Pisa
V. Roma, 67, 56100, Pisa, Italy

39. Indocyanine green angiography in central serous chorioretinopathy

U. MENCHINI, G. VIRGILI, P. LANZETTA and E. FERRARI

(Udine, Italy)

Introduction

The pathogenesis of central serous chorioretinopathy (CSC) is still under discussion. Using indocyanine green angiography (ICG-A), numerous authors have observed hyperfluorescent lesions related to choroidal hyperpermeability, thus giving new support to the hypothesis of a choroidal pathogenesis for CSC[1-6]. Delayed choroidal perfusion has also been observed[1,6], leading to the hypothesis that capillary or venous congestion after ischemia in one or more choroidal lobules might be the cause of choroidal hyperpermeability.

Here we report the findings obtained with ICG-A in a large group of patients, analysing above all the images which are seen in the late phases.

Results

Ninety consecutive patients with CSC were examined, with an average of 48 years (22–75 years) and average duration of CSC of 63.6 months (1–240 months). A total of 127 eyes were affected by one of the forms of the disease. Forty-eight presented with acute CSC, 21 had had one episode that had completely regressed and 58 presented with chronic CSC. The images obtained with ICG-A were compared with the fluorescein angiographic findings.

In 85 out of 99 (85.9%) eyes which presented one or more leakage points on the fluorescein angiogram, ICG-A revealed a corresponding hyperfluorescence by dye diffusion[1-6]. These spots appeared during the early minutes and were brightest in the latest phases. Areas of hyperfluorescence with characteristics analogous to those previously described[1-6], related to choroidal hyperpermeability, were observed in all cases (127 eyes) and in nine fellow eyes with no signs of CSC on the fluorescein angiogram.

One hundred and three eyes showed hypofluorescent lesions that became progressively more distinct in the course of the examination. The great majority of the lesions corresponded to areas of alteration to the retinal pigment epithelium that were visible during fluorescein angiography as hyperfluorescent lesions owing to window defect or less frequently by hyperpigmentation. During ICG-A, these hypofluorescent lesions appeared after 10–20 min and

G. Coscas and F. Cardillo Piccolino (eds.), Retinal Pigment Epithelium and Macular Diseases, pp. 243–246.
© *1998 Kluwer Academic Publishers.*

became more distinct after 30–60 min. The morphology of the hypofluorescent lesions presented clearly defined edges. Spaide *et al.*[5] reported that areas of RPE atrophy appeared hypofluorescent in ICG-A. They observed that the fluorescence of the underlying larger choroidal vessels seemed normal, thus excluding a masking of fluorescence, which is in agreement with our results. The authors believed that the hypofluorescence in areas of RPE atrophy was due to choriocapillaris hypoperfusion, resulting from the decreased amount of trophic factors produced by atrophic RPE. They also noticed that the areas with relatively intact choriocapillaris demonstrated hyperpermeability and areas with RPE atrophy remained hypofluorescent, suggesting that the choriocapillaris must be present for choroidal vascular hyperpermeability to occur. In contrast, we observed that areas of hyperpermeability and areas of late hypofluorescence may be partially superimposed. This may indicate that atrophy of the choriocapillaris is not the cause, or the only cause, of the hypofluorescence related to RPE atrophy. It is difficult to explain what these lesions might represent because of the limited knowledge available on the dynamics and interactions of ICG with ocular tissues *in vivo*. An interaction between ICG and pigment epithelium could be hypothesized to explain this dynamic behaviour, such as a staining of normal RPE. Matsubara *et al.*[7] observed ICG staining of the retinal pigment epithelium in pigmented rats. According to this hypothesis, the normal pigment epithelium could bring about part of the fluorescence seen on indocyanine green angiography at a stage when choroidal fluorescence is fading because of the reduced concentration of ICG in the blood. A chronic alteration of the pigment epithelium could therefore lead to a progressive hypofluorescence due to lack of staining with characteristics similar to the hypofluorescence described. Alternatively, an alteration of the binding of ICG to proteins of the Bruch's membrane could be hypothesized, but this structure can neither be studied by clinical or fluorangiographic examination in CSC, nor is any clinico-pathological correlation available.

Fluorescein angiography showed RPE atrophic tracts in at least one eye of 22 patients. A total of 31 tracts were examined. On ICG-A, the tracts displayed two features, which appear to be linked to their stage of development (Fig. 1). In an early stage with limited RPE atrophy, the tract is hyperfluorescent owing to subretinal diffusion of ICG in correspondence to the neuroepithelial detachment (11 tracts). At a later stage with marked RPE atrophy, this hyperfluorescence is replaced by hypofluorescence due to advanced damage to the RPE (20 tracts).

The role of ICG-A in the treatment of and formulation of a prognosis for CSC needs to be evaluated with further studies. At present, this method is of interest mainly for the opportunity it offers to study the choroidal alterations manifested in the course of the disease. Our study indicates how alterations of the pigment epithelium may be correlated to characteristic late images obtained with ICG-A.

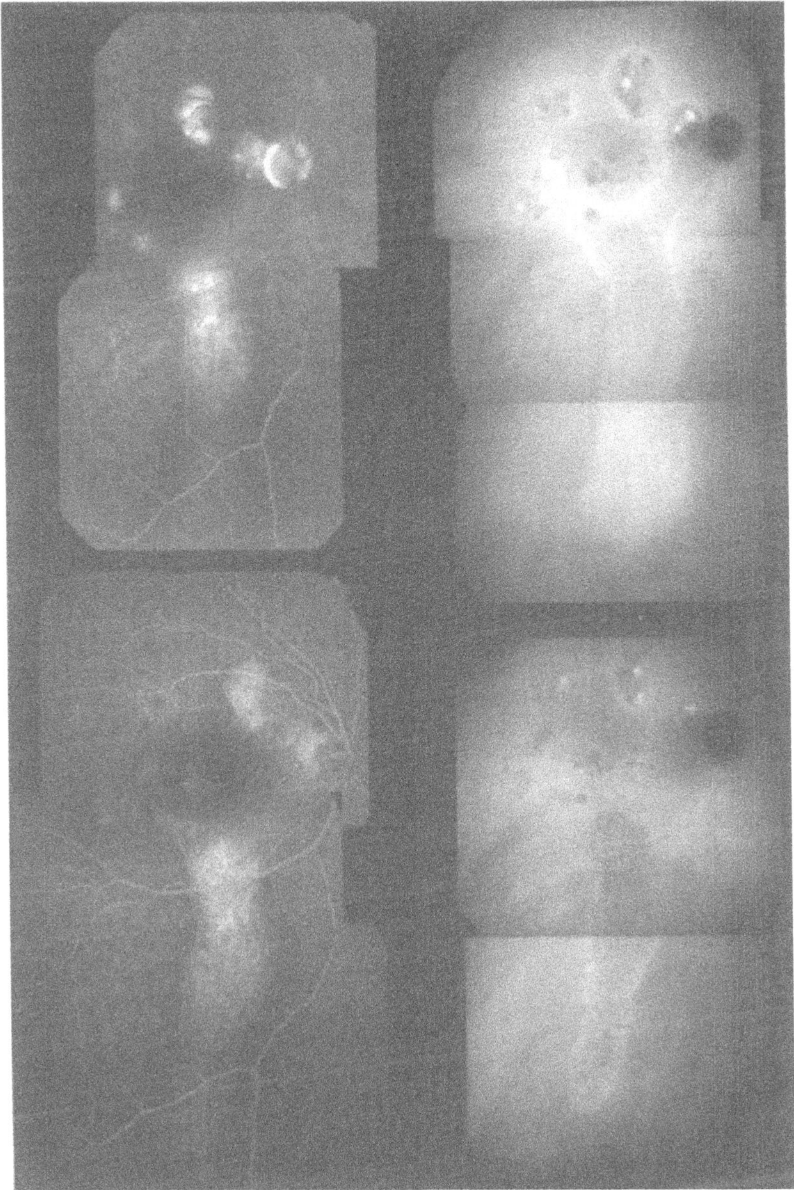

Fig. 1. Fluorescein angiographic aspect (top left) of a RPE tract in an early stage of development with minimal RPE atrophy and some hyperfluorescence due to pooling of dye in the neuroepithelial detachment, that is also seen with ICG angiography after about 1 h (top right). After 3 years, the amount of RPE atrophy has increased with fluorescein angiography (bottom left) as well as the hypofluorescence with ICG angiography in the late phases (bottom right).

References

1. Scheider, A., Nasemann, J.E., Lund, O.-E. Fluorescein and indocyanine green angiographies of central serous choroidopathy by scanning laser ophthalmoscopy. Am J Ophthalmol. 1993; 115: 50–56.
2. Cardillo Piccolino, F., Borgia, L. Central serous chorioretinopathy and indocyanine green angiography. Retina. 1994; 14: 231–242.
3. Guyer, D.R., Yannuzzi, L.A., Slakter, J.S., Sorensen, J.A., Ho, A., Orlock, D. Digital indocyanine green videoangiography of central serous chorioretinopathy. Arch Ophthalmol. 1994; 112: 1057–1062.
4. Cardillo Piccolino, F., Borgia, L., Zinicola, E., Zingirian, M. Indocyanine green angiographic findings in central serous chorioretinopathy. Eye. 1995; 9: 324–332.
5. Spaide, R.F., Hall, L., Haas, A. *et al.* Indocyanine green videoangiography of older patients with central serous chorioretinopathy. Retina. 1996; 16: 203–213.
6. Prunte, C., Flammer, J. Choroidal capillary and venous congestion in central serous chorioretinopathy. Am J Ophthalmol. 1996; 121: 26–34.
7. Matsubara, T., Uyama, M., Takhashi, K. *et al.* Localization of indocyanine green in the choroid and retina, histological proof. Presented at the International Symposium on Fluorescein Angiography. Le Chateau Frontenac, Quebec, Canada. June 20–24, 1994; Abstract book page 44.

Department of Ophthalmology
University of Udine
V.le Venezia 410, 33100 Udine, Italy

40. Follow-up evaluation of indocyanine green angiographic findings in central serous chorioretinopathy

L. BORGIA, F. CARDILLO PICCOLINO, E. ZINICOLA
and M. ZINGIRIAN

(Genova, Italy)

Introduction

Observations with indocyanine green (ICG) angiography by our group and other authors suggest a primary involvement of the choroid in central serous chorioretinopathy (CSC)[1–3]. The main result of our studies was the constant observation of areas of dye diffusion in the choroid in correspondence with the pigment epithelial alterations that characterize CSC[3]. We proposed zonal hyperpermeability of the choriocapillaris as the primary lesion in CSC, leading to degenerative alterations of the retinal pigment epithelium and passage of fluid in the subretinal space[3].

In this study we verified our previous results by analysing the ICG angiographic findings in a large number of patients and investigated possible changes of the ICG angiographic pattern in patients with CSC.

Patients and methods

A total of 176 patients with acute or chronic active or inactive CSC were examined in the last 3 years at the Retina Service of the University Eye Clinic of Genoa. On the basis of clinical history, fundus examination and fluorescein angiography the cases were classified as acute CSC (98), healed CSC (17) and chronic CSC (61). Each patient underwent digital ICG videoangiography utilizing the Topcon IMAGEnet H1024 Digital Imaging System (Ijssel, The Nederlands). Forty-eight patients, 32 with acute CSC and 16 with chronic CSC, were re-examined every 3–6 months for a follow-up period of 6–39 months (mean 16 months). Fifteen of these patients received laser photocoagulation of the leaking points. On the ICG angiograms we evaluated choroidal filling, choroidal vascular permeability and alterations of the retinal pigment epithelium. In patients with follow-up we looked for any changes in the ICG angiographic findings obtained at the first examination.

G. Coscas and F. Cardillo Piccolino (eds.), Retinal Pigment Epithelium and Macular Diseases, pp. 247–251.
© *1998 Kluwer Academic Publishers.*

Results

ICG angiographic findings

The ICG behaviour at the leaking points was essentially analogous to that of fluorescein. However when fluorescein leakage was low the subretinal diffusion of ICG could be hardly distinguished from the background fluorescence.

Small pigment epithelial detachments were present in 40 (27.5%) patients: 15 (17.6%) with acute and in 25 (52%) with chronic CSC. The detachments of the retinal pigment epithelium became fluorescent in the first minutes of the ICG examination. The dye was then gradually eliminated from the sub-epithelial space, leaving residues along the border of the detachment. In the more advanced angiographic phases the pigment epithelial detachments appeared as hypofluorescent areas surrounded by a hyperfluorescent ring.

One or more areas of choroidal staining became evident from 3 to 5 min after dye injection in all patients except two (98.6%) with inactive disease. This was observed beneath all leaking points, all areas of pigment epithelial decompensation and all pigment epithelial detachments. Such staining also occurred in some regions where degenerative changes of the retinal pigment epithelium were visible with fluorescein angiography and/or biomicroscopy.

Dye diffusion progressed in a centrifugal way from the area first stained, and in 2–5 min extended over double this area. Shifting of ICG in the choroid was particularly evident and rapid, with a wash-out phenomenon, in corre-spondence with the pigment epithelial detachments and in several areas where alterations of the retinal pigment epithelium appeared as dark spots during the most advanced angiographic phases. In many areas of choroidal staining, as background fluorescence faded, these hypofluorescent spots of varying size and irregular shape became more and more visible. They were more evident and numerous in patients with recurrent or chronic disease.

Follow-up findings

During the follow-up period subretinal exudation and fluorescein leaking points disappeared in the 15 eyes that underwent photocoagulation and in another 12 eyes that had not been treated. In five patients new leaking points were found during the follow-up examinations.

In the 48 cases followed with periodic examinations the areas of dye diffusion in the choroid were always present and did not show significant variations. They persisted also when the leaking points had disappeared spontaneously or after photocoagulation (Fig. 1). During follow-up we did not detect any areas of choroidal staining which had not been present at the first observation.

In the patients in whom new leaking points appeared, they were situated in correspondence of choroidal areas where dye diffusion was already evident at the first angiographic examination (Fig. 2).

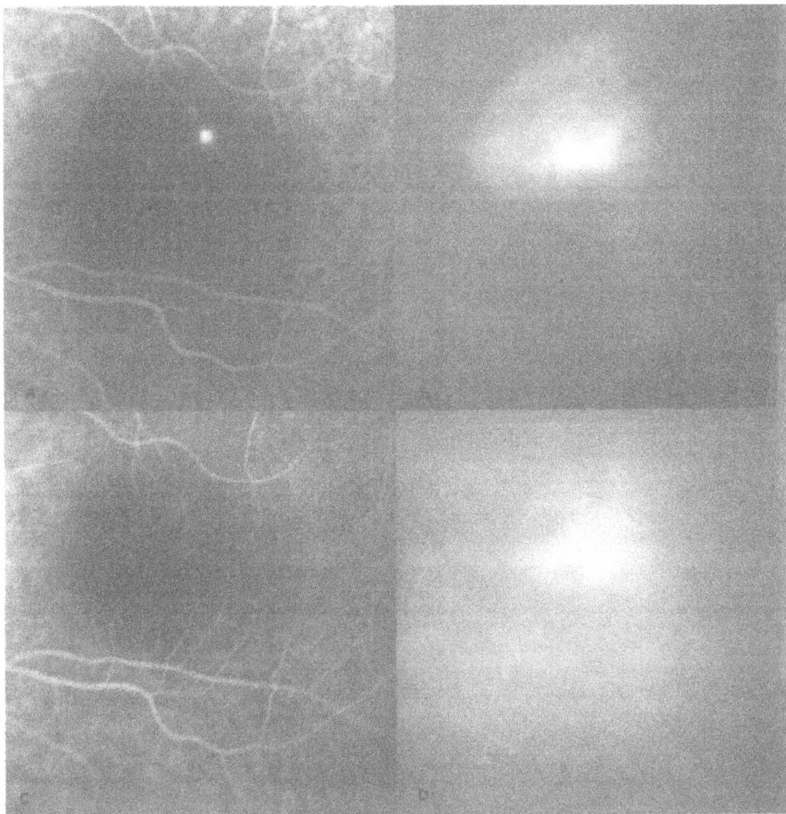

Fig. 1. Central serous chorioretinopathy with resolution of the subretinal but not of the choroidal exudation. (a, b) Fluorescein and indocyanine green (ICG) photographs taken at the initial examination. (c, d) Fluorescein and ICG photographs taken about 18 months years later.

At the follow-up examinations hypofluorescent spots were unchanged in all cases except for three in which some patches appeared slightly enlarged. In one eye we progressively observed the presence of a leak, of a pigment epithelial detachment after regression of the leak and of dark spots after regression of the detachment.

Conclusions

The results of this study greatly support the concept, expressed by Gass[4] many years ago and recently taken up again by our group and others[1-3,5], that an abnormal permeability of the choriocapillaris in CSC precedes the alterations of the retinal pigment epithelium and presumably is the cause of

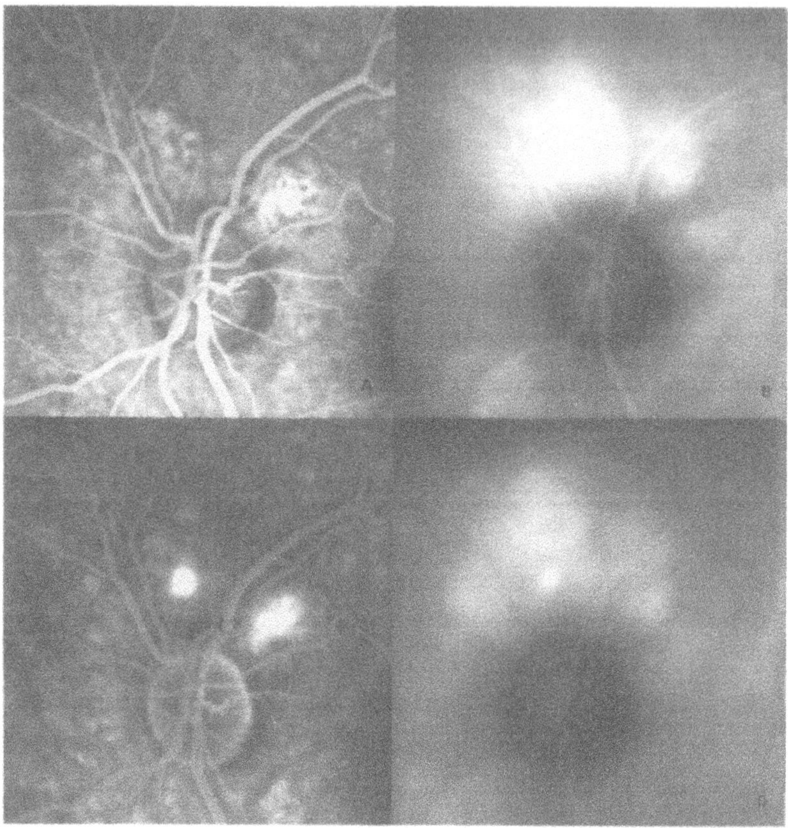

Fig. 2. Central serous chorioretinopathy with a leaking point in correspondence of a preexisting area of choriocapillaris hyperpermeability. (a, b) Fluorescein and indocyanine green (ICG) photographs taken at the initial examination. (c, d) Fluorescein and ICG photographs taken 1 year later.

these alterations. A massive focal exudation in the choroid could reach the subretinal space with a rate of flow so high to overwhelm the fluid transport of the retinal pigment epithelium. On the basis of our observation we also propose that when the zonal hyperpermeability of the choriocapillaris corresponds to a local condition of particulary elevated blood flow retinal pigment epithelial detachments can occur. The immobility of the choroidal angiographic pattern observed in our cases also suggests that the causative factor of vascular hyperpermeability acts in a lasting and constant manner in patients with CSC. Another possible hypothesis is that a temporary 'moxa' may produce long lasting or irreversible damage to the endothelium of the choriocapillaris.

References

1. Hayashi, K., Hasegawa, Y., Tokoro, T. Indocyanine green angiography of central serous chorio-retinopathy. Int Ophthalmol. 1986; 9: 37–41.
2. Scheider, A., Nasemann, J.E., Lund, O.E. Fluorescein and indocyanine green angiography of central serous chorioretinopathy by scanning laser ophthalmoscopy. Am J Ophthalmol. 1993; 115: 50–56.
3. Cardillo Piccolino, F., Borgia, L. Central serous chorioretinopathy and indocyanine green angiography. Retina. 1994; 14: 231–242.
4. Gass, J.D.M. Pathogenesis of disciform detachment of the neuroepithelium. II Idiopatic central serous choroidopathy. Am J Ophthalmol. 1967; 63: 587–592.
5. Cardillo Piccolino, F., Borgia, L., Zinicola, E., Zingirian, M.. Indocyanine green angiographic findings in central serous chorioretinopathy. Eye. 1995; 9: 324–332.

Department of Ophthalmology
University of Genoa
Via S. Luca d'Albaro, 37/3
16146 Genova, Italy

41. Long-term follow-up in patients with chronic central serous chorioretinopathy

D. PAULEIKHOFF and A. WESSING

(Essen, Germany)

Purpose

Chronic central serous chorioretinopathy (CSCR) can be seen in young patients with multiple areas of central RPE changes in combination with focal or diffuse leakage not related to choroidal neovascularization. Previous history of acute CSCR is suspected and the recovery as well as the prognosis for visual acuity and the development of new lesions is uncertain. In order to evaluate the long-term visual prognosis in patients with chronic CSCR and to describe the clinical and angiographic varieties as well as the possibilities of laser treatment a re-evaluation of patients with chronic CSCR diagnosed between 1980 and 1990 was performed.

Methods

Thirty-six patients were included in this study (mean age 43 years, range 30–64, five female, 31 male) with a mean follow-up of 36 months (range 1–15 years). Angiographic changes and visual acuity were analysed during follow-up.

Results

The initial visual acuity was between 0.2 and 1.0. The areas of initial central RPE atrophy and the number of leakage spots varied largely between patients and bilateral disease was found in 27 patients (75%). Recurrences of CSCR during follow-up could be seen in 12 patients (33%). Visual loss at the final examination could be observed in 26 patients (70%). It was significantly correlated with enlargement of central RPE changes and the appeerence of recurrences. Patients with focal photocoagulation treatment of areas with leakage demonstrated less visual loss and fewer recurrences compared with untreated patients.

G. Coscas and F. Cardillo Piccolino (eds.), Retinal Pigment Epithelium and Macular Diseases, pp. 253–254.
© 1998 Kluwer Academic Publishers.

Conclusions

Because chronic CSCR is often associated with bilaterality and larger areas of RPE changes, this disease must be differentiated from patients with unilateral acute CSCR. Only a small number of patients with acute CSCR may develop chronic CSCR. Initial extension of central RPE changes and the status of the second eye may help to differentiate the two CSCR entities. In chronic CSCR enlargement of central RPE changes and the appearence of recurrences are important prognostic factors for the development of visual loss during follow-up. Laser treatment of areas with leakage may reduce this visual loss and the risk of recurrences.

Department of Ophthalmology
University of Essen
Germany

42. Indocyanine green angiography in multifocal posterior pigment epitheliopathy

M. UYAMA, H. MATSUNAGA, T. MATSUBARA, I. FUKUSHIMA,
K. IWASHITA, T. KIMOTO, H. YAMADA and Y. NAGAI

(Osaka, Japan)

Introduction

This paper describes the clinical features and pathophysiology of a peculiar type of non-rhegmatogenous, exudative retinal detachment, which was called bullous retinal detachment by Gass[1], and which is an unusual manifestation of central serous chorioretinopathy (CSC). We propose the term, multifocal posterior pigment epitheliopathy (MPPE), for this clinical entity[2]. This disease has previously been called as multiple serous chorioretinopathy[3] and idiopathic exudative retinal detachment[4], among others[5].

The clinical course and features are characterized by bilateral bullous retinal detachment in the lower periphery and flat serous retinal detachment in the posterior pole with multiple retinal exudations[1,5]. Exudations are commonly ring-shaped and slit lamp biomicroscopy reveals that these are the result of oedema in the deep sensory retina, not true exudates.

Most patients have a history of recurrences of CSC in one eye for several years as a prodromal to this disease. At the beginning of this disease, or at the initial stage, serous retinal detachment with retinal exudations appears in the posterior pole in one or both eyes. Thereafter, evolution of the disease is relatively rapid in both eyes. Bullous retinal detachment with multiple exudations appears in the evolutional stage. Shift of the subretinal fluid is marked. Three to 6 months later, the disease usually regress gradually, but some subretinal fibrosis remains. Patients are usually 30–40 years of age, and the condition is four times more prevalent in males than in females.

Fluorescein angiography in this disease reveals profused leakages from the choroid into the subretinal space at pinpoint sites in the posterior pole. Each leakage site corresponds to the retinal exudations.

Laser photocoagulation of the leakage sites is the only effective treatment in MPPE. The pathophysiology and aetiology of this disease are still obscure and no exact pathology has yet been reported. From these clinical manifestations, we suggest that damage to the retinal pigment epithelium (RPE) may be a primary lesion, and that this disease and central serous chorioretinopathy are at both ends of the same spectrum.

G. Coscas and F. Cardillo Piccolino (eds.), Retinal Pigment Epithelium and Macular Diseases, pp. 255–262.
© 1998 Kluwer Academic Publishers.

In CSC, indocyanine green ICG fluorescence angiography demonstrated extravascular leakage in the choroidal vessels, and suggested that hyperpermeability in the choroidal vessels may be the primary cause in CSC[8-12]. In MPPE, Iida[13] also demonstrated similar findings in ICG angiography. We confirm these reports and suggest a cause of MPPE.

Patients and methods

All patients fulfilled the criteria of MPPE, showing clinical characteristics mentioned above[1,5]. Diagnosis was made with binocular ophthalmoscopy and fluorescence fundus angiography.

During the past 3 years (1993–1995), we studied 42 eyes of 24 cases of MPPE and performed ICG angiography in our clinic. Patients were aged 30–63 (average 50 years) in age. Seventeen were (71%), and 18 (75%) were bilaterally affected. ICG angiography were performed by Topon camera or Rodenstock SLO.

Results

In patients with MPPE with exudative retinal detachment, fluorescein angiography showed, in the early phase, multiple pinpoint leakages corresponding to the retinal exudations. In the middle to late phase, profound leakages from the choroid into the subretinal space at the leakage sites were remarkable (Figs. 1, 2).

ICG angiography, in the early phase, showed dilatation of the choroidal veins in 15% of patients. In the middle phase (1–5 min after ICG injection) extravascular leakages from the choroidal vessels were remarkable (Fig. 3). In the late phase (15–20 min after ICG injection), marked diffuse hyperfluorescence was seen in the choroid in 90% of patients (Fig. 4). In some cases, ICG leaked through RPE into the subretinal space.

These abnormal ICG findings were seen in the posterior pole, diffusely and widely. Diffuse hyperfluorescence close to the leakage points in fluorescein angiography were most remarkable. Hypofluorescence or delayed perfusion in the background fluorescence in the early phase in ICG angiography was seen in only 10% of cases. Dilation and tortuosity in the choroidal vein were seen in the early phase of ICG angiography in 15% of all cases.

Laser photocoagulation of leakage sites detected by fluorescein angiography effectively stopped leakage from the choroid, and retinal exudations and retinal detachment subsided thereafter. All cases were cured completely by laser photocoagulation, after which performed fluorescein and ICG angiography were repeated.

Fluorescein angiography showed that all leakages from the choroid into the subretinal space disappeared. ICG angiography in the middle phase,

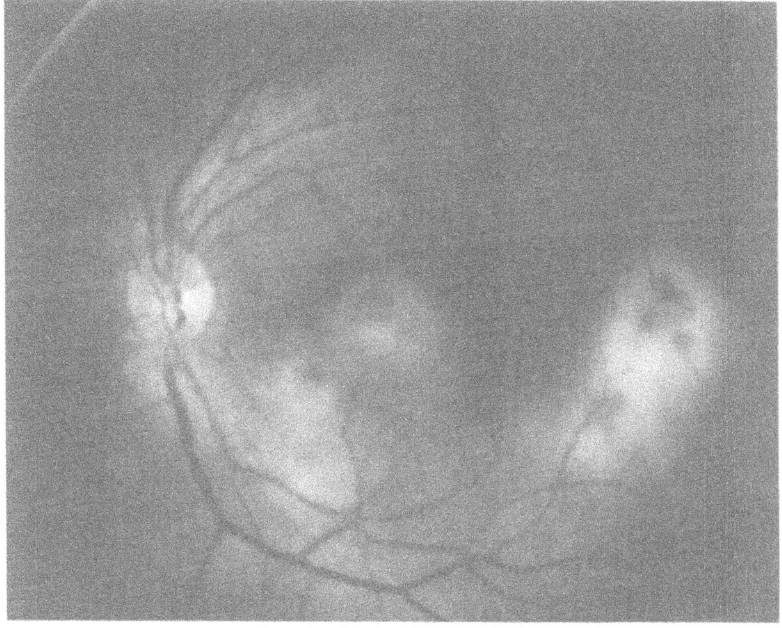

Fig. 1.   Fundus photograph of a 32-year-old man with multifocal posterior pigment epitheliopathy (MPPE). Flat diffuse serous retinal detachment and multiple retinal exudations are seen.

however, showed that extravascular leakage from the choroidal vessels still remained, and in the late phase, diffuse marked hyperfluorescence persisted.

Discussion

In MPPE, ICG angiography revealed the following findings:

1. In the early phase, dilatation of the choroidal vein and delayed perfusion in the choroidal circulation in only some cases.
2. In the middle phase, marked extravascular leakages from the choroidal vessels in almost all cases.
3. In the late phase, marked diffuse staining by ICG in the choroid in almost all cases 90%. These findings were seen from the posterior pole to the equator.

Iida[13] demonstrated that extravascular leakages from the choroidal vessels in MPPE was due to increased permeability of these vessels, and he suggested that this may be the primary cause of this disease.

In CSC, Hayashi[8], Scheider[9], Piccolino[10], Guyer[11] and Iida[12] showed extravascular leakage from the choroidal vessels in the middle phase of ICG

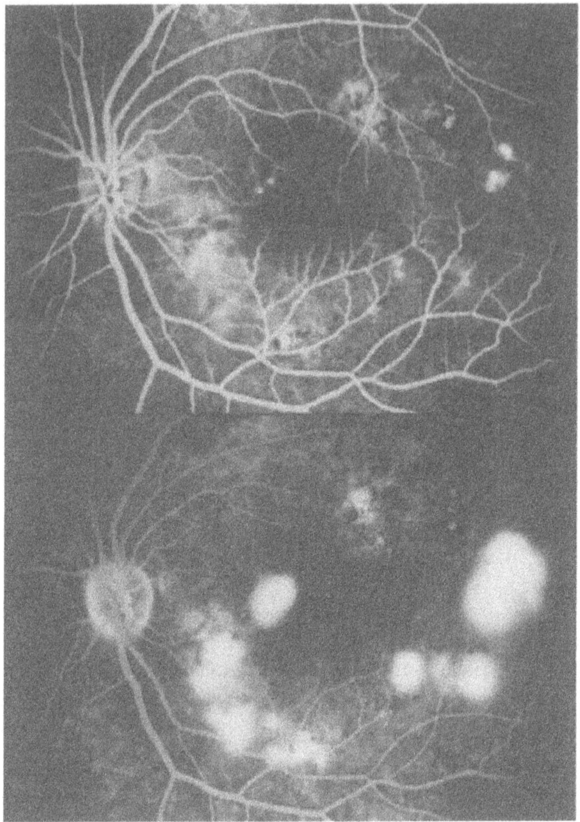

Fig. 2. Fluorescein fundus angiography of the same patient as Fig. 1. Upper: In the early phase, many pinpoint leakages at the retinal pigment epithelium, which correspond to the retinal exudations. Bottom: In the late phase, marked leakages from the choroid into the subretinal space are seen.

angiography, with tissue staining in the choroid in the late phase. This suggests that the primary lesion in this disease may be in the choroidal vessels. These findings in CSC were similar to that in MPPE. In MPPE, however, abnormal findings were more widespread and appeared diffusely in the posterior pole. In CSC, abnormalities in the choroid which were demonstrated by ICG angiography were localized in a small area and less remarkable.

The middle phase of ICG angiography showed marked extravascular leakage from the choroidal vessels. These leakages seemed to be due to hyperpermeability of the choroidal vessels, probably from the choriocapillaris. In our experiments to prove localization of ICG in the choroid[14], background fluorescence in the late phase of ICG angiography was a manifestation of

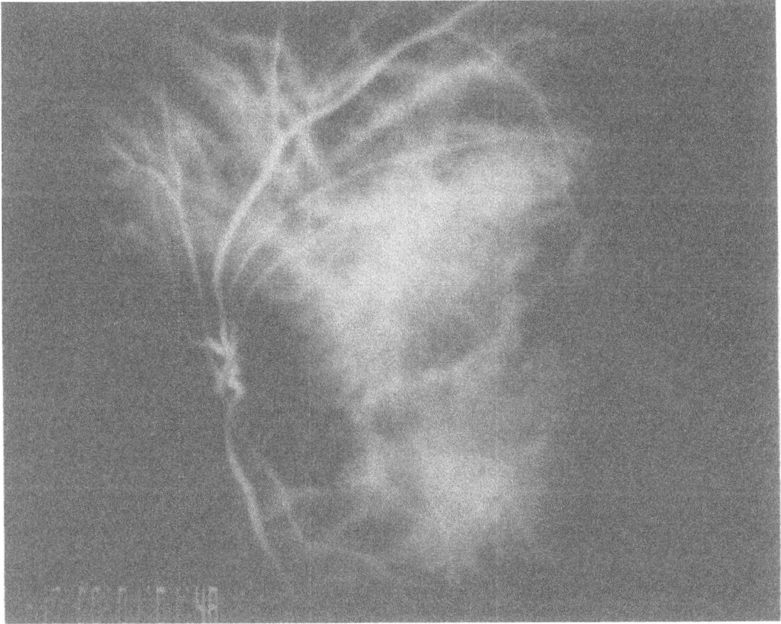

Fig. 3.   ICG angiography of the same patient as Fig. 1. In the middle phase (1 min), hyperfluorescence due to extravascular leakage in the choroid is diffuse and widespread.

pooling of ICG in the choroidal stroma-derived leakage from the choriocapillaris. The marked hyperfluorescence in the late phase of ICG angiography was, therefore, interpreted as a manifestation of excess pooling of ICG in the choroidal stroma from the hyperpermeable choriocaprellaris. Hayashi[8] demonstrated congestion of the choroidal vein in ICG angiography; however, these findings were seen in a small number of eyes by Iida[13] and us. Thus, we did think this finding may not be essential.

From these ICG angiographic findings of MPPE, we can suggest the following model for the pathophysiology of MPPE (Fig. 5).

1. The primary cause of this disease must be hyperpermeabity in the choroidal vessels, probably in the choriocapillaris. Excess fluids then accumulate in the choroidal stroma, derived from extravasation from the choroidal vessels. These pathologies are subclinical and potentially without clinical manifestations.
2. This pathology damages the RPE, and initiators such as high dose steroids or renal insufficiency promote damage of the RPE[15].
3. Destruction of the outer blood retinal barrier occurs as a result of damage to the RPE, and fluid in the choroid leaks into the subretinal space through damaged RPE.

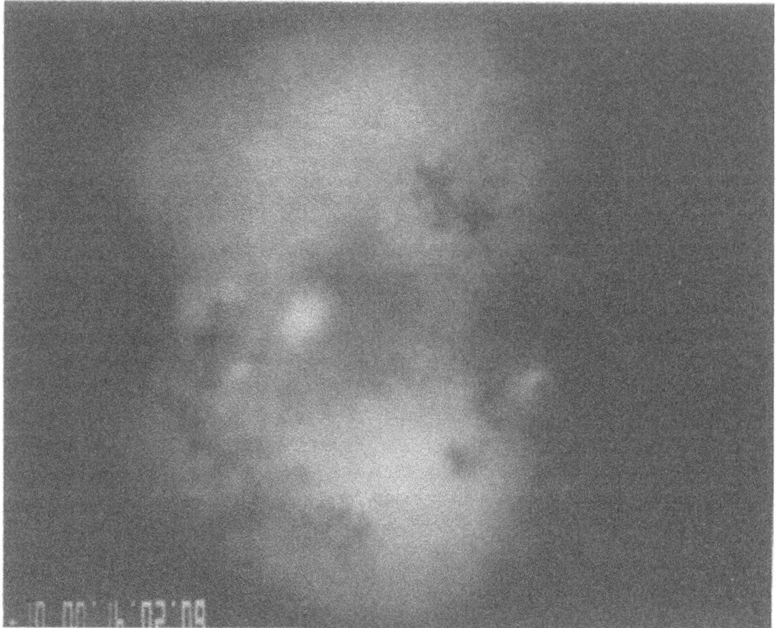

Fig. 4. In the late phase 15 min diffuse, marked hyperfluorescence is seen in the posterior pole, suggesting increased permeability in the choriocapillaris in the posterior pole.

4. Active fluid movement from the retina outwards across the RPE[16,17] is inhibited by damage of the RPE.
5. These processes result in fluid accumulating in the subretinal space, and the disease develops to give clinical manifestation of MPPE.

The pathophysiology of MPPE has a great similarity to that of CSC. Before ICG angiography became available, fluorescein angiography suggested that the primary cause of CSC as well as MPPE may be damage to the RPE. However, ICG angiography suggests that the primary cause of these diseases may be in the choroidal vessels, particularly in their hyperpermeability. Damage to the RPE may be secondary. There are many similarities between MPPE and CSC, such as fluorescein and ICG angiography appearances, effect of laser photocoagulation treatment and prevalence in middle-aged males, but there also are multiple differences, including massive, profound and many leakages in fluorescein angiography, bullous retinal detachment, retinal exudations, and involvement in both eyes in MPPE.

From those facts, we conclude that CSC and MPPE are at the both ends of the same spectrum, but MPPE is a distinct clinical entity.

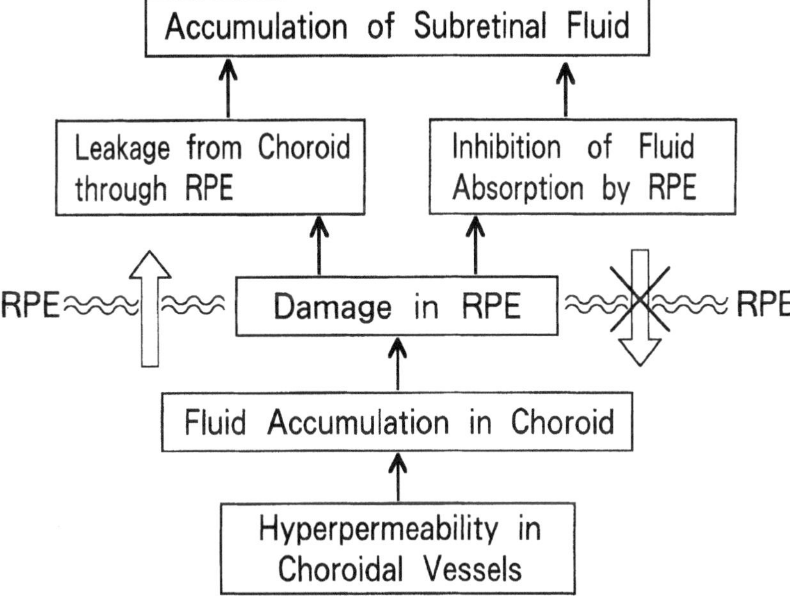

Fig. 5. Pathophysiology of MPPE (schema), primary cause may be hyperpermeability in the choriocapillaris, and damage to the retinal pigment epithelium may be secondary.

References

1. Gass, J.D.M. Bullous retinal detachment, an unusual manifestation of indiopathic central serous choroidopathy. Am J Ophthalmol. 1973; 75: 810–821.
2. Uyama, M., Tsukahara, I., Asayama, K. Multifocal posterior pigment epitheliopathy, clinical features and treatment with photocoagulation. Jpn J Clin Ophthalmol. 1977; 31: 359–372.
3. O'Connor, P.R. Multifocal serous choroidopathy. Ann Ophthalmol. 1975; 7: 237–245.
4. De Bustros, S., Michels, R.G., Rice, T.A., Knox, D.L. Treatment of idiopathic exudative retinal detachment. Retina. 1984; 4: 158–162.
5. Tsukahara, I., Uyama, M. Central serous choroidopathy with bullous retinal detachment. Graefes Arch Klin Exp Phthalmol. 1978; 206: 169–178.
6. Benson, W.E., Shields, J.A., Annesley, W.H. et al. Idiopathic central serous chorioretinopathy with bullous retinal detachment. Ann Ophthalmol. 1980; 12: 920–924.
7. Matsunaga, H., Nishimura, T., Uyama, M. Recent cases of multifocal posterior pigment epitheliopathy. Jpn J Clin Ophthalmol. 1992; 46: 729–733.
8. Hayashi, K., Hasegawa, Y., Tokoro, T. Indocyanine green angiography of central serous chorioretinopathy. Int Ophthalmol. 1986; 9: 37–41.
9. Scheider, A., Nasemann, J.E., Lund, O.E. Fluorescein and indocyanine green angiographies of central serous choroidopathy by scanning laser ophthalmoscopy. Am J Ophthalmol. 1993; 115: 50–56.
10. Piccolino, F.C., Borgia, L. Central serous chorioretinopathy and indocyanine green angiography. Retina. 1994; 14: 231–242.
11. Guyer, D.R., Yannuzzi, L.A., Slakter, J.S. et al. Digital indocyanine green videoangiography of central serous chorioretinopathy. Arch Ophthalmol. 1994; 112: 1057–1062.
12. Iida, T., Muraoka, K., Hagimura, N. et al. Choroidal lesions of central serous chorioretinopathy by indocyanine green angiography. Jpn J Ophthalmol. 1994; 48: 1583–1593.

13. Iida, T., Hagimura, N., Otani, T. et al. Choroidal vascular lesions in serous retinal detachment viewed with indocyanine green angiography. J Jpn Ophthalmol. 1996; 100: 817–824.
14. Matsubara, T. Histological localization of indocyanine green in the retina and choroid. Jpn J Clin Ophthalmol. 1995; 49: 25–33.
15. Kishimoto, N., Uyama, M., Fukushima, I. et al. The effect of corticosteroid on the repair of the retinal pigment epithelium. Acta Soc Ophthalmol Jpn. 1993; 97: 360–369.
16. Spitznas, M. Pathogenesis of central serous retinopathy: a new working hypothesis. Graefe's Arch Clin Exp Ophthalmol. 1986; 224: 321–324.
17. Marmor, M.F. New hypotheses on the pathogenesis and treatment of serous retinal detachment. Graefe's Arch Clin Exp Ophthalmol. 1988; 226: 548–552.

Department of Ophthalmology
Kansai Medical University
Moriguchi, Osaki 570
Japan

43. Idiopathic serous pigment epithelium detachment and indocyanine green angiography

A. GIOVANNINI, B. SCASSELLATI-SFORZOLINI,
E. D'ALTOBRANDO and C. MARIOTTI

(Ancona, Italy)

Introduction

Serous pigment epithelium detachment (PED) is a non-specific reaction of the retinal pigment epithelium (RPE) to trauma affecting its adhesion with Bruch's membrane. Idiopathic PED or of the young is a subgroup of central serous chorioretinopathy with onset before 50 years of age, in the absence of retinal and/or choroidal alterations. The aim of our study was to analyse the choroidal alterations, detected by indocyanine green angiography (ICGA), associated with idiopathic PED.

Materials and methods

Forty-two eyes of 26 consecutive patients (17 males and nine females; age 26–48 years; mean age 37.4) affected by idiopathic PED were studied. The follow up was 1–43 months (mean 21 months). The patients included in our study had no sign of general or other ocular diseases. All patients underwent a complete ophthalmic examination; retinography, fluorescein angiography (FA) and ICGA were performed in both eyes of each patient. FA and ICGA were performed with a high definition videoangiography system (Topcon Imagenet H1024).

Results

On FA an early, complete and homogeneous filling of the PED was observed in all patients; the hyperfluorescence increased in the late phases with well defined edges (Figs 1–3). ICGA always showed early, complete and homogeneous filling of the PED with well defined margins and a peak of fluorescence during the middle phases. The ICGA pattern in the late phases changed with the size of the detachment[1]. PED bigger than one optic disk in diameter showed a hyperfluorescence in the late phases of ICGA, surrounded by a ring of brighter hyperfluorescence (Fig. 1). A wash-out of ICG was observed in

G. Coscas and F. Cardillo Piccolino (eds.), Retinal Pigment Epithelium and Macular Diseases, pp. 263–267.
© *1998 Kluwer Academic Publishers.*

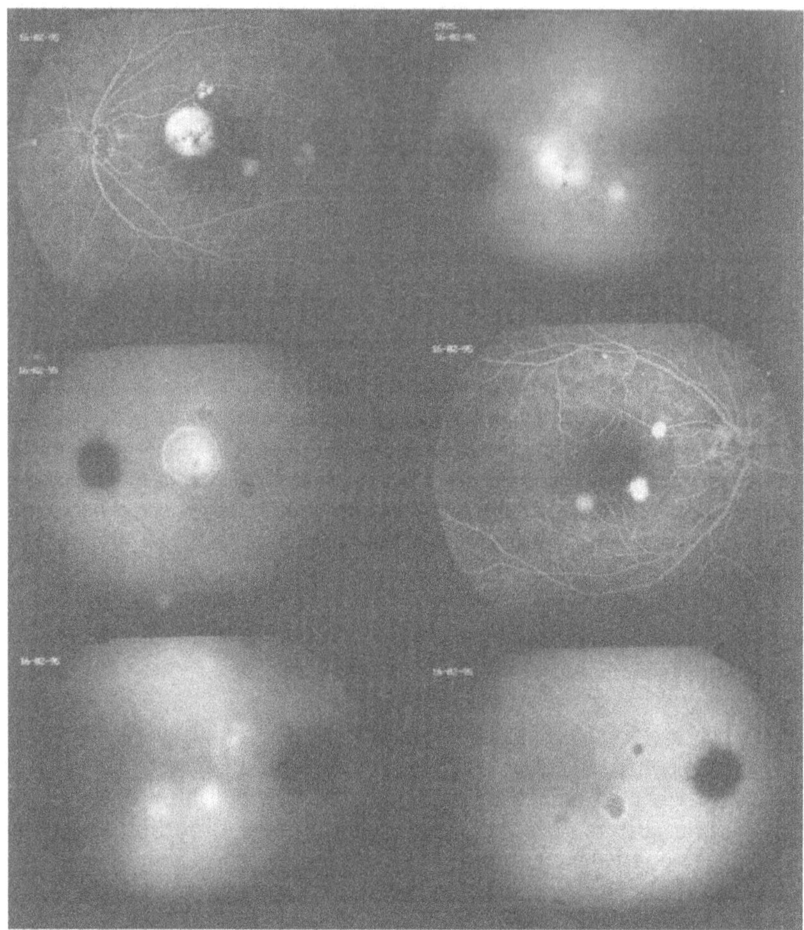

Fig. 1. Bilateral idiopathic PED in a 41-year-old male. (A) FA: multiple PED can be observed. (B) Middle phase of ICGA: the PED are hyperfluorescent; the leakage of dye can be seen around the detachments. (C) Late phase of ICGA: the PED bigger than one optic disk diameter is still hyperfluorescent with well defined margins, surrounded by a ring of brighter hyperfluorescence; the smaller ones (arrow) show a late wash out of the dye with a hyperfluorescent ring. (D) The FA shows multiple PED smaller than one optic disk diameter in the fellow eye. (E) In the middle phases of ICGA a choroidal leakage can be observed around the detachments. (F) The typical ICG pattern in the late phases is clearly visible (arrows).

PED smaller than one optic disk in diameter. In the late phases a hypofluorescent area surrounded by a hyperfluorescent ring was visible (Figs 1, 3). Sometimes the PED was no more visible in the late phases.

In 35 eyes (83.3%) and five unaffected eyes choroidal permeability alterations, similar to that of CSC, were seen on ICGA in the middle phases

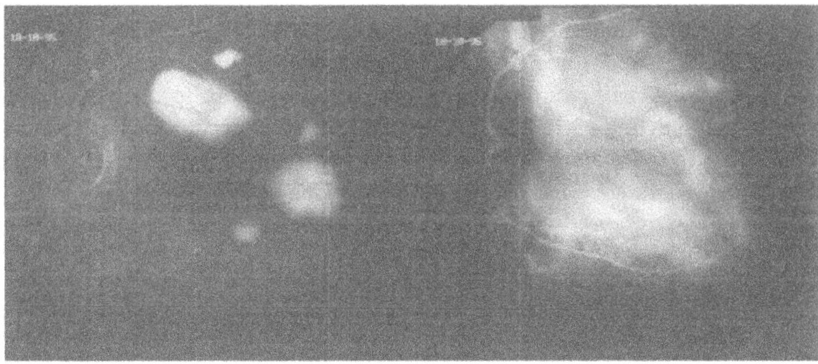

Fig. 2. Left eye of a 45-year-old male with multiple idiopathic PED. (A) FA: six PEDs are visible. (B) Early phase of ICGA: dilatation of the choroidal veins is evident (arrows).

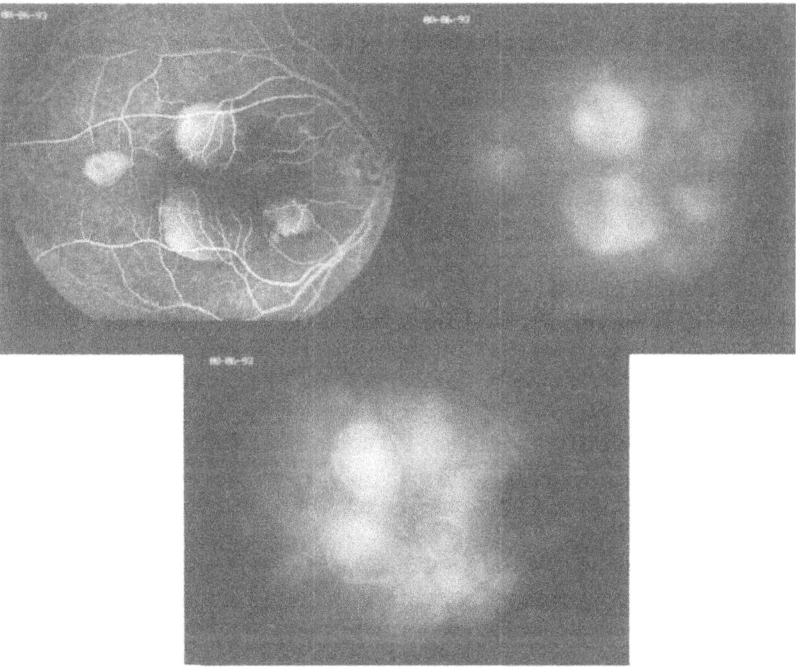

Fig. 3. Right eye of a 34-year-old female with multiple idiopathic PED. (A) FA: multiple PEDs are evident. (B) Middle phase of ICGA: a widespread choroidal hyperpermeability is evident. (C) Late phase of ICGA: the bigger detachments are still hyperfluorescent while the smaller ones are hypofluorescent with or without a hyperfluorescent ring.

(Fig. 1), sometimes the leakage was multifocal, involving the choroid far from the sites of detachment (Fig. 3). In 16 eyes (38.1%) ICGA showed irregular dilatation of the choroidal veins in the area of the detachments (Fig. 2); in two cases the same finding was also present in the unaffected eye. In 17 eyes (40.5%) focal delays of the choroidal perfusion were observed near the detachments, but in the majority of cases the choroidal filling was complete within 8 s. During follow-up no choroidal neovascularization developed in any affected or fellow eyes.

Discussion

ICGA showed areas of choroidal hyperpermeability associated with idiopathic PED in 34 eyes (82.9%) and in two unaffected fellow eyes: these data are similar to those of CSC[2-6].

The ICG filling of idiopathic PED and the observation of areas of choroidal leakage suggest that a widespread alteration in choroidal permeability may involved in the pathogenesis of idiopathic PED. That supports the hypothesis of Gass[7,8], that idiopathic PED is secondary to choroidal exudation. In fact ICG is highly bound to plasma proteins and diffuses in the early and middle phases only when altered permeability of the choroidal vessels is present.

The visualization in 16 eyes (39%) of irregular dilatation of the choroidal veins adjacent to the detachments is further evidence that alterations at the level of the choroidal vessels may be important in the pathogenesis of the disease. Prünte and Flammer[9] made the same observation on 32 patients affected by CSC. These authors hypothesized that increased choroidal permeability would be the consequence of localized capillary and venous congestion in the choroid, resulting in increased exudation of fluid and plasma proteins (together with protein bound ICG) from the choriocapillaris. Prünte and Flammer[9] presumed that focal ischaemia of choroidal lobules could be the primary abnormality of CSC; in our patients we observed focal areas of delayed choroidal filling in the same area as the PED in 40.5% of the affected eyes. As in CSC, where the data are controversial[2-6,9], it is difficult to establish a relationship between idiopathic PED and delayed choroidal filling.

The ICG study supports the hypothesis of Lewis that idiopathic PED is a variant of CSC[10], this is confirmed by our study on 26 patients affected by idiopathic PED.

Our observations could add new information on the pathogenesis of idiopathic PED and on the possible correlations between this disease and CSC. These hypotheses remain speculative and further studies on larger series are needed to confirm our findings.

References

1. Giovannini, A, Scassellati Sforzolini, B., Tittarelli, R. Indocyanine angiographic findings in idiopathic serous pigment epithelium detachment. Invest Ophthalmol Vis Sci. 1994; 35: 1507.

2. Hayashi, K., Hasegawa, Y., Tokoro, T. Indocyanine green angiography of central serous chorioretinopathy. Int Ophthalmol. 1986; 9: 37–41.
3. Scheider, A., Nasemann, J.E., Lund, O.E. Fluorescein and Indocyanine green angiographies of central serous choroidopathy by scanning laser ophthalmoscopy. Am J Ophthalmol. 1993; 115: 50–56.
4. Cardillo Piccolino, F., Borgia, L. Central serous chorioretinopathy and indocyanine green angiography. Retina. 1994; 14: 231–242.
5. Cardillo Piccolino, F., Borgia, L., Zinicola, E., Zingirian, M. Indocyanine green angiographic findings in central serous chorioretinopathy. Eye. 1995; 9: 324–332.
6. Guyer, D.R., Yannuzzi, L.A., Slakter, J.S., Sorenson, J.A., Ho, A., Orlock, D. Digital indocyanine green videoangiography of central serous chorioretinopathy. Arch Ophthalmol. 1994; 112: 1057–1062.
7. Gass, J.D., Norton, E.W.D., Justice, J. Serous detachment of the retinal pigment epithelium. Trans Am Acad Ophthalmol Otolaryngol. 1966; 70: 990–1015.
8. Gass, J.D.M. Pathogenesis of disciform detachment of the neuroepithelium. Am J Ophthalmol. 1967; 63: 573–615.
9. Prünte, C., Flammer, J. Choroidal capillary and venous congestion in central serous chorioretinopathy. Am J Ophthalmol. 1996; 121: 26–34.
10. Lewis, M.L. Idiopathic serous detachment of the retinal pigment epithelium. Arch Ophthalmol. 1978; 96: 620–624.

Department of Ophthalmology
University of Ancona
Ospedale di Torrette
60020 Ancona, Italy

44. Propranolol and nimodipine in the treatment of acute and chronic central serous choroidopathy

F. BANDELLO, A. MALEGORI, F. MAGONIO and R. BRANCATO

(Ferrara and Milan, Italy)

Introduction

The pathogenesis of central serous choroidopathy (CSC) is still unknown. In the past an important role of retinal pigment epithelium had been assumed by many authors[1-4]. Routinary use of indocyanine green (ICG) angiography has recently demonstrated disturbances in choroidal haemodynamics in most cases of CSC[5-7], with late hyperfluorescence noted in the great majority of studies. Such hyperfluorescence has been interpreted as secondary to an increase of blood flow[7] or to ischaemic damage of the choriocapillaris[5,6]. Scheider *et al.*[6] described early hypofluorescence in the same affected areas and speculated that the reduction of blood supply could be a primary stage of CSC pathogenesis. On the basis of these features a pathogenesis of the disease similar to that of migraine could be assumed:

1. Reduction of blood supply;
2. Ischaemic damage to choriocapillaris;
3. Increased protein concentration in the extracellular space;
4. Accumulation of fluid in the extracellular space.

Beta-blockers and calcium channel blockers are the most effective drugs in the chronic treatment of migraine and are routinary used for the therapy of this condition[8-11]. We performed a double-blind study to evaluate the usefulness of propranolol (a non-selective beta-blocker) and nimodipine (a calcium channel blocker with selective action on intracranial vessels) in patients with acute and chronic decompensation of retinal pigment epithelium.

Patients and methods

After informed consent, all patients affected by acute or chronic CSC, examined in our Department between November 1994 and May 1996 were evaluated for inclusion in the study.

The inclusion criteria were age over 18, with acute or chronic decompensation of retinal pigment epithelium. Exclusion criteria were diabetes, asthma, heart or hepatic diseases, hypertension, allergy to fluorescein or iodine media, and other pharmacologic therapies.

G. Coscas and F. Cardillo Piccolino (eds.), Retinal Pigment Epithelium and Macular Diseases, pp. 269–273.
© *1998 Kluwer Academic Publishers.*

Twelve patients with acute and 42 with chronic CSC (16 and 78 eyes, respectively) were included in the study. The clinical characteristics of the included patients are summarized in Table 1. Each patient underwent first a medical examination and then a complete ophthalmologic evaluation, fluorescein as well as ICG angiography. Thereafter patients were randomly allocated to 2 weeks therapy with propranolol, nimodipine or placebo. Dosage was 20 mg three times a day for propranolol and 40 mg three times a day for nimodipine. At the end of the therapy patients underwent a further complete ophthalmologic evaluation, fluorescein and ICG angiographies.

Of the 12 patients affected by acute CSC, two (three eyes) were treated with propranolol, five (eight eyes) with nimodipine and five (five eyes) with placebo. In the group with chronic CSC, 14 patients received propranolol (26 eyes), 14 received nimodipine (25 eyes) and 14 received placebo (27 eyes).

Visual acuity, positive scotomatas and metamorphosias were the functional parameters considered. Number of leaking points and amount of leakage were the parameters examined on fluorescein angiograms. The dynamics of choroidal circulation (perfusion defects in the early phases, number and extension of the hyperfluorescences in the late phases) was examined on ICG angiograms. Considering these parameters an overall judgment of improvement, worsening or stability was assigned to each eye for fluorescein as well as for ICG angiography. Clinical evaluation and interpretation of the results were carried out unaware of the treatment employed. Fisher's exact test was used for stastical analysis of the results, and all adverse reactions were recorded.

Results

Eyes showing improvement, stability or worsening of visual acuity at the end of the study are described in Table 2. Comparing improved eyes with the worsened or unchanged ones showed no stastically significant difference between patients treated with the two drugs or placebo in either the acute and chronic group.

Eyes showing an improvement on fluorescein or ICG angiograms after therapy are reported in Tables 3 and 4 respectively. In the acute CSC group

Table 1. Clinical characteristics of the patients included in the study.

	Acute CSC	*Chronic CSC*
Age	43 (ds: 7.72)	45 (ds: 8.40)
Sex (males)	9 (75%)	38 (90%)
Visual acuity	0.72 (ds: 0.25)	0.68 (ds: 0.32)
Disease duration (years)	0.28 (ds: 0.26)	3.29 (ds:3.57)

Table 2. Modification of visual acuity after treatment.

	Propranolol		Nimodipine		Placebo	
	Improved	*Unchanged, worsened*	*Improved*	*Unchanged, worsened*	*Improved*	*Unchanged, worsened*
Acute CSC	0	3	2	6	2	3
Chronic CSC	3	23	4	21	5	22

Table 3. Evolution of fluorescein angiography picture after therapy.

	Propranolol		Nimodipine		Placebo	
	Improved	*Unchanged, worsened*	*Improved*	*Unchanged, worsened*	*Improved*	*Unchanged, worsened*
Acute CSC	1	2	3	5	3	2
Chronic CSC	5	21	4	21	0	27

Table 4. Evolution of ICG picture after therapy.

	Propranolol		Nimodipine		Placebo	
	Improved	*Unchanged, worsened*	*Improved*	*Unchanged, worsened*	*Improved*	*Unchanged, worsened*
Acute CSC	1	2	1	7	1	4
Chronic CSC	4	22	2	23	1	26

analysis of fluorescein and ICG angiograms showed no statistically significant difference between patients taking placebo and the two drugs. In the chronic group, however, fluorescein angiography demonstrated a significant difference between eyes treated with propranolol ($p = 0.023$) and nimodipine ($p = 0.047$) compared with those treated with placebo.

Adverse reactions are shown in Table 5. They were always very mild, except

Table 5. Side effects registered during treatment.

Propranolol	Nimodipine
Asthenia (4)	Migraine (1)
Arterial hypotension (2)	Hot flush (2)
Sexual impotence (2)	Mouth dryness (1)
Bradycardia (1)	Dizziness (1)
Somnolence (1)	
Weight gain (1)	

in four cases in whom therapy had to be discontinued (two cases of sexual impotence and one of bradicardia with propranolol and one case of migraine with nimodipine).

Discussion

In 1966 Potts[12] demonstrated the role of the adrenergic system in the regulation of macular circulation. Yannuzzi[13], in 1986, described a relationship between CSC and type A behaviour, characterized by increased activity of adrenergic system. These observations induced Avci and Deutmann[14] to start a clinical experience on the treatment of acute and chronic CSC with a beta-blocker. In their study, published in 1993, all six patients treated wih metoprolol showed a significant improvement of symptoms and no relapse of the disease during treatment. Moreover improvements in ICG angiography quality of these last years have demonstrated disturbances of choroidal circulation in patients affected by acute and chronic CSC[5-7]. CSC pathogenesis may be somewhat similar to that of migraine, and the use of beta blockers and calcium channnel blockers seems reasonable.

We decided to study separately patients with the acute and the chronic form of the disease since these two clinical forms appear quite different from many points of view, including natural history, prognosis and, probably, response to treatment. This decision, however, led to a small number of patients in each group, especially with typical CSC. Moreover tendency to spontaneous regression, a typical characteristic of this form, made it difficult to analyse the results of this group. Since this form of the disease shows an acute course, the effects of treatment will appear different depending on whether clinical observation is started at the beginning or towards the end of the episode.

Considering patients with the chronic form, evaluation of fluorescein angiograms showed a therapeutical efficacy of both propranolol and nimodipine. The same results was not observed evaluating ICG frames or visual acuity. It seems likely that these latter parameters were not able to detect mild modifications of chronic lesions such as those presented by most patients included in the study.

In conclusion, our results confirm only partially the first very positive experience referred by Avci and Deutmann with metoprolol and further investigations are necessary to confirm the utility of these drugs in the treatment of CSC.

References

1. Maumenee, A.E. Symposium: macular diseases. Pathogenesis. Trans Am Acad Ophthalmol Otolaryngol. 1965; 69: 691–699.

2. Gass, J.D.M. Pathogenesis of the disciform detachment of the neuroepithelium. II. Idiopathic central serous choroidopathy. Am J Ophthalmol. 1967; 63: 587–615.

3. Spitznas, M. Pathogenesis of central serous retinopathy: a new working hypothesis. Graefe's Arch Clin Exp Ophthalmol. 1986; 224: 321–324.

4. Marmor, M.F. New hypotheses on the pathogenesis and treatment of serous retinal detachment. Graefe's Arch Clin Exp Ophthalmol. 1988; 226: 548–552.

5. Hayashi, K., Hasegawa, Y., Tokoro, I. Indocyanine green angiography of central serous chorioretinopathy. Int Ophthalmol. 1986; 9: 37–41.

6. Scheider, A., Nasemann, J.E., Lund, O.E. Fluorescein and indocyanine green angiographies of central serous choroidopathy by scanning laser ophthalmoscopy. Am J Ophthalmol. 1993; 115: 50–56.

7. Cardillo Piccolino, F., Borgia, L. Central serous chorioretinopathy and indocyanine green angiography. Retina. 1994; 14: 231–242.

8. Diamond, S., Millstein, E. Current concepts of migraine therapy. J Clin Pharmacol. 1988; 28: 193–199.

9. Diamond, S., Solomon, G.D. Pharmacologic treatment of migraine. Ration Drug Ther. 1988; 22: 1–6.

10. Spierings, E.L.H. Clinical and experimental evidence for a role of calcium entry blockers in the treatment of migraine. Ann NY Acad Sci. 1988; 522: 676–689.

11. Greenberg, D.A. Calcium channel antagonists and the treatment of migraine. Clin Neuropharmacol. 1988; 9: 311–328.

12. Potts, A.M. An hypothesis on macular diseases. Trans Am Acad Ophthalmol Otolaryngol. 1966; 70: 1058.

13. Yannuzzi, L.A. Type A behavior and central serous chorio-retinopathy. I. Clinical findings. Trans Am Ophthalmol Soc. 1986; 84: 799–845.

14. Avci, R., Deutman, A.S. Die Behandlung der zentralen serösen Choroidopathie mit dem Betarezeptorenblocker Metoprolol (Vorläufige Ergebnisse). Klin Monatsbl Augenheilk. 1993; 202: 199–205.

R. Brancato
Department of Ophthalmology and Visual Sciences
Scientific Institute H S. Raffaele
Via Olgettina 60, 20132 Milano, Italy

45. Photic maculopathy in a patient under treatment with clomipramine and bright light therapy

L. LOBEFALO, L. MASTROPASQUA, A. LIBERATOSCIOLI,
L. COLANGELO, E. D'ANTONIO and P.E. GALLENGA

(Chieti, Italy)

Introduction

Seasonal affective disorder (SAD), first described by Rosenthal *et al.*[1], is characterized by recurrent episodes of winter depressions with summer remissions. Symptoms of SAD include increased sleep, fatigue, carbohydrate craving and dysphoric mood. It is estimated that in the USA this syndrome affects about 11 million people at syndromal levels and about 25 million people at subsyndromal levels[2].

In the last few years, the use of artificial bright light for the treatment of winter depression and various circadian rhythm disturbances has been reported[3]. Some parameters of interest for the therapeutic use of light include light intensity, disease duration, exposure time and, in particular, light wavelength. Most studies of light therapy have used full-spectrum fluorescent lights. Light sources used for this therapy include both full-spectrum fluorescent light, emitting small amounts of ultraviolet (UV) light, and incandescent light sources with negligible UV emission[4].

The evidence that prolonged exposure even to small amounts of UV radiation may induce retinal damage, has led several authors to underline the potential risk of this therapy[4,5]. We report a case of bilateral photic retinopathy after bright light therapy for SAD in a patient treated with clomipramine.

Case report

In January 1995, a 35-year-old man, came to our observation for a bilateral reduction of visual acuity and a positive central scotoma. This patient suffered from no systemic disease apart from a clinical history of depression, matching DSM-III-R diagnostic criteria for recurrent major depression, seasonal pattern, and was undergoing a 2-week bright light therapeutic cycle. When observed for the first time, the patient had undergone five daily sessions each lasting 60 min between 6.00 and 8.00 p.m. Light treatment had been performed

G. Coscas and F. Cardillo Piccolino (eds.), Retinal Pigment Epithelium and Macular Diseases, pp. 275–278.
© *1998 Kluwer Academic Publishers.*

with full-spectrum fluorescent light (Vitalities, Durotest Canada Inc., Toronto, Canada) at 5000 lux. During treatment, the patient did not discontinue his current medication (clomipramine 100 mg per day).

At first observation, best corrected visual acuity was 40/200 (ETDRS chart) in both eyes and a marked reduction of contrast sensitivity at all frequencies was found (Vistech 6500 chart); Amsler grid test showed the presence of a bilateral central scotoma. Central visual field (Humphrey perimeter; program 10-2) showed normal data with the exception of a bilateral marked reduction of foveal threshold (RE 11 dB; LE 9 dB). Both maculae demonstrated the loss of the foveolar reflex and the presence of a central yellowish-white lesion, with surrounding orange-red halo at the level of the retinal pigment epithelium (Fig. 1a, b). Fluorescein angiography revealed no foveal staining or leakage.

The patient was treated with 8 mg methylprednisolone per day intravenously for 3 days. One month later visual acuity was 20/20 in both eyes. Contrast sensitivity and foveal threshold showed only a slight impairment; a small positive central scotoma was detected using Amsler grid test. In both eyes foveolar reflex was absent, but there was no sign of other lesions.

During the following year a further slight functional impairment was still present and contrast sensitivity at high frequencies and central scotoma persisted. An electroretinogram 1 year after the first presentation was normal.

Discussion

We report bilateral photic maculopathy developing in a patient who had been treated for 5 days with light therapy. To our knowledge this is the first report of ocular damage secondary to bright light therapy. An important factor in the development of photic maculopathy is that the patient did not discontinue

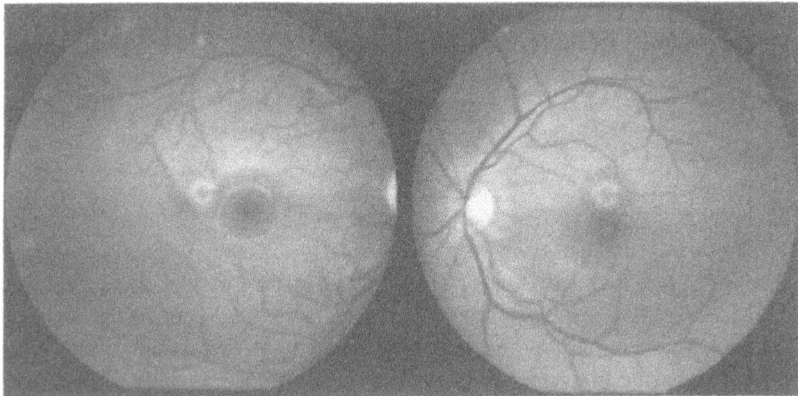

Fig. 1a, b. Ophthalmoscopic appearance showing bilateral central yellow white lesions with surrounding orange-red discoloration.

the concurrent clomipramine medication. This tricyclic antidepressant agent could be an active photosensitizer: the presence of three fused aromatic rings gives this drug long-lived triplet states, low oxidation potential status and the possibility to transfer energy to ground state oxygen[6]. Moreover, several polycyclic aromatic compounds, both antipsychotic and antidepressant agents, have a high affinity for melanin[6-8] and the extensive accumulation of drugs by melanin appears the most important factor governing the long-term therapeutic/toxicological activities[9]. Furthermore, high-affinity binding sites for antidepressant tricyclic drugs were detected in chicken and pig retinas[10]. The anticholinergic effect of clomipramine on the pupil size could increase the potential risk of retinal hazard, thus having a cumulative effect with photosensitization.

Our patient had undergone routine ophthalmologic examination by his private consultant 3 months before starting therapy and no retinal abnormalities had been found. On the basis of this evidence, we suggest that photic maculopathy could be related to light therapy and clomipramine photosensitizing effect.

Many authors[2,5,11,12] have underlined the potential risk of bright light therapy, recommending ophthalmologic examination before therapy in all forms of light therapy, even when there is no history of eye complaints. We agree with this statement, but the absence of retinal abnormalities is not sufficient to avoid retinal complication related to light therapy, as demonstrated in our case report. Levitt *et al.*[13] reported the usefulness of bright light therapy in the treatment of recurrent major depression in 10 subjects who had not discontinued medications, including imipramine and amitriptyline. In this study the light parameters, intensity and type of source, were similar to that used in our case, i.e. fluorescent light at 5000 lux for 1 h or, in non-responders, for 2 h per day for 2 weeks. However, in this series, no ophthalmologic examination was performed before or after therapy, so it is not possible to determine whether this treatment caused any retinal damage. In a selected group of patients treated with bright light therapy, Gallin *et al.*[2] found no ocular abnormalities after short-term or long-term treatment. However, the light parameters in the latter study were very different from those in our case, using a higher illuminance but minimizing the ultraviolet radiation, and current treatment with psychotropic or photosensitizing medications was an exclusion criterion.

Another factor which might have contributed to the development of photic maculopathy is that our patient was exposed for a long time to outdoor light and that there was a very clear sky during the last few days before the development of symptoms.

In conclusion, we suggest that several co-factors led to the development of photic retinopathy in this case and, as suggested by Terman *et al.*[14], bright light therapy in association with photosensitizing drugs may induce retinal damage.

References

1. Rosenthal, N.E., Sack, D.A., Gillin, A.J. *et al.* Seasonal affective disorder: a description of the syndrome and preliminary findings with light therapy. Arch Gen Psychiatry. 1984; 41: 72–80.
2. Gallin, P.F., Terman, M., Remè, C.E., Rafferty, B., Terman, J.S., Burde, R.M. Ophthalmologic examination of patients with seasonal affective disorder, before and after bright light therapy. Am J Ophthalmol. 1995; 119: 202–210.
3. Parry, B.L., Berga, S.I., Mostofi, N., Sependa, P.A., Kripke, D.F., Gillin, J.C. Morning versus evening bright light treatment of late luteal phase dysphoric disorder. Am J Psychiatry. 1989; 146: 1215–1217.
4. Buchanan, A., Clark, M.C., Remick, R.A. Ultraviolet versus non-ultraviolet light therapy for seasonal affective disorder. J Clin Psychiatry. 1991; 52: 213–216.
5. Vanselow, W., Dennerstein, L., Armstrong, S., Lockie, P. Retinopahty and bright light therapy. Am J Psychiatry. 1991; 148: 1266–1267.
6. Lerman, S. Photosensitizing drugs and their possible role in enhancing ocular toxicity. Ophthalmology. 1986; 93: 304–318.
7. Meier-Ruge, W. Drug induced retinopathy. CRC Crit Rev Toxicol. 1972; 32: 352–380.
8. Persad, S., Menon, A., Basu, P.K., Haberman, H.F. Binding of imipramine, 8-methoxypsoralen, and epinephrine to human blue and brown melanins. J Toxicol Cutan Ocul Toxicol. 1986; 5: 125–132.
9. Salazar-Bookman, M.M., Wainer, I., Patil, P.N. Relevance of drug-melanin interactions to ocular pharmacology and toxicology. J Ocul Pharmacol. 1994; 10: 217–239.
10. Kari, E., Tuomisto, L., Airaksinen, M.M., Leino, M. [^{3}H]Imipramine binding in the retinas of chickens and pigs. Exp Eye Res. 1988: 47: 679–688.
11. Waxler, M., James, R.H., Brainard, G.C., Moul, D.E., Oren, D.A., Rosenthal, N.E. Retinopathy and bright light therapy. Am J Psychiatry. 1991; 149: 1610–1611.
12. Remè, C.E., Terman, M. Does light therapy present an ocular hazard? Am J Psychiatry. 1992; 149: 1762–1763.
13. Levitt, A.J., Joffe, R.T., Kennedy, S.H. Bright light augmentation in antidepressant nonresponders. J Clin Psychiatry. 1991; 52: 336–337.
14. Terman, M., Remè, C.E., Rafferty, B., Gallin, P.F., Terman, J.S. Bright light therapy for winter depression: potential ocular effects and theoretical implications. Photochem Photobiol. 1990; 51: 781–792.

Institute of Ophthalmology
'G. D'Annunzio' University
via Gran Sasso 100, Chieti I-66100, Italy

46. Dexamethasone treatment for solar retinopathy: long-term follow-up

L. LOBEFALO, L. MASTROPASQUA, G. DE NICOLA,
A.P. D'AURELIO, G. DELLA LOGGIA and P.E. GALLENGA

(Chieti, Italy)

Introduction

The damaging effect of light on the retina has received considerable attention. Visual loss associated with sungazing has been reported since the time of Plato, eclipse watching being the major cause of solar retinopathy. It has also been described in sunbathers, pilots, military recruits, in patients with mental illness and following religious rituals[1,2]. The aim of this 8-year case-control study was to evaluate the short- and long-term effects of solar retinopathy in a group of patients, who during the same religious ritual gazed at the sun in the effort to witness an apparition.

Patients and methods

Eighty-seven patients (31 male, 56 female: mean age 37.12 ± 7.51 years) were observed at the University Eye Clinic of Chieti from February 28th to March 1st 1988. All patients reported blurred vision and central scotoma; in 72 cases symptoms were bilateral. All patients had gazed at the sun at about noon on February 28th 1988 in an attempt to witness an apparition. There was a clear sky and no patient was wearing tinted lenses or filters. At first observation patients were randomly divided into two groups matched for age, sex and time of sunlight exposure (Table 1): group A comprised 32 patients (59 eyes) (nine male, 23 female: mean age 35.64 ± 6.47) treated with intravenous dexamethasone (8 mg/day) for 4 days and then with Deflazacort

Table 1. Exposure time in the three groups.

	Group A	Group B	Group C
<1 min	14	12	9
1–3 min	13	16	7
>3 min	5	6	5
Patients (no of eyes)	32 (59)	34 (65)	21 (35)

3×3 contingency tables: exposure time $p = 0.841$.

G. Coscas and F. Cardillo Piccolino (eds.), Retinal Pigment Epithelium and Macular Diseases, pp. 279–283.
© *1998 Kluwer Academic Publishers.*

30 mg/day for 10 days. Group B comprised 34 patients (65 eyes) (12 male, 22 female: mean age 37.51 ± 8.14) treated with Deflazacort 30 mg for 15 days. The remaining 21 patients (35 eyes; 10 male, 11 female; mean age 38.74 ± 7.95; group C) refused treatment and were used for this study as controls. All the other enrolled subjects signed their informed consent. The research followed the tenets of the Declaration of Helsinki and was approved by the Ethical Committee of the Medical Faculty of the University of Chieti.

Patients were followed up for 8 years, and the following parameters were measured at baseline, after 7 days, 1 month and at the end of the study: best corrected visual acuity, contrast sensitivity 3, 12 and 18 cps (Vistech 6500 chart), Amsler grid, colour vision test (Farnsworth 100 HUE; normal range was the age-corrected total error score as suggested by Verriest[3]), foveal threshold (mean of three tests; Humphrey 640 HFA perimeter) and colour retinography (Kowa RC-XF fundus camera). Fluorescein angiography (Kowa RC-XF fundus camera) was performed only in those patients showing the greatest functional impairment. Fluorescein angiography was performed after rapid injection of 2 ml 20% sodium fluorescein into the antecubital vein. Angiograms were taken with ASA400 black and white film.

Statistical analysis

Statistical analysis was performed with SPSS software package (Release 6.0, 444 N. Michigan Av. Chicago, Illinois, USA). To evaluate the intergroup differences at baseline and at each control, one-way ANOVA for visual acuity and foveal threshold and 3×2 contingency tables for colour vision, Amsler grid and contrast sensitivity tests were used. Intragroup modifications during the follow-up were evaluated by ANOVA for repeated measures (visual acuity and foveal threshold) and by 3×2 contingency tables (colour vision, Amsler grid and contrast sensitivity tests).

Results

Exposure time in the three subgroups is reported in Table 1. At baseline both corrected visual acuity and foveal threshold were similar in the three groups (Table 2). Further, no significant differences were found as regards the number of subjects with colour vision, Amsler grid test and contrast sensitivity values outside the normal range (Table 3). Seven days after exposure, visual acuity and foveal threshold in group A were significantly higher than in the other two groups (Table 2). Fewer subjects in group A had abnormal contrast sensitivity at high frequencies ($p < 0.001$), Amsler grid ($p = 0.003$) and colour vision test results ($p = 0.007$, Table 3).

One month after exposure and at the end of the follow-up visual acuity, foveal threshold, contrast sensitivity at low and middle sensitivity and Amsler grid test were similar in the three subgroups (Tables 2, 3). Colour vision

Table 2. Visual acuity and foveal threshold in the three groups during the study.

	Group	Baseline	1 week	1 month	8 years	p
Visual acuity	A	7.25 ± 1.67	$9.25 \pm 1.57^{a,b}$	9.81 ± 0.47	9.85 ± 0.45	<0.001
	B	7.29 ± 1.87	8.31 ± 2.12	9.68 ± 0.92	9.74 ± 0.76	<0.001
	C	7.34 ± 1.45	8.24 ± 2.03	9.60 ± 1.12	9.66 ± 1.16	<0.001
Foveal threshold	A	32.05 ± 3.73	$33.49 \pm 2.90^{c,d}$	33.92 ± 2.20	34.03 ± 1.53	0.008
(dB)	B	31.08 ± 3.83	31.97 ± 3.27	33.42 ± 2.12	33.82 ± 1.39	0.017
	C	31.86 ± 2.52	31.31 ± 3.02	33.57 ± 1.50	33.86 ± 1.44	0.012

[a] $p = 0.006$ vs group B.
[b] $p = 0.008$ vs group C.
[c] $p = 0.007$ vs Group B.
[d] $p < 0.001$ vs group C.

Table 3. Patients showing abnormal data at contrast sensitivity, colour vision and Amsler grid tests in the three groups during the study.

	Group	Baseline	1 week	1 month	8 years
Contrast sensitivity (eyes with abnormal data)					
3 cps/sec	A	15	3	1	4
	B	21	5	2	6
	C	8	2	1	2
12 cps	A	42	17	7	5
	B	48	29	9	7
	C	27	18	6	3
18 cps	A	50	22	9	5
	B	58	40 $p < 0.0001$	22 $p = 0.037$	17 $p = 0.018$
	C	28	27	12	10
Colour vision test (eyes with age-corrected abnormal data)					
TES	A	30	17	11	9
	B	37	31 $p = 0.007$	24 $p = 0.014$	12
	C	23	19	16	7
Amsler grid test (eyes with positive scotoma)					
	A	59	28	11	6
	B	65	47 $p = 0.003$	16	8
	C	35	27	9	4

showed abnormal age-corrected values in more subjects in groups B and C than in group A ($p = 0.014$) after 1 month, while no difference between the subgroups was found at the end of the study (Table 3). Abnormal contrast sensitivity values at 18 cps were found both at 1 month and at the end of the follow-up in more patients in groups B and C than in group A ($p = 0.037$ after 1 month and $p = 0.018$ after 8 years; Table 3). During the follow-up all the three groups showed significant improvement of visual function, particularly of visual acuity and foveal threshold (Table 2).

During the study one patient in group B developed inner lamellar macular hole in one eye, while 13 patients (four in group A, five in group B and four in group C) showed defects of retinal pigment epithelium.

Discussion

Solar retinopathy is due to a combination of thermal and photochemical injury. Variability in the clinical appearance and severity of solar retinopathy probably arises from differences in exposure parameters, environmental conditions and patients[4,5]. In our study the environmental conditions were the same for every patient, having all patients gazed the sun at the same day time (around noon) and at the same site on February 28th 1988; the two subgroups were similar for age, sex and time of sunlight exposure, differing for medical treatment established at the time of exposure only. For these reasons, the long-term results of this study can be related to the different therapy used in the evaluated subgroups. High dose intravenous treatment with dexamethasone seems to be more effective than oral steroids or no therapy in improving visual function in the short-term. These data are in agreement with several experimental procedures in a rat model[6,7]: these reports demonstrated that high doses of methylprednisolone or dexamethasone ameliorate light-induced photoreceptor degeneration in rats and that this effect is dose-dependent. Furthermore, Rosner[8] demonstrated that this effect is dose dependent and that no beneficial effect is observed when treatment is delayed for 24 h. In the present report this latter aspect was not considered and it is under evaluation.

In the long term, contrast sensitivity at high frequencies was the only test that showed significant differences between subgroups, with a higher sensitivity in patients treated with intravenous dexamethasone than the others. All the other tests, e.g. visual acuity, foveal threshold, colour vision, Amsler grid and contrast sensitivity at low and middle frequencies, showed similar results at the end of follow-up in all subgroups. In conclusion, the effect of dexamethasone after solar retinopathy is first related to the rapid improvement of visual function, probably related to his potent antioxidant activity, through the inhibition of lipid peroxidation[9,10]. Even though this treatment, in long-term follow-up, differs from the other treatment regimens only for data relative to contrast sensitivity at high frequencies, according to the experimental studies, it seems a useful treatment for this condition. Further evidence, particularly relative to the effect in relation to delaying treatment, is necessary to fully demonstrate its real efficacy.

References

1. Hope-Ross, M., Travers, S., Mooney, D. Solar retinopathy following religious rituals. Br J Ophthalmol. 1988; 72: 931–934.

2. De Nicola, G.C., Mastropasqua, L., Lobefalo, L., Ciancaglini, M., Calogiuri, M.T. Solar Maculopathy: long-term evolution. Ann Ott Clin Ocul. 1990; 116: 781–786.
3. Verriest, G., Van Laethem, J., Uvijls, A. A new assessment of the normal ranges of the Farnsworth-Munsell 100-hue test scores. Am J Ophthalmol. 1982; 93: 635–642.
4. Mainster, M.A. Foveomacular retinitis. Clinical and physical considerations. In: Zingirian, M., Cardillo Piccolino, F. (eds.). Retinal pigment epithelium. Amsterdam: Kugler & Ghedini Publications, 1988: 153–157.
5. Dhir, S., Gupta, A., Jain, S. Eclipse retinopathy. Br J Ophthalmol. 1981; 65: 42–45.
6. Fu, J., Lam, T.T., Tso, M.O.M. Dexamethasone ameliorates retinal photic injury in albino rats. Exp Eye Res. 1992; 54: 583–594.
7. Rosner, M., Fu, J., Tso, M.O.M, Lam, T.T. Methylprednisolone ameliorates retinal photic injury in rats. Arch Ophthalmol. 1992; 110; 857–861.
8. Rosner, M., Lam, T.T., Tso, M.O.M. Therapeutic parameters of methylprednisolone treatment for retinal photic injury in a rat model. Res Commun Clin Pathol Pharmacol. 1992; 77: 299–311.
9. Hall, E.D., Braughler, J.M. Acute effects of intravenous glucocorticoid pretreatment on the *in vitro* peroxidation of cat spinal cord tissue. Exp Neurol. 1981; 73: 321–324.
10. Hall, E.D., Braughler, J.M. Central nervous system trauma and stroke. Free Rad Biol Med. 1989; 6: 303–313.

Institute of Ophthalmology
'G. D'Annunzio' University
via Gran Sasso 100, Chieti I-66100, Italy

47. Subretinal fibrosis in Stargardt's disease

J.J. DE LAEY and F. MEIRE

(Ghent, Belgium)

Introduction

Fundus flavimaculatus (Stargardt's disease) is a bilateral, symmetrical and progressive macular dystrophy, that usually starts between the ages of 6 and 20 years and rapidly leads to loss of central vision. Although the fundus may initially appear normal, atrophic macular changes appear. The macular dystrophy is frequently associated with fundus flavimaculatus flecks, the number of which usually increases with time. These flecks are more dense in the posterior pole but are classically absent in the peripapillary region. They gradually decrease in number towards the equator of the fundus. The central atrophy becomes gradually more apparent, giving rise to an aspect of central choroidal sclerosis. The flavimaculatus flecks may eventually fade.

A characteristic fluoroangiographic sign is the dark choroid or so-called choroidal silence first described in 1971 by Bonnin[1]. This phenomenon results probably from the accumulation of abnormal material in the retinal pigment epithelium over the whole posterior pole. Klien and Krill were the first to demonstrate on histopathology, the presence of an abnormal substance within the retinal pigment epithelium[2]. Later studies suggested that this abnormal material is lipofuscin, which acts as an optical filter by absorbing short wave lengths[3–7].

Other fundus changes have also been described in Stargardt's disease, including pallor of the optic disc, attenuated retinal vessels, occasionally pigmentation in the form of bone spiculae in the retinal periphery, lesions with an aspect of cicatricial chorioretinitis, retinal pigment epithelial hyperplasia, subretinal neovascularization and subretinal fibrosis[5,8–12]. An asymmetrical presentation of fundus flavimaculatus has been described in a patient with unilateral myopia[13].

At the Third Meeting of the European Macular Group in Athens, the first author reported on three patients with Stargardt's disease and massive subretinal fibrosis. Two patients presented the classic ophthalmoscopic and fluoroangiographic appearance of Stargardt's disease in one eye and dense orange subretinal material in the posterior pole of the fellow eye. During the follow-up period the abnormal material disappeared, leaving subretinal fibrosis and localized retinal pigment epithelial hypertrophy. In one of these two patients, an ocular contusion occurred in the eye with abnormal material, eight days

G. Coscas and F. Cardillo Piccolino (eds.), Retinal Pigment Epithelium and Macular Diseases, pp. 285–290.
© 1998 Kluwer Academic Publishers.

before the first consultation. The left fundus of a third patient was characterized by an area of subretinal fibrosis in the midperiphery. It was presumed that the abnormal material was lipofuscin and that this possibly represented an exaggerated response to a minor trauma.

Intrigued by these observations, we retrospectively analysed the ophthalmoscopic features of 56 patients with Stargardt's disease, seen in the Eye Department of the University of Ghent in the past 15 years. We found two other patients with subretinal fibrosis and a history of ocular trauma.

Case reports

Case 1

This 18-year-old patient was diagnosed as suffering from Stargardt's disease at the age of 7 years. One year later her left eye was struck by a chestnut. She was seen for the first time in the department of ophthalmology 10 years after the trauma. The left eye presented a contusion cataract, whereas the lens of the right eye was clear. The vision was reduced to finger counting in both eyes. Electrophysiological tests corresponded to a cone-rod dystrophy. The right fundus presented a pale optic disc and an atrophic macular region. In the left eye a similar atrophic macular lesion was noticed, but the fundus was mainly characterized by the presence of marked subretinal fibrosis surrounding the optic disc and the macular region. These lesions were associated with an area of retinal pigment epithelial hyperplasia situated inferotemporally to the macula. The region immediately surrounding the optic disc appeared normal (Fig. 1).

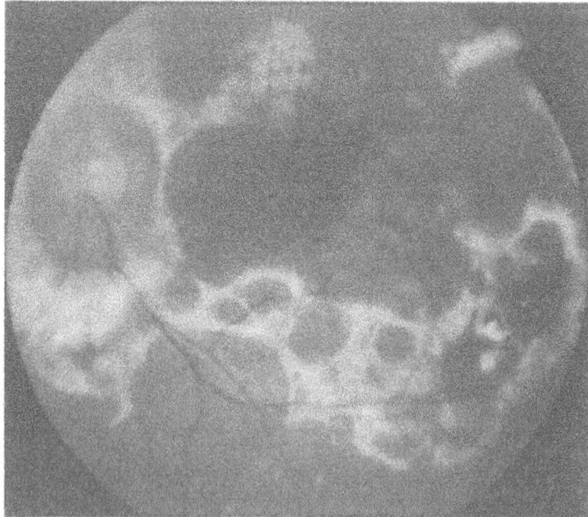

Fig. 1. Case 1. Fundus photography of the left eye 10 years after contusion.

Case 2

This boy was seen for the first time at the age of 10 years with a visual acuity of 2/10 in the right eye and 3/10 in the left eye. Colour vision testing revealed an acquired red-green dyschromatopsia. On ophthalmoscopy pigmentary changes were seen in the macular area of both eyes as well as fundus flavimaculatus flecks, which were especially numerous around the macula. Subretinal fibrosis was not present. The photopic ERG showed slightly reduced responses for red light, whereas the scotopic ERG was normal. The EOG Arden ratios were subnormal (145% right eye; 130% left eye). At the age of 14 years the vision was further reduced to 1/10 in the right eye and 2/10 in the left eye. In March 1995 he received a ball on the right temporal region and experienced a sudden vision loss in the right eye. He was examined in the Department of Ophthalmology 10 days later. The anterior segments of both eyes appeared normal. Vision was reduced to 3.5/100 in the right eye and to 1.7/10 in the left eye. Ophthalmoscopy showed subretinal fibrosis surrounding the right optic disc and extending linearly in the inferotemporal direction and also in the inferonasal direction. Patches of subretinal fibrosis were also present at the temporal side of the macula and superonasally to the disc. A few small retinal haemorrhages were visible around the disc. The left eye also presented patchy subretinal fibrosis around the macula, although less extensive than in the right eye. On fluorescein angiography the fundus flavimaculatus flecks and the macular dystrophy were obvious. No choroidal rupture could be detected around the right optic disc. There was some masking effect due to the subretinal fibrosis but remarkably little staining of the fibrosis except close to the optic disc. The disc showed an increased late fluorescence (Fig. 2). In the left eye hyperfluorescence was noted corresponding to the patches of subretinal fibrosis.

Five months later, the ophthalmoscopic appearance of the right eye was essentially unchanged, except for the disappearance of the retinal haemorrhages and a more dense appearance of the subretinal fibrosis. Fluorescein angiography showed an intense staining of the different areas with subretinal fibrosis. The late fluorescence of the disc was normal. Subretinal vessels could not be detected (Fig. 3). The vision remained reduced to less than 1/60 in the right eye and to 1.5/10 in the left eye.

Discussion

These two patients with Stargardt's disease present marked subretinal fibrosis after an ocular trauma. In the first patient the trauma was sufficient to produce a contusion cataract. Unfortunately the patient was only seen 10 years after the trauma and we have no accurate description of the fundus in the first days after the eye had been traumatized. The second patient presented 10 days after a possible indirect ocular contusion and although the fellow eye also

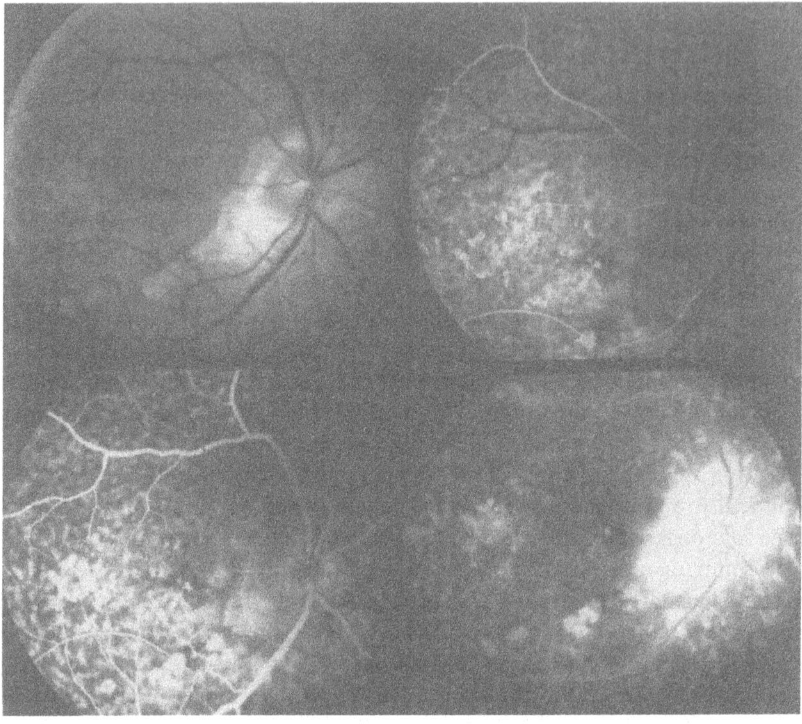

Fig. 2. Case 2. Red free and fluoroangiography of the right fundus 10 days after the trauma.

presented some patches of subretinal fibrosis, the fibrosis was much more marked at the affected side. The location of the fibrosis suggested possible choroidal ruptures, although fluorescein angiography was not typical for that diagnosis. Fundus pictures taken 5 years before the accident did not reveal the presence of subretinal fibrosis in either eye.

Our two patients present striking similarities to three cases discussed previously[14], in particular the unilaterality or at least the marked asymmetry of the subretinal fibrosis. In two of these three cases the subretinal fibrosis was preceded by the presence of diffuse subretinal material in the posterior pole. This subretinal material was considered to represent massive hyperlipofuscinosis possibly as a consequence of a trauma. Such orange material was not found in the two cases presented here. Del Buey *et al.*[15] reported a young girl with Stargardt's disease who sustained a contusion in one eye. Whereas the fundus before the trauma was similar in both eyes, marked subretinal fibrosis was observed in the traumatized eye a few weeks later. The authors suggest that the fibroglial reaction could have been induced by the liberation of growth factors from the diseased retinal pigment epithelium[15].

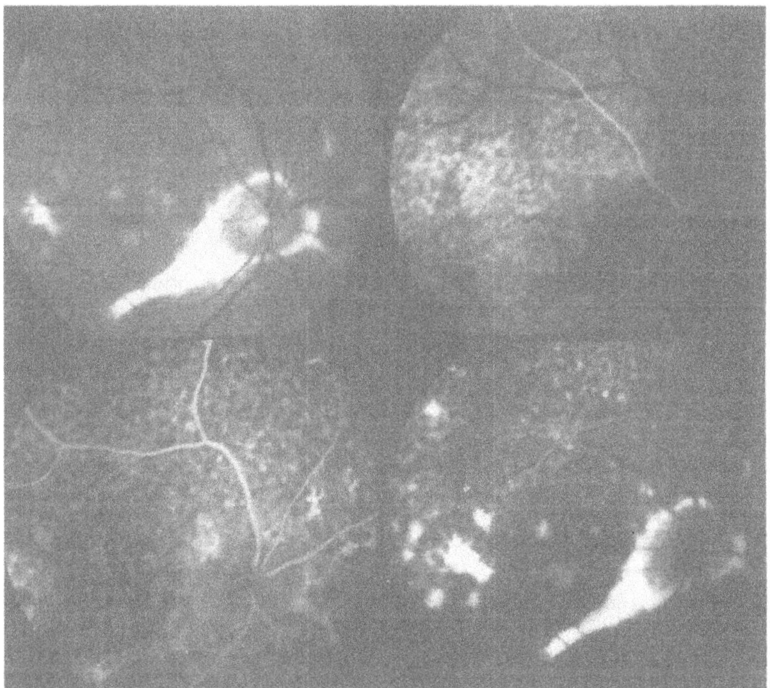

Fig. 3. Case 2. The same eye as Fig 2, 5 months later.

Subretinal fibrosis may be related to subretinal neovascularization, a complication known to occur in Stargardt's disease/fundus flavimaculatus. However in our cases no subretinal new vessels could be detected and the fibrosis was too extensive to be the consequence of a localized problem.

Subretinal fibrosis can also be observed in uveitis[16] and is thought to result from an autoimmune mediated inflammation, with local antibody production possibly to retinal pigment epithelial structures[17]. Parodi[12] suggested that the subretinal fibrosis in fundus flavimaculatus may represent the result of retinal pigment epithelium metaplasia, as a non-specific response to an inflammation.

Conclusion

The unilaterality or at least the marked asymmetry of the subretinal fibrosis in these two observations and in the three cases published previously[14] suggest that some external factor could be responsible. In three of these five cases we have reasons to believe that a (mild) trauma induced the mechanism which lead to subretinal fibrosis. The exact mechanism is still questionable. It can however be suspected that a direct or indirect ocular trauma will have a far more devastating effect in eyes with Stargardt/fundus flavimaculatus. Such a trauma could result in massive hyperlipofuscinosis as observed in exceptional cases or directly in extensive subretinal fibrosis.

Children with Stargardt's disease should be advised to wear protective goggles on the playground or during sports.

References

1. Bonnin, P. Le signe du silence choroidien dans les dégénérescences tapétorétiniennes centrales examinées sous fluorescéine. Bull Soc Ophtalmol Fr. 1971; 71: 348–351.
2. Klein, R., Lewis, R.A., Meyers, S.M., Meyers, F.L. Subretinal neovascularization associated with fundus flavimaculatus. Arch Ophthalmol. 1978; 96: 2054–2057
3. Birnbach, C.D., Järvaläinen, M., Possin, D.E., Milam, A.H. Histopathology and immuno-chemistry of the neurosensory retina in fundus flavimaculatus. Ophthalmology. 1994; 101: 1211–1219.
4. Eagle, R.C. Jr., Lucier, A.C., Bernardino, J.B. Jr., Yanoff, M. Retinal pigment epithelial abnor-malities in fundus flavimaculatus: a light and electron microscopic study. Ophthalmology. 1980; 87: 1189–2000.
5. Leveille, A.S., Morse, P.H., Burch, J.V. Fundus flavimaculatus and subretinal neovasculariza-tion. Ann Ophthalmol. 1982; 14: 331–334.
6. Lopez, P.F., Maumenee, I.H., de la Cruz, Z., Green, W.R. Autosomal dominant fundus flavimaculatus. Clinicopathologic correlation? Ophthalmology. 1990; 97: 798–809.
7. Steinmetz, R.I., Gartner, A., Maguire, J.I., Bird, A.C. Histopathology of incipient fundus flavimaculatus. Ophthalmology. 1991; 98: 953–956.
8. De Laey, J.J., Leys, A., Van Hyfte, R. Retinal pigment hypertrophy and chorioretinal dystro-phies. Bull Soc Belge Ophtalmol. 1987; 223: 67–73.
9. Deutman, A.F. The Hereditary Dystrophies of the Posterior Pole of the Eye. Assen: van Gorcum and Co, 1971: 107–117.
10. Franceschetti, A., François, J., Babel, J. Les Hérédo-dégénerescences Chorio-rétiniennes. Paris: Masson, 1963: 426–4764.
11. Klien, B.A., Krill, A.E. Fundus flavimaculatus: clinical, functional and histopathologic obser-vation. Am J Ophthalmol. 1967; 64: 3–23.
12. Parodi, M.B. Progressive subretinal fibrosis in fundus flavimaculatus. Acta Ophthalmol. 1994; 72: 260–264.
13. Lafaut, B.A., van Egmond, J., De Laey, J.J. Asymmetric fundus flavimaculatus/Stargardt's disease associated with unilateral myopia. Int. Ophthalmol. 1996; 19: 235–255.
14. De Laey, J.J., Verougstraete, C. Hyperlipofuscinosis and subretinal fibrosis in Stargardt's disease. Retina. 1995; 15: 399–406.
15. del Buey, M.E., Huerva, V., Minguez, E., Cristobal, J.A., Iturbe, F., Palomar, A. Posttraumatic reaction in a case of fundus flavimaculatus with atrophic macular degeneration. Ann Ophthalmol. 1993; 25: 219–221.
16. Palestine, A.G., Nussenblatt, R.B., Parver, L.M., Knox, D.L. Progressive subretinal fibrosis in uveitis. Br J Ophthalmol. 1984; 68: 667–673.
17. Palestine, A.G., Nussenblatt, R.B., Chan, C.C., Hooks, J.J., Friedman, L., Kuwabara, T. Histopathology of the subretinal fibrosis and uveitis syndrome. Ophthalmology. 1985; 92: 838–844.

Department of Ophthalmology
University Hospital
Ghent, Belgium

48. Age-related geographic atrophy and pattern dystrophy of the RPE

M.F. MARMOR
(Stanford, USA)

Introduction

The pattern dystrophies are a group of hereditary disorders characterized by granular and reticular pigment patterns in the macula and periphery[1,2]. They typically have a clinical course that is relatively benign, with good visual acuity and few electrophysiologic changes except for a borderline or slightly reduced electro-oculogram. Some older family members have been observed with geographic atrophy, but it is unclear whether these cases represent progression of the dystrophy or independent age-related pathology.

We have had the opportunity to re-examine members of a large dominant pedigree with pattern dystrophy 20 years after their initial evaluation[3]. At issue is not only whether geographic macular atrophy may be a late concern in pattern dystrophy, but the implications of this finding for the pathophysiology of age-related atrophic macular degeneration.

Methods

Four patients, presently aged 35–73 years, were re-examined 20 years after initial evaluation. Two additional older individuals, aged 61 and 69, were evaluated from the same dominant pedigree. Fundus photographs and fluorescein angiograms were obtained for comparison with previous results. Electroretinography (ERG) and electro-oculography (EOG) were performed in accordance with current international standards[4,5].

Results

The original propositus, now aged 62, showed no change in visual acuity over 20 years (20/25 in each eye), and her EOG remained stable with a light/dark ratio of 1.8. However, her fundus, which 20 years previously showed irregular granular and reticular pigmentation, now showed discrete geographic patches of RPE and choriocapillary atrophy nasal and temporal to the fovea (Fig. 1). She was aware of paracentral scotomas corresponding to these lesions. Over

G. Coscas and F. Cardillo Piccolino (eds.), Retinal Pigment Epithelium and Macular Diseases, pp. 291–296.
© *1998 Kluwer Academic Publishers.*

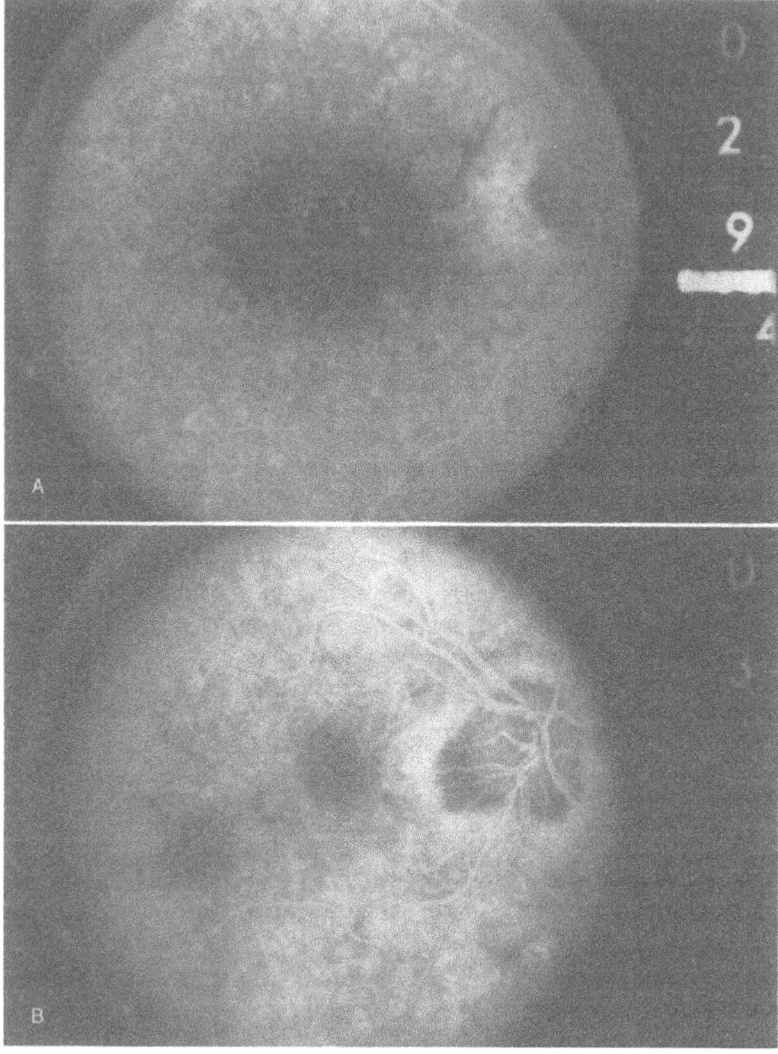

Fig. 1. Fluorescein angiograms from the propositus. (A) Age 42. There is a dense granular pigment pattern in the macula. (B) Age 62. Much of the pigment has dispersed and there are parafoveal zones of RPE and choriocapillary atrophy. From Ref. 3.

the 20 year interval, she developed a mild tritan colour deficiency and mild (0.3 log unit) elevation of her dark-adaptation threshold. She also showed a significant change in her electroretinogram: her cone and rod b-waves were normal when first examined, but 20 years later her b-wave amplitudes were roughly 30% below the minimum of the normal range for both cones and rods.

Two of her children, now aged 35 and 38, were re-examined after 20 years. Their acuity was 20/20 and their EOG light/dark ratios remained slightly reduced. They showed no loss of colour vision, dark-adaptation or ERG. However, both showed considerable dispersion of the pigmentary patterns that were present 20 years ago (Fig, 2), and some diffuse thinning of RPE pigmentation (although without any discrete areas of choriocapillary loss).

A cousin of the propositus, now 73 years old, had also been examined 20 years previously. His acuity remained excellent over the 20 years, and measured 20/20–25 at the most recent examination. Electrophysiology had not been performed previously, and he now showed an EOG light/dark ratio of 1.65, and ERG b-waves for both cone and rod systems that were at the borderline between normal and subnormal. His fundus showed considerable thinning of RPE pigmentation relative to 20 years previously, and there were small patches of geographic atrophy temporal to the fovea.

Two other affected family members aged 61 and 69 showed diffuse RPE atrophy in the maculae, without choriocapillary loss. Visual acuity ranged from 20/25 to 20/50, and the ERG b-waves were borderline subnormal.

Discussion

The pattern dystrophy in this family has followed a relatively benign course over the past 20 years, insofar as all of the family members studied have retained good visual acuity. However, there has been clear progression of fundus lesions, with gradual loss of the pigmentary patterns and the development of diffuse RPE thinning and atrophy. In the older individuals, beginning patches of choriocapillary atrophy were beginning to develop: these raise concern that visual acuity may become affected as these individuals reach their mid-seventies and eighties. Indeed, the mother of the propositus, when examined at age 80 in the original report, had geographic atrophy and 20/200 visual acuity.

The results also show that the disease is not limited to the RPE. The EOG remained relatively stable in these patients, but the ERG which was normal in all family members examined 20 years ago, was now borderline or subnormal in the older individuals. The dysfunction is not severe, nor associated with peripheral field loss, and yet the finding clearly shows that a degree of photoreceptor dysfunction occurs in this disease over time. The ERG results also indicate that the disease is a diffuse one throughout the retina, and not limited to the macula alone (in which case the full-field ERG would not be abnormal).

The aetiology of pattern dystrophy is unknown. Some patients with a similar phenotype have been found to have a mutation in the coding sequence of the RDS gene[6], but the propositus in our family did not show this mutation. Nevertheless, it is clear that a phenotype of RPE pigmentary changes can

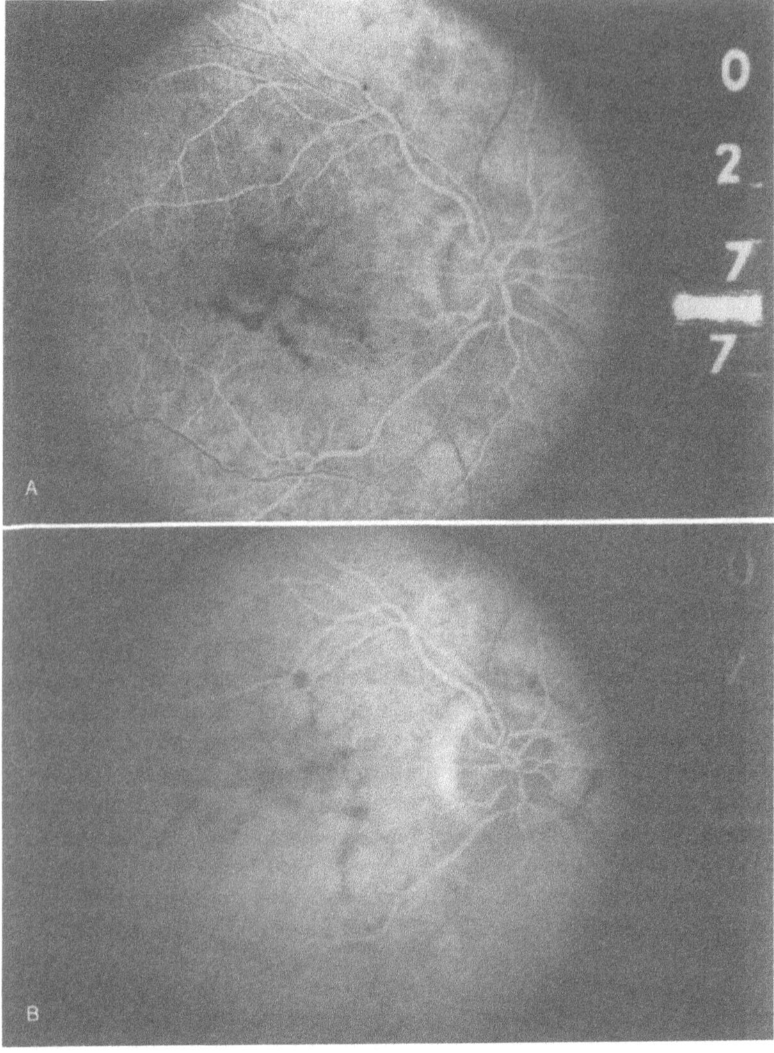

Fig. 2. Fluorescein angiograms from the son of the propositus. (A) Age 19. There is a dense reticular pattern in the central macula. (B) Age 38. The pattern has faded and there is diffuse thinning of the RPE. From Ref. 3.

result from a retinal mutation (as well as, presumably, one in the RPE). The gradual loss of ERG signal in our family could signify retinal pathology, but could also represent dysfunction secondary to RPE dysfunction.

Geographic atrophy of the macula is part of the spectrum of age-related macular degeneration, and is probably a relatively non-specific finding that

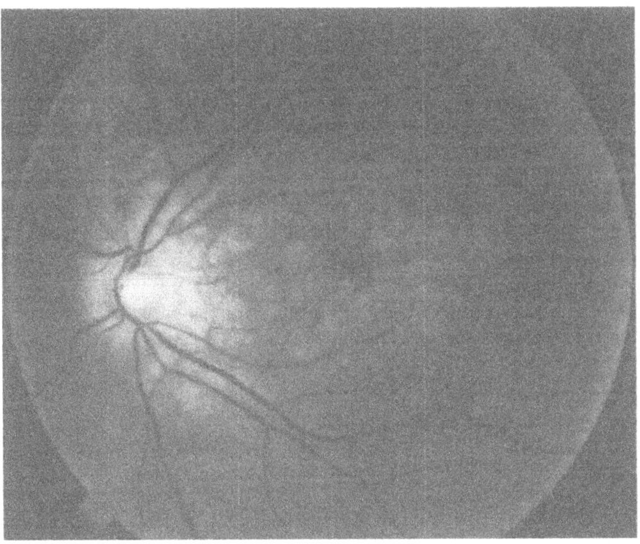

Fig. 3. Fundus photograph from an affected cousin of the propositus, age 69. The eye showed geographic RPE atrophy without choriocapillary loss. Visual acuity in this eye was 20/50. From Ref. 3.

may have many aetiologies. In this family, the RPE depigmentation and atrophy seems clearly associated with the pattern dystrophy. The atrophic changes begin in this family at ages far below that normally associated with age-related macular degeneration. It is not clear whether the atrophic changes are a direct result of the metabolic dystrophy, or whether the dystrophy is simply predisposing these retinas to an early or greater susceptibility to age-related changes. There may be an analogy to the atrophy that can progress or develop many years after exposure to some retinal toxins such as thioridazine or chloroquin[7].

The converse question can also be asked: could some patients that have been considered to have age-related macular degeneration actually be showing late manifestations of pattern dystrophy? Early pattern dystrophy can easily be missed, since it is largely asymptomatic at younger ages and the fundus changes are not necessarily obvious. As the mechanisms of pattern dystrophy become better understood, they may give clues to the pathophysiology of age-related disease. The finding of geographic atrophic macular degeneration in older individuals may warrant consideration of whether the family has a hereditary disease such as pattern dystrophy.

References

1. Marmor, M.F., Byers, B. Pattern dystrophy of the pigment epithelium. Am J Ophthalmol. 1977; 84: 32–44.

2. Hsieh, R.C., Fine, B.S., Lyons, J.S. Pattern dystrophy of the pigment epithelium. Am J Ophthalmol. 1976; 13: 112–116.
3. Marmor, M.F., McNamara, J.A. Pattern dystrophy of the retinal pigment epithelium and geographic atrophy of the macula. Am J Ophthalmol. 1996; 122: 382–392.
4. Marmor, M.F., Zrenner, E. (for the International Society for Clinical Electrophysiology of Vision). Standard for clinical electroretinography (1994 update). Doc Ophthalmol. 1995; 89: 199–210.
5. Marmor, M.F., Zrenner, E. (for the International Society for Clinical Electrophysiology of Vision). Standard for clinical electro-oculography. Doc Ophthalmol. 1993; 85: 115–124.
6. Nichols, B.E., Sheffield, V.C., Vandenburgh, K., Drack, A.V., Kimura, A.E., Stone, E.M. Butterfly-shaped pigment dystrophy of the fovea caused by a point mutation in codon 167 of the RDS gene. Nature Genet. 1993; 3: 202–207.
7. Marmor, M.F. Is thioridazine retinopathy progressive? Relationship of pigmentary changes to visual function. Br J Ophthalmol. 1990; 74: 739–742.

Department of Ophthalmology
Stanford University Medical Center
Stanford, CA 94305-5308
USA

49. Bilateral ocular toxoplasmosis: a clinical case

G. DI MARZIO, P. CAPONE, L. DI MARZIO, B. RICCI,
G. DI BONAVENTURA, G. MORBIDUCCI and L. DI NORSCIA

(Atri, Italy)

Introduction

Toxoplasma gondii, an intracellular parasite, frequently causes ocular infections[1]. The natural host of this zoonosis is the cat, in which the protozoan ends its enteroepithelial cycle[2]. Several mammals and birds can be infected and they then become a source of infection.

T. gondii appears in three forms: tachyzoites (invasive form), bradyzoites (latent infection) and oocysts (infections form). Man is an accidental host who becomes infected through ingestion of raw or insufficiently cooked contaminated foods[3], oocyte ingestion[4] or by transplacental transmission[5]. Systemic, ocular aquired and congenital forms of toxoplasmosis have been described; a particular form is present in immunodeficient patients.

Ocular toxoplasmosis appears as a necrotic focal retinitis, involving the inner layers of the retina: the whitish soft lesion has surrounding oedema. An inflammatory process of the vitreous body, with inflammatory cells, can also occur and a vasculitis often co-exists. Fifty percent of cases are bilateral and the macular area is involved in 80%.

The main symptoms, present in almost all the patients, include visual loss by macular involvement, miodesopsia, metamorphopsia, photophobia and sometimes pain[6]. Secondary complications of toxoplasmosis include cataract, glaucoma, macular cystic oedema, rear synechia and vasculitis[7].

The diagnosis of ocular toxoplasmosis is based on ophthalmoscopic evidence of the ocular lesions and the demonstration of the organism in ocular tissues. Serological methods are preferred because of their high sensitivity, specificity and easy execution. The most used diagnostic tests are Sabin-Feldman, complement fixation reaction, haemagglutination, ELISA and indirect immunofluorescence.

The current therapeutic strategy consist of a triple drug combination, pyrimetamine, sulphadiazine and corticosteroids; in some cases clindamycin is used[8]. In 1992 Opremcak *et al.*[9] treated 16 patients with *Toxoplasma* retinochoroiditis with trimethoprim-sulfamethoxazole, with resolution of disease and improved vision in all clinical cases.

Because of the severe complications of these drugs some authors have used alternative treatments such as cryotherapy and laser photocoagulation[10,11]. The goal is to destroy the cysts and/or to denature the antigenic proteins responsible for late hypersensitivity reactions.

G. Coscas and F. Cardillo Piccolino (eds.), Retinal Pigment Epithelium and Macular Diseases, pp. 297–299.
© 1998 Kluwer Academic Publishers.

Laser treatment is not without complications, and vitreoretinal membranes, retinal and/or vitreous haemorrhages and subretinal vessels can be observed. A combination of pars plana vitrectomy and endophotocoagulation has been proposed[12].

Case report

The 13-year-old child was admitted to paediatric units on several occasions. His mother reported that he liked to eat raw meat. At 4 months old he was admitted because of 'acute enteritis with pharingitis'. Laboratory tests were normal. A second admission at 5 years old followed cranial trauma. Laboratory tests were normal. A fundus examination of both eyes showed no pathological findings. In 1992 he was seen with 'bronchopneumonic infiltrate of the upper right lobe with the nettle rash following antibiotic therapy (Ceftibufen)'. Laboratory tests were normal.

In May 1993 he was admitted to our Ophthalmological Unit because of visual reduction in right eye, which was worsening. When he was admitted to hospital the vision in the right eye was 20/200 and 20/20 in the left eye. The front segment was normal. Fundus examination showed no blood vessels and no optic disc alterations. An active retinochoroiditis focus, half papillary diameter wide, situated below the macula, with surrounding oedema, was found in the right eye. In the left eye two retinochoroiditis foci, situated below the superior vascular arcade, with a small active lateral focus, were seen.

All laboratory tests, except the anti-*Toxoplasma gondii* levels, were normal. The patient's mother had been investigated for *Toxoplasma* infection during pregnancy and no sign of infection was detected. A fluorangiography confirmed a diagnosis of ocular toxoplasmosis.

Treatment consisted of triamcinolone, clorphenamine, trimethopim, sulphamethoxazole and corticosteroids. Two months later the ophthalmoscopic seeing was improved with right eye vision of 20/25. In 1994 the patient had a new reduction of vision in the right eye, following a viral infection, and he was admitted once again to our unit. The anterior segment was normal in both eyes. Vision was 20/60 in the right eye and 20/20 in the left eye. The right eye fundus showed, at the posterior pole, a retinal haemorrhage with surrounding oedema involving the macula. In the left eye the fundus examination showed an infectious focus reactivation which was treated with photocoagulation. Fluorangiography confirmed the hypothesis of infectious focus reactivation in right and left eye. The previous treatment strategy was changed to roxitromicine and ofloxacine. No further infectious focus reactivations occurred.

References

1. Gass, J.M.D. Stereoscopic Atlas of Macular Diseases: Diagnosis and Treatment, 2nd edn. St. Louis: CV Mosby Co., 1987.

2. De Carneri, I. Parassitologia generale e umana. In: Diseases of the Retina, pp. 656–660.
3. Shoukrey, N., Tabbara, K.F. Eye related parasitic diseases. In Tabbara K.F., Hyndiuk, R.A. (eds). Infections of the Eye. Boston, Little, Brown & Co 1966.
4. Frenkel, J.K. Toxoplasmosis. Pediatr Clin North Am. 1985; 32: 917–932.
5. Couvreur, J., Desmonts, G. Congenital and maternal toxoplasmosis: a review of 300 congenital cases. Dev Med Child Neurol. 1962; 4: 519–530.
6. Friedman, C.T., Knox, D.L. Variations in recurrent active toxoplasmic retinochoroiditis. Arch Ophthalmol. 1969; 81: 481–493.
7. Quinland, P., Jabs, D.A. Ocular toxoplasmosis. In: Ryan (ed.) Retina. 1989; 563–574.
8. Lam, S., Tessler, H.H. Quadruple therapy for ocular toxoplasmosis. Can J Ophthalmol. 1993; 28: 58–61.
9. Opremcak, E.M., Scales, D.K., Sharpe, M.R. Trimethoprim-sulfamethoxazole therapy for ocular toxoplasmosis. Ophthalmology. 1992; 99: 920–925.
10. Dobbie, J.G. Cryotherapy in the management of toxoplasma retinochoroiditis. Trans Am Acad Ophthalmol Otolaryngol. 1968; 72: 364–367.
11. Sthealy, L.P. Laser treatment of toxoplasmosis. Ann Ophthalmol. 1989; 21: 36–38.
12. Obana, A. *et. al.* A case of ocular toxoplasmosis treated with vitrectomy and endophotocoagulation. Jpn J Clin Ophthalmol. 1991; 45: 983–986.

Ocular Division Hospital
'S. Liberatore' Atri
A.U.S.L. TE, Italy

50. Indocyanine green angiography of drusen

G. COSCAS, J. ARNOLD, M. QUARANTA, D. KUHN
and G. SOUBRANE

(Créteil, France)

Introduction

Age-related maculopathy (ARM) is a chronic degenerative disease affecting primarily the retinal pigment epithelium, Bruch's membrane and the choriocapillaris. Drusen, considered to be an early sign of ARM, are multiple, yellowish, usually discrete, slightly elevated, variably sized deposits. Moreover drusen, especially when large, soft and confluent, have been identified as a risk factor for the blinding complications, chiefly choroidal neovascularization, of age-related maculopathy (ARM).

Histopathologically, ARM is defined as the presence of membranous debris on both aspects of the basement membrane of the retinal pigment epithelium (RPE) associated with a continuous layer of basal laminar deposit beneath the macula. Drusen are deposits of extracellular material lying between membrane of retinal pigment epithelium and the inner collagenous zone of Bruch's membrane.

A refined classification of drusen, based not only on clinical features including evolution over time but also on histopathology, notes that there appear to be four main categories of drusen:

(1) isolated hard drusen;
(2) drusen which show evidence of their derivation from clusters of hard drusen: a group which included hard cluster-derived drusen, and a group which included soft cluster-derived drusen;
(3) membranous drusen, consisting of focal collections of a diffuse deposit of membranous debris, termed basal linear deposit;
(4) regressing drusen.

Purpose

Indocyanine green angiographic features of the early stages of age-related macular degeneration are controversial. This study was undertaken to analyse the indocyanine green angiographic findings of drusen.

G. Coscas and F. Cardillo Piccolino (eds.), Retinal Pigment Epithelium and Macular Diseases, pp. 301–302.
© *1998 Kluwer Academic Publishers.*

Methods

Eyes with all types of drusen but without exudative complications of age-related macular degeneration were included. In a prospective study, 69 eyes of 53 consecutive patients with drusen, but without exudative complications of age-related macular degeneration were studied. Drusen were classified into the four groups described above. An additional category was constituted by reticular pseudodrusen that could be associated with drusen of either group. Results of contact lens biomicroscopy and fluorescein angiography were compared with findings on indocyanine green angiography.

Results

Isolated hard drusen and hard cluster-derived drusen were hyperfluorescent during indocyanine green angiography. By contrast, all sizes of soft drusen derived from clusters of hard drusen were hypofluorescent throughout the angiogram. Membranous drusen, visible on biomicroscopy and fluorescein angiography, were not visible during indocyanine green angiography. Regressing drusen may show hyperfluorescence at the early stages of indocyanine green angiography but associated calcium and pigmentation were hypofluorescent. Reticular pseudodrusen were visible on red-free photographs; on mid- and late-phase indocyanine green angiography using the scanning laser ophthalmoscope only, reticular pseudodrusen appeared as a pattern of hypofluorescent dots.

Conclusion

The indocyanine green angiographic findings add to and support the clinico-pathological classification of drusen. Indocyanine green angiography may help to distinguish the different types of drusen and may thus be of use in evaluating the risk of progressive age-related macular degeneration in patients with drusen.

Clinique Ophtalmologique Universitaire de Créteil
40 avenue de Verdun
94010 Créteil, France

51. A clinicopathological study of drusen types

J. SARKS and S. SARKS

(Sydney, Australia)

Drusen are known to be associated with the more severe manifestations of age-related macular degeneration, eyes with large, soft or confluent drusen being at greatest risk. Clinical grading systems have therefore been developed which define drusen ophthalmoscopically as hard or soft based on their size and their margins. Small hard drusen, which only become visible in the fundus when at least 30 µm in diameter, are round, yellowish deposits with well defined borders. The alternative designation of drusen as soft is based on poorly defined edges and a softer appearance, characteristics which in turn appear related to drusen size, drusen over 125 µm and most of those over 63 µm being regarded as soft. However, on fluorescein angiography and pathological examination intermediate types can be recognized which shed light on their evolution. The aim of this study was to trace the lifecycle of drusen on the basis of clinical documentation, with up to 20 years follow up, together with pathological correlation in many cases.

On histopathological examination drusen are deposits of extracellular material lying between the basement membrane of the retinal pigment epithelium (RPE) and the inner collagenous zone of Bruch's membrane. Deposits in this location may be focal or diffuse and there appear to be two corresponding pathways of drusen formation.

Drusen developing as focal deposits can be classified morphologically as follows[1]:

1. Small hard drusen. These may occur at a young age, have a hyalinised amorphous structure and may occur in any part of the fundus. They often occur in clusters and represent the building blocks of most larger drusen.
2. Hard clusters. These are formed by fusion of the small hard drusen within a cluster. They are larger deposits which may have a soft clinical appearance and hence have also been termed soft distinct drusen[2], but fluorescein angiography demonstrates the constituent small drusen.
3. Soft clusters. Breakdown of the amorphous material into smaller particles results in a soft indistinct appearance in which the small drusen are no longer distinguishable. These soft clusters may appear in middle age on a background of small hard drusen (Fig. 1) and tend to become confluent. They commonly lead to the atrophic form of age-related macular degeneration.

G. Coscas and F. Cardillo Piccolino (eds.), Retinal Pigment Epithelium and Macular Diseases, pp. 303–305.
© *1998 Kluwer Academic Publishers.*

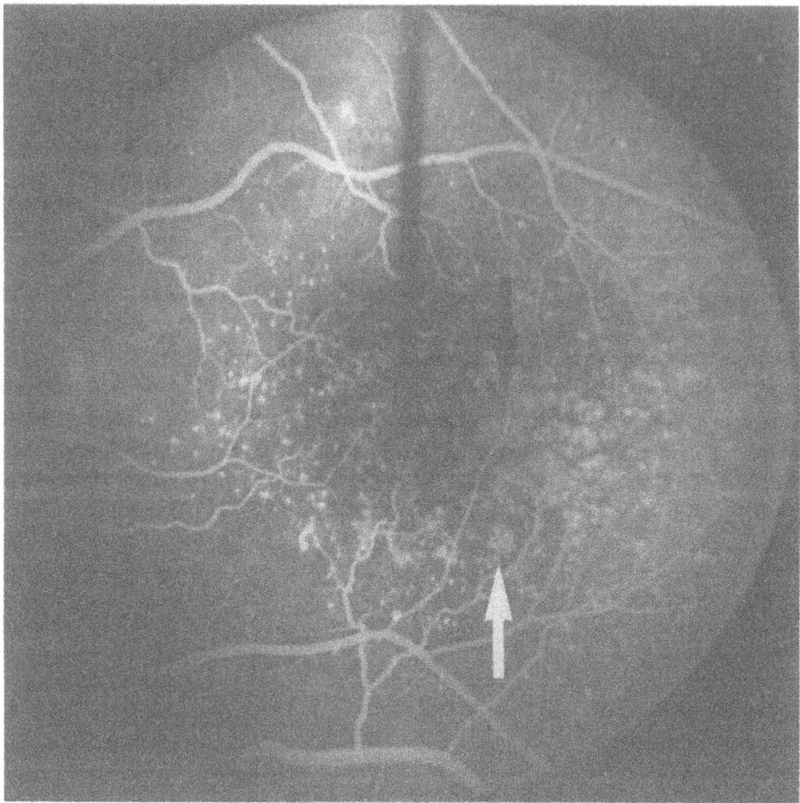

Fig. 1. Fluorescein angiogram of left eye of man aged 58, showing evolution of cluster of small hard drusen into larger soft drusen. The small drusen are initially discrete, then become aggregated into clusters (white arrow). Closer to the fovea they form clusters in which the individual drusen are more difficult to distinguish. Those clusters at the margin of the fovea have become homogeneous on fluorescein angiography (black arrow).

4. Drusenoid detachments of the RPE. Larger confluent drusen may also develop a cystic appearance, termed drusenoid detachments of the RPE if $>1000\,\mu$m in size. These appear in addition to contain fluid, probably because lipid in Bruch's membrane interferes with the action of the RPE pump.

The second pathway is that of soft membranous drusen. Late in the seventh decade diffuse deposits appear, comprising the basal laminar deposit internal to the basement membrane of the RPE and membranous debris external to the basement membrane. Soft membranous drusen develop as accentuations of this layer of membranous debris, which has also been termed the basal linear deposit[3]. They are usually shallower and less prominent than the soft clusters but carry a high risk of choroidal neovascularization. Changes noted at this stage are the presence of macrophages and giant cells in relation to focal thinning of Bruch's membrane and activation of the underlying choroidal capillaries. This is the earliest evidence of choroidal neovascularization and it may remain entirely confined to the choroid[4], or small vessels may bulge into Bruch's membrane. Further progress possibly depends on the opening of a cleavage plane by the membranous debris[5], underlining recent attempts to reduce the amount of soft drusen material by gentle prophylactic laser[6] in order to limit spread.

Unfortunately the current classification of drusen as hard and soft does not reflect whether they represent a focal or diffuse disturbance. Although considerable refinement is obviously required, the above scheme attempts to grade drusen according to their pathogenesis and so more accurately reflect their clinical implications.

There are other drusen types which are recognized, but which are not part of this scheme. Regressing drusen: both focal and diffuse drusen types may undergo regression, assuming a whiter and harder appearance with irregular margins and pigment clumping over the surface. Ultimately the drusen may fade completely to leave multifocal patches of atrophy which can contain glistening calcium deposits. Basal laminar drusen are material internal to the basement membrane of the RPE. They characteristically present as a dominantly inherited dystrophy of very small radially arranged deposits. Reticular drusen refers to a yellowish lobular pattern commonly observed in the outer macular region that does not fluoresce and is best seen in blue or red-free light[7]. No debris has been found to correspond with this picture and the term pseudodrusen seems more appropriate at the present time.

References

1. Sarks, J.P., Sarks, S.H., Killingsworth, M.C. Evolution of soft drusen in age-related macular degeneration. Eye. 1994; 8: 269–283.
2. Klein, R., Klein, B.E.K., Linton, K.L.P. Prevalence of age-related maculopathy. The Beaver Dam Eye Study. Ophthalmology. 1992; 99: 933–943.
3. Green, W., Enger, C. Age-related macular degeneration histopathologic studies. Ophthalmology. 1993; 100: 1519–1535.
4. Killingsworth, M.C. Angiogenesis in early choroidal neovascularization secondary to age-related macular degeneration. Graefe's Arch Clin Exp Ophthalmol. 1995; 233: 313–323.
5. Sarks, J.P., Sarks, S.H., Killingsworth. M.C. Morphology of early choroidal neovascularisation in age-related macular degeneration: correlation with activity. Eye. In press.
6. Sarks, S.H., Sarks, J.P., Arnold, J.J., Gillies, M.C., Walter, C.J. Prophylactic perifoveal laser treatment of soft drusen. Aust NZ J Ophthalmol. 1996; 24: 15–26.
7. Mimoun, G., Soubrane, G., Coscas, G. Macular drusen. Fr J Ophthalmol. 1990; 13: 511–530.

Prince of Wales Hospital
Sydney, Australia

52. Histopathological features of drusen and age-related macular degeneration

J.B. HARLAN and W.R. GREEN

(Bethesda, USA)

Introduction

Age-related macular degeneration (ARMD) is the most prevalent cause of legal blindness in the geriatric population in the USA[1]. The clinical course, histological characteristics and methods of treatment have been described extensively[2-9]. We review the key histopathological features of ARMD and describe the salient features present after treatment with laser photocoagulation and submacular surgery.

Drusen

Drusen are localized deposits located between the basement membrane of the retinal pigment epithelium (RPE) and the remainder of Bruch's membrane. A classification scheme was developed by Bressler *et al.*[8] taking into account the different clinical and histological features. Types of drusen defined include diffuse, hard, soft, small, large, calcified, cuticular, nodular and semisolid.

Diffuse drusen represent a sign of diffuse RPE disease. Diffuse drusen is solely a histopathological term describing diffuse thickening of the inner aspect of Bruch's membrane, usually within the entire central macular region. Diffuse drusen are clinically detectable only by secondary changes, which include RPE hypopigmentation and atrophy, pigment clumping, soft (large) drusen, drusenoid RPE detachments, RPE detachments, choroidal neovascularization and, ultimately, disciform scarring[4,8,9]. Transmission electron micrographic studies disclosed two types of sub-RPE deposits. Basal laminar deposits are material visualized on TEM which is mostly composed of wide-spaced collagen, located between the plasma membrane and the basement membrane of the RPE (Figs 1, 2). The second type, basal linear deposit (Figs 1, 3), consists of granular and vesicular electron-dense, lipid-rich material located external to the basement membrane of the RPE, in the inner collagenous zone of Bruch's membrane. The origin of basal linear deposit is unknown, although it has been suggested that it is released from the RPE via the basal plasma membrane.

Distinguishing between basal laminar and basal linear deposit may be

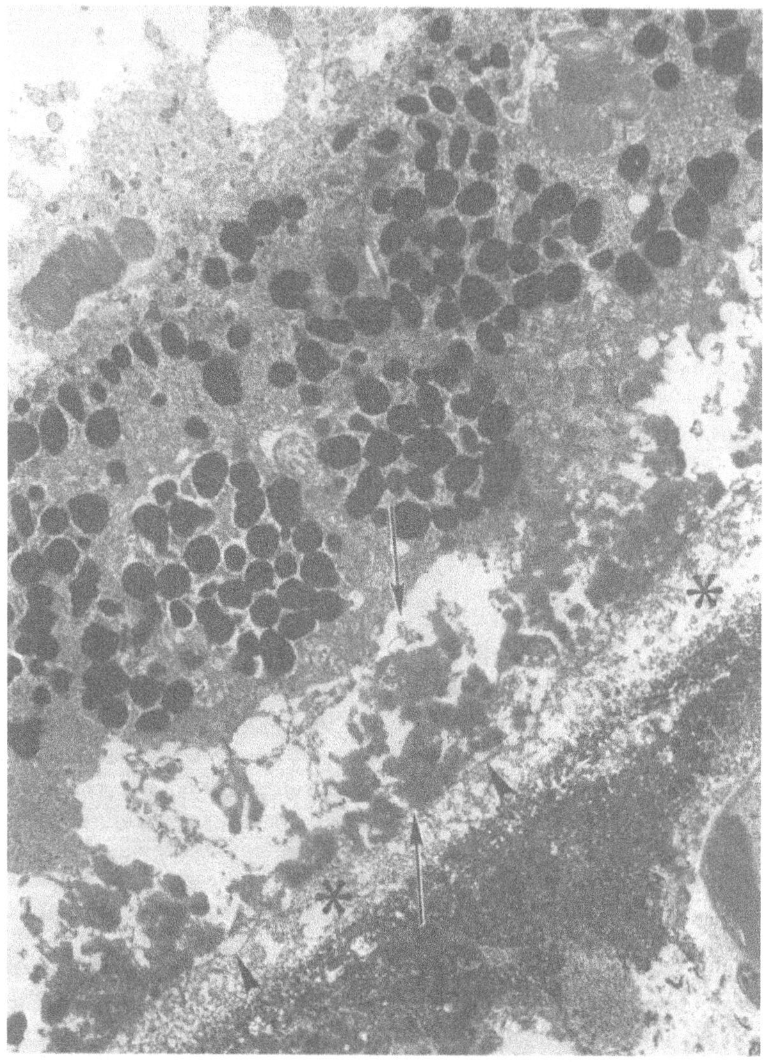

Fig. 1. Ultrastructural appearance of a 5.0 μm thick layer of basal laminar deposit (between arrows) located between the RPE and its basement membrane (arrowheads). A 3.3 μm thick layer of basal linear deposit (asterisks) is located between the basement membrane of the RPE and the remainder of Bruch's membrane.

difficult by light microscopy, and both are often present in the same eye. With the periodic acid–Schiff stain, the inner aspect of basal laminar deposit has a brush-like appearance and is located internal to the RPE basement membrane.

Basal laminar deposit, along with the RPE and its basement membrane,

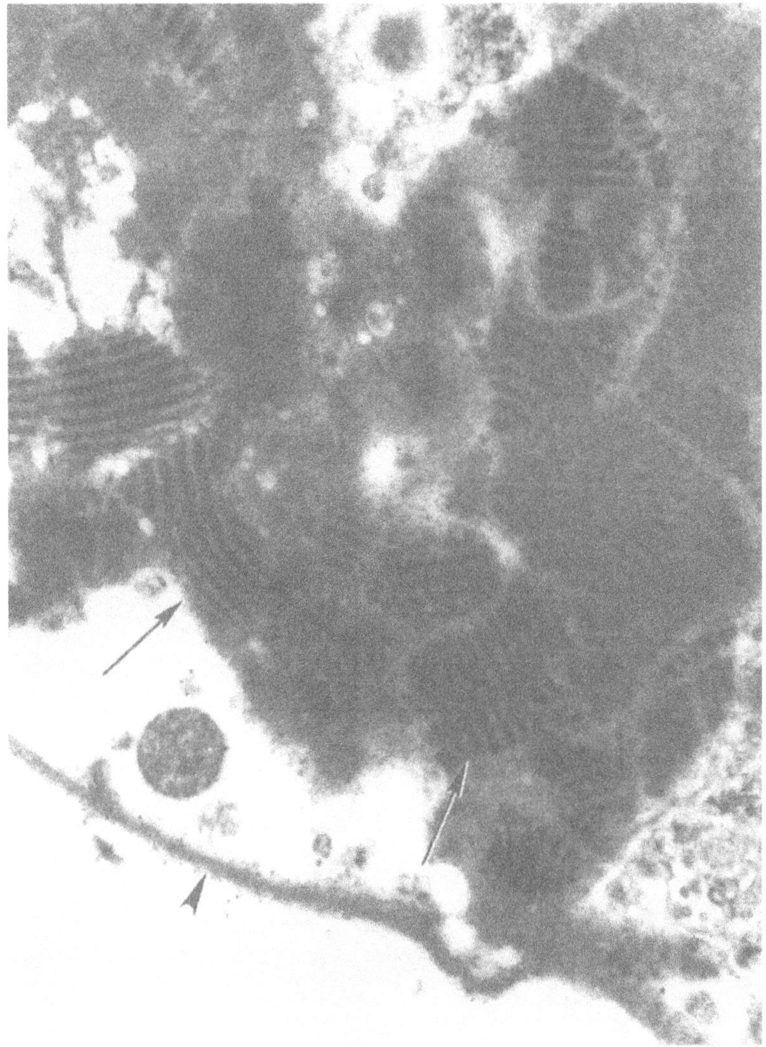

Fig. 2. At higher power the basal laminar deposit is mostly composed of wide-spaced collagen (arrows) with a diameter of up to 1.0 µm and a periodicity of 10.0 nm located internal to the RPE basement membrane (arrowhead) (× 30 000).

may become detached by a proteinaceous material. Localized detachments of this type correspond to soft drusen (drusen with amorphous, poorly demarcated boundaries and usually > 63 µm in size), and large detachments are clinically evident as 'drusenoid detachments' and serous detachments of the RPE. A similar progression may occur with basal linear deposit, with a

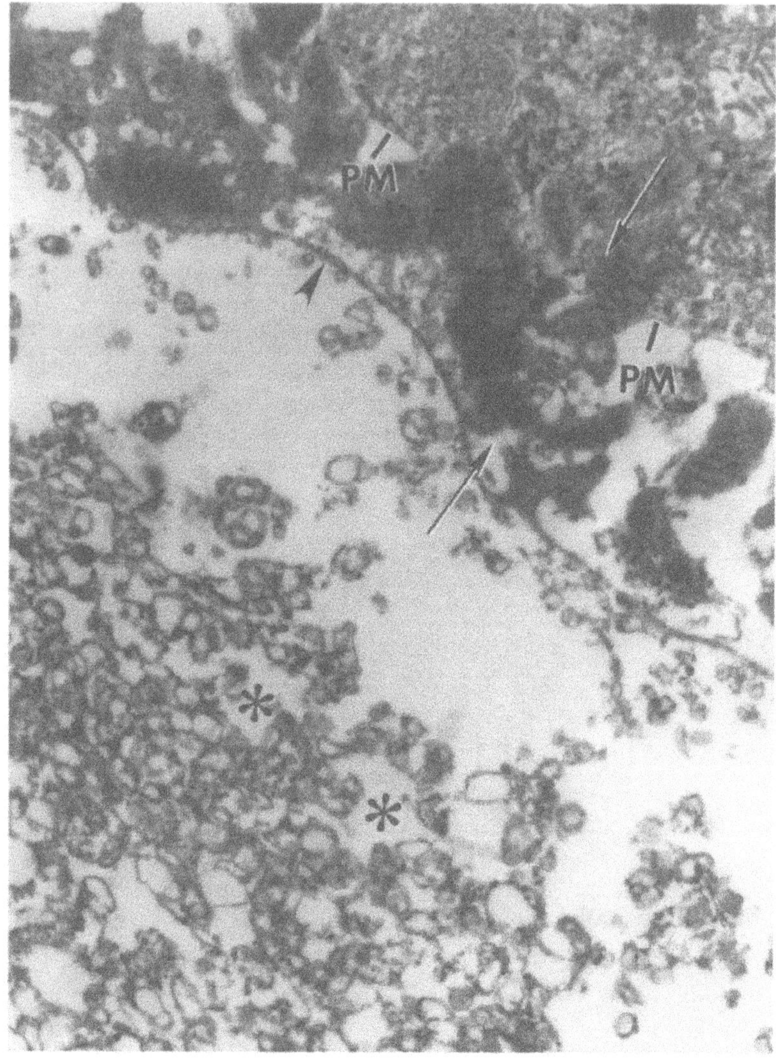

Fig. 3. At higher power the basal linear deposit (asterisks) is mostly composed of coated and non-coated vesicles located external to the RPE basement membrane (arrowhead). A thin layer of basal laminar deposit (between arrows) is located between the RPE plasma membrane (PM) and basement membrane (arrowhead) (× 20 100).

tendency for cleavage to develop between the basal linear deposit and the remainder of Bruch's membrane, leading to a detachment of the RPE. When the detachment is localized, a soft druse is observed clinically. Larger detachments correspond clinically to serous RPE detachment[9].

In essence, the term 'soft drusen' actually describes at least three distinct morphological scenarios: a localized detachment of the RPE with basal laminar deposit in an eye with diffuse basal laminar deposits; a localized detachment of RPE and basal linear deposit in an eye with diffuse basal laminar and basal linear deposits; and a localized detachment due to the localized accumulation of basal linear deposit but without diffuse basal linear deposits[8,9]. Clearly more direct clinicopathological correlative studies of large drusen are needed.

Kenyon *et al.*[10] described one unusual case of diffuse drusen in a 46-year-old woman characterized by marked diffuse thickening of the inner portion of Bruch's membrane with uniform internal nodularity. This deposit consisted of a curious reticulum of curvilinear membranous profiles on TEM. The authors postulated that this unusual accumulated material might represent either an extreme elaboration of the basal plasma membrane and basement membrane by the RPE or, alternatively, an extracellular proliferation of plasma membrane and basement membrane materials secreted by the pigment epithelial cells. This unique type of diffuse drusen with superimposed highly uniform internal nodularity is termed 'cuticular' drusen[9]. Clinically, cuticular drusen appear as numerous, small, uniform, discretely round, slightly raised, yellow lesions at the level of the RPE which fluoresce discretely on angiography[8].

Within the classification scheme of Bressler *et al.*, the term 'large druse' corresponds clinically to a yellowish lesion at the level of the RPE greater than 64 µm in size, usually with poorly demarcated boundaries. Histopathologically, there is generally little distinction between soft and large drusen. The terms small and hard are both used to describe nodular drusen which appear clinically as sharp, discrete lesions with well demarcated boundaries, usually less than 64 µm in size. Histopathologically, nodular drusen are localized accumulations of hyaline material along the inner aspect of Bruch's membrane with attenuation of the overlying RPE. The pathogenesis of nodular drusen is not known. Some authors found evidence that nodular drusen are formed by the extrusion of a portion of the RPE cell[11]. Another theory implicated lipoidal degeneration of the RPE cells as a mechanism[12–15]. The term calcified drusen describes drusen which appear clinically as glistening yellow lesions, usually associated with RPE atrophy. Histopathologically, all types of drusen may have calcification. The term semisolid drusen is a histopathological term used by Sarks[6] to describe drusen that contain hyaline material (as in nodular drusen) in which the material has fragmented. When numerous contiguous areas of this change are apparent the appearance may be similar to, although not quite as extensive as, diffuse drusen.

A recent comprehensive histopathological evaluation of 760 eyes with ARMD in the Eye Pathology Laboratory of the Wilmer Institute revealed that basal laminar deposit, basal linear deposit and diffuse drusen were important positive associations with choroidal neovascularization, disciform scarring and visual loss. Nodular (hard, small) drusen were not associated with these degenerative changes and were thus not considered as an important risk factor for vision loss in ARMD[9].

Retinal pigment epithelial abnormalities

Abnormalities of the RPE, clinically apparent as generalized or focal pigment mottling, include pigment epithelial cell attenuation, atrophy, hypertrophy, hyperplasia, and pigment clumping. Using terminology proposed by Bressler *et al.*, the RPE abnormalities present in ARMD fall into four basic categories: focal hyperpigmentation; non-geographic atrophy; geographic or areolar atrophy; and lipidized RPE[8].

Focal hyperpigmentation of the RPE, observed clinically as focal clumps of pigmentation, appears histologically as clumps of pigmented cells in the subretinal space or outer layers of the retina[8]. Non-geographic atrophy, clinically associated with hyperpigmentation, appears histologically as mottled areas of hypopigmentation or atrophy of the RPE overlying a diffusely thickened inner aspect of Bruch's membrane from basal laminar and linear deposits. Geographic or areolar atrophy, appearing clinically as well demarcated areas of atrophy in which the underlying choroidal vasculature may be more apparent, appears histologically as well-demarcated areas of RPE atrophy in which the underlying choriocapillaris may be sclerosed with thickening of the intercapillary septae and/or atrophy of the choriocapillaris. Basal laminar and basal linear deposits are usually present. In older lesions the basal linear and, to a lesser degree, the basal laminar deposits may partially or completely disappear. Areolar atrophy is accompanied by loss of photoreceptors which are metabolically dependent on the RPE. Although vascular insufficiency of the choriocapillaris might play a role in the pathogenesis of areolar atrophy, the histopathology of areolar atrophy is clearly distinct from the type of atrophy caused by choroidal vascular insufficiency. In diseases classically attributed to choriocapillary insufficiency, such as cobblestone degeneration and healed Elschnig spots, the outer portion of the inner nuclear layer of the retina is usually affected. In areolar atrophy, however, the entire inner nuclear layer of the retina remains intact[4]. Finally, lipidization of the RPE, observed clinically as discrete, pinpoint areas of hypopigmentation, histologically are individual RPE cells with loss of pigment and intracellular accumulation of lipid. This lipoidal RPE degeneration is also included in the histologic definition of small or hard drusen[8].

RPE detachment

Serous detachment of the RPE is a form of exudative or wet ARMD. Basal laminar and basal linear deposits are frequently the predisposing factor to the splitting of Bruch's membrane, creating an intra-Bruch's membrane detachment, with the plane of serous and/or haemorrhagic detachment occurring between the thickened inner portion of Bruch's membrane and the remainder of Bruch's membrane[4,7,8]. A localized detachment of the RPE is part of the histological definition of a soft druse, and the coalescence of several soft drusen is all that is necessary for an apparent clinical progression from soft drusen to drusenoid detachment, and serous detachment of the RPE. Areolar atrophy may then follow the resolution of these serous detachments[4,7,8].

Choroidal neovascularization

Choroidal neovascularization starts with capillary-like vessels that extend through the outer layer of Bruch's membrane and into the sub-RPE area, usually in association with basal laminar or basal linear deposits, alone or in combination. The process is complex and the pathophysiology is poorly understood. Vessel ingrowth may involve metabolic factors released from tissues, mechanical factors acting on the walls of blood vessels, physical and chemical properties of the extravascular matrix, pericyte–endothelial cell interactions, and various peptide signalling molecules, such as fibroblast growth factor, vascular endothelial growth factor and transforming growth factor β. Early neovascularization may be associated with cellular breakdown of Bruch's membrane with the presence of multinucleated giant cells. Dastgheib and Green[16] observed numerous foreign body giant cells intimately associated with Bruch's membrane in a case of ARMD. Cytoplasmic extension of some of these giant cells was present on both the inner and outer surfaces of Bruch's membrane and at the margin of several defects in Bruch's membrane. This granulomatous reaction to Bruch's membrane is thought to play a role in the pathogenesis of choroidal neovascularization, by creating points of minimal or absent resistance in Bruch's membrane through which new blood vessels can preferentially pass[16]. Ingrowth of choroidal capillaries through defects in Bruch's membrane eventually lead to proliferation of fibrovascular tissue in the sub-RPE space.

Ophthalmoscopic signs of choroidal neovascularization include a subretinal membrane, haemorrhagic detachment of the retina and/or RPE, intraretinal or subretinal exudates in the absence of vascular disease, subretinal pigment epithelial ring lesions, and serous detachment of the RPE, particularly when associated with an indentation or notch of the margin of the RPE detachment or radial chorioretinal folds surrounding the RPE detachment. The neovascular tissue may be clinically apparent on fluorescein angiography as a lacy network of vessels at the level of the RPE. The vessels classically have a sea-fan or cartwheel pattern during the early phases of angiography. In the later phases of angiography, there is leakage of fluorescein from the neovascular membrane into the subretinal space with loss of the sea-fan or cartwheel character. Visualization of the membrane is made more difficult by overlying blood, exudate or RPE detachment. So called occult choroidal neovascularization (also referred to as ill-defined, poorly defined, poorly demarcated, or fluorescein leakage of undetermined origin) may be associated with the presence of blood or exudate at the margin of an RPE detachment. Angiographic clues to the presence of occult choroidal neovascularization include an area of hypofluorescence or non-fluorescence on angiography corresponding to a meniscus of blood, a localized zone of hyperfluorescence or 'hot spot' within the RPE detachment during the early phases of angiography, the absence of late staining of the notched border of the RPE detachment, the presence of an irregular elevation of the RPE which stains often and leaks fluorescein dye in the late transit frames, and the presence of areas of late-phase leakage at the level of the outer retina that do not correspond to distinct areas of hyperfluorescence in the early or midphase frames[17,18]. It has been estimated that between 50%[19–21] and 87%[22] of choroidal neovascularization due to ARMD consists of vessels which are not classic or well defined, but rather occult or poorly defined.

Chang *et al.*[23] reported the success of indocyanine green videoangiography in the identification of occult CNV not visualized with conventional fluorescein angiography. A detailed postmortem histological study of the involved eye revealed a thin vascular subretinal pigment epithelial choroidal neovascular membrane associated with diffuse basal laminar deposit, demonstrating for the first time a clinicopathological correlation of occult CNV identified by ICG videoangiography. The theoretical advantage of ICG over fluorescein is that the spectral absorption and emission characteristics of the ICG molecule, which derive from operating within the longer, near infra-red spectrum, make it easier for the ICG fluorescence to penetrate through exudation, pigment, haemorrhage and lens opacities. Because the ICG molecule is also quickly and almost totally bound to serum proteins, it tends not to leak as readily from the choriocapillaris or abnormal vessels and accumulate within serous cavities and tissue spaces to obscure basic pathological changes[23].

Disciform scar

Choroidal neovascularization located between a thickened inner layer of Bruch's membrane and the remainder of Bruch's membrane tends to leak and bleed, causing serous or haemorrhagic detachment of the RPE and the inner aspect of Bruch's membrane along an intra-Bruch's membrane plane of splitting. In such a setting, fibrous tissue proliferation occurs with the development of a fibrovascular scar between the two layers of Bruch's membrane. A second component of scarring may develop between the neurosensory retina and the detached and thickened inner layer of Bruch's membrane. This inner component of the scar usually results from RPE hyperplasia and is not vascularized. The outer, intra-Bruch's membrane fibrocellular component of the scar, often containing spindle-shaped cells with myoblastic features, may contract, ripping the inner layer of Bruch's membrane with the RPE. The two separate inner and outer components of the disciform scar may then become continuous through these torn areas[4,7,8]. Green and Enger[9] analysed disciform scars in 310 eyes and found that 48.1% of eyes had two-component scars. The two components were continuous in 6.8% of eyes at tears in the RPE and basal laminar deposit.

Vascularization of disciform scars usually originates in the choroid, but some scars receive a contribution from the retinal vasculature. In the series studied by Green and Enger[9], vascularization from the choroid was present in 74.5% of cases with vascular contribution from the retina present in 2.6% of cases. No apparent neovascularization was present in 25.5% of eyes with disciform scars. Disciform scars in this group were generally small and thin. Photoreceptor cell degeneration was also progressively greater as the diameter and thickness of the disciform scar increased[9].

Patients with a disciform scar may develop complications such as extensive intra- and subretinal exudation along with serous and/or haemorrhagic detachments of the adjacent retina and/or RPE. The sub-RPE haemorrhage may resorb, dissect under the retina or, rarely, break into the vitreous cavity. El Baba *et al.*[24] studied several cases of ARMD complicated by massive subretinal and/or vitreous haemorrhage and found that in such cases, the origin of the haemorrhage appeared to be from disciform scars that were vascularized from the choroid. Rupture of large choroidal vessels extending into the disciform scar accounted for massive haemorrhage erupting through all layers and into the vitreous. Three cases demonstrated the presence of large choroidal vessels emerging into the disciform scar through defects in Bruch's membrane with rupture of the vessel walls. The authors postulated that the process must begin with an initial bleeding event or exudation from neovascular tissue which in turn causes a serous and/or haemorrhagic detachment of the RPE. This process extends under the disciform scar, a fibrovascular membrane fed by choroidal arteries and veins, until it reaches a point where a feeder artery and vein emerge from the choroid. Further serous and haemorrhagic detachment may then lead to pressure necrosis of the choroidal artery and ultimately rupture with massive haemorrhage. The massive haemorrhage dissects under the RPE and erupts through the RPE and into the subretinal space. In some instances, the haemorrhage may disrupt the retina and extend into the vitreous. The authors also found that patients with disciform scars who were taking anticoagulants and antithrombotic medications appeared to be at risk for such haemorrhagic complications[24].

Laser treatment of CNV – clinicopathological correlations

The Macular Photocoagulation Study for ARMD demonstrated that laser photocoagulation of extrafoveal choroidal neovascularization (posterior boundary of CNV 200 μm from the foveal centre) substantially reduces the risk of severe visual loss[25]; that patients with juxtafoveal CNV (posterior boundary 1–199 μm from the foveal centre) clearly benefit from photocoagulation[26]; and that eyes with subfoveal CNV fare better with treatment that with no treatment[27]. Laser treatment is thought to control the neovascular process by stimulating the formation of a chorioretinal scar, which presumably re-establishes the blood–ocular barrier. Factors and substances released by stimulated retinal pigment epithelium or other cells may play a role in containment and resolution of CNV[28].

Despite the proven benefits of argon blue-green laser photocoagulation in treatment of CNV in ARMD, there are limitations in regard to its use. Because absorption of the blue component of argon blue-green laser by xanthophyll is about 60%, treatment of lesions very close to the foveal avascular zone or in the papillomacular bundle can result in transretinal destruction. This transretinal destruction causes retinal whitening, which serves to make further treatment ineffective and interferes with an adequate fluorescein angiographic evaluation of the post-treatment status of the CNV membrane. The inner retinal damage created is also believed to lead to an increased incidence of more severe scarring and secondary macular distortion. Krypton red and argon green laser photocoagulation are theoretically better for the treatment of juxtafoveal and subfoveal choroidal neovascular membranes because these wavelengths are much less absorbed by xanthophyll (argon green, 18% krypton red, <1%). However, even with krypton red, repeated treatment in the same area may result in full-thickness retinal destruction[30]. The MPS group recently evaluated the use of argon green vs. krypton red laser for treatment of subfoveal CNV and found no clinically and statistically significant differences between these two forms of treatment in the management of eyes with subfoveal CNV[29].

Green and associates[30,31] have studied a number of post-mortem eyes with treated choroidal neovascular membranes in the setting of ARMD. In three cases, the choroidal neovascularization associated with ARMD was obliterated by photocoagulation, but a new or additional unrecognized area of neovascularization was observed histopathologically. Two of these new areas of neovascularization had been noted clinically. In one case, the new vessels originated in the retina. In a fourth case[30], CNV was treated with argon green and krypton red lasers on four separate occasions until it was clinically considered to have been eliminated. Histopathological evaluation revealed the presence of residual vessels in the scar and in the subretinal pigment epithelial area along the nasal margin of the krypton red treated area. Krypton red-treated areas revealed sparing of the inner retinal layers, whereas transretinal scarring was present in the argon green-treated areas. In a fifth case, an eye with CNV was treated by krypton red laser on two occasions with complete obliteration of the lesion by clinical standards. Histopathological analysis disclosed the origin of the neovascularization to be in the subfoveal area outside the treatment zone, demonstrating incomplete treatment and clinically unrecognized persistence of the neovascular membrane[31].

Unfortunately, persistent or recurrent choroidal neovascular membranes occur frequently after laser treatment and adversely affect visual acuity. The Macular Photocoagulation Study Group has reported a CNV recurrence rate of 59% in cases of ARMD[32]. Most recurrences occurred within 1 year after treatment and were located on the foveal side of the membrane. It is difficult in the clinical setting to determine whether post-laser CNV represents persistent, inadequately treated neovascularization or whether it represents a new site of neovascularization contiguous to the area of treatment. Detailed histopathological study, utilizing serial sections through the area of interest, allows one to be more precise about the nature and origin of neovascular tissue. Histopathologically, CNV may be persistent or recurrent and still be clinically undetectable[31]. It is also very likely that multiple sources of subretinal pigment epithelial neovascularization, as noted on histological studies, account for the high incidence of contiguous persistence and recurrences of CNV.

Another recognized effect of laser treatment is the increase in size of the photocoagulation lesion in the post-treatment period. This effect is independent of laser wavelength, and is thought to occur due to a variety of possible mechanisms: (1) subclinical thermal damage to the RPE and delayed atrophy at the periphery of a photocoagulation lesion; (2) extension of RPE atrophy due to post treatment inflammation, oedema and scarring such that intact RPE adjacent to the treated RPE may be involved in the reparative process, undergoing constant degeneration; (3) because of a moving blood column, vessel effects from laser photocoagulation may be located downstream from the actual exposure site, creating choroidal ischaemia adjacent to the site of laser treatment with subsequent atrophy of the overlying RPE and photoreceptor cell layer. Dastgheib *et al.*[33] studied this phenomenon in an eye with ARMD treated with krypton red laser for extrafoveal CNV and found expansion of RPE atrophy in the area of clinically visible lesion expansion. Histological study revealed an area of laser treatment surrounded by a zone of RPE atrophy with loss of the overlying photoreceptor layer. Expansion of RPE atrophy beyond the area of initial treatment was present and was associated with loss of the overlying photoreceptor layer. This has obvious implications for juxtafoveal laser application. In this particular case, the expansion of RPE atrophy increased the linear dimension of the laser lesion by as much as 40% during the 3 year post-laser follow-up period prior to post-mortem examination[33].

Clinicopathological correlation of submacular surgery in ARMD

Given that the majority of choroidal neovascular membranes do not meet the MPS criteria for laser photocoagulation due to their size, location or ill-defined borders, attention has recently turned to submacular surgery as an alternative therapy.

Rosa *et al.*[46] recently studied an eye of a patient with ARMD who underwent submacular membranectomy and had retention of good visual acuity for almost 4 years following surgery despite recurrent choroidal neovascularization treated with krypton laser photocoagulation and mild expansion of the laser lesion over time. Histological examination of an eye obtained post-mortem revealed a 2.75 × 2.1 mm RPE defect with overlying photoreceptor cell atrophy centred on the temporal parafoveal area and extending just into the nasal perifoveal area. The RPE was intact near the centre of the fovea. A 0.6 × 0.1 mm subretinal pigment epithelium fibrovascular membrane was present 0.4 mm temporal to the fovea, with an area of RPE hyperplasia and vascularization originating from the retina. Basal laminar deposit was present in the region of the fovea and nasal parafoveal area. In the region of the macula treated with krypton red laser for recurrent CNV, the inner retina was nicely preserved, including the nerve fibre layer, ganglion cell layer and much of the inner nuclear layer. A thin subretinal fibrocellular membrane was present in this area[46].

Hsu and associates[47] studied an eye which underwent submacular membranectomy for CNV associated with ARMD after two unsuccessful laser photocoagulation treatments. Histopathological study of the excised subfoveal membrane disclosed a thin two-component fibrovascular membrane with the larger component internal to residual RPE and basal laminar deposit. Photoreceptor outer segments were present on the internal surface of the membrane near one margin. Histological study of the post-mortem globe revealed a very thin 1.5 mm subfoveal sub-RPE fibrovascular membrane with loss of the photoreceptor cell layer in a central 0.5 mm area. Two sources of choroidal vessels were present in this membrane. Given the presence of RPE in the surgically excised specimen, it was felt that this membrane represented a new CNVM which developed during the post-surgical period. Attenuated RPE was present internal to the membrane, except over the central portion where it was absent for about 0.5 mm, suggesting that RPE had partially migrated across the region of denuded RPE for about 0.5 mm in the periphery of the lesion. The photoreceptor cell layer was totally lost over the central third of the membrane and was moderately lost over the remaining two-thirds. The preservation of the photoreceptor cells in this case corresponded to the intactness of the underlying RPE, with tapering of the photoreceptor cell layer over areas of mild RPE attenuation, total loss of photoreceptors over areas of marked RPE attenuation, and preservation of photoreceptors over intact RPE. This clearly demonstrates the important role of the RPE in photoreceptor function and preservation. This clinicopathological study demonstrates that submacular surgery for recurrent CNV in the setting of ARMD was effective in this case, with repopulation of two-thirds of the area of membranectomy by extension of attenuated RPE from neighbouring areas. There was, however, persistence or recurrence of CNV, moderate atrophy of the overlying retina with total loss of the photoreceptor cells over the central 0.5 mm portion of the recurrent membrane, and moderate loss of photoreceptor cells over the remaining area[47].

Histopathological studies[35–45] of the excised membrane have often revealed a two-component membrane separated by residual RPE and basal laminar deposit.

Conclusion

Age-related macular degeneration is the leading cause of severe visual loss in North America. ARMD occurs in the setting of diffuse RPE disease. The exact aetiology is not known, but postulated to be multifactorial, with contributions from genetic factors, environmental stresses such as blue solar radiation and cigarette smoking, iris colour, and race[48]. The histopathology of ARMD has been extensively studied and characterized. Diffuse RPE disease becomes manifest in the form of diffuse drusen, which in turn may be associated with soft drusen, focal and generalized RPE detachment, and RPE abnormalities which include pigment mottling, pigment clumping, attenuation, hypertrophy, atrophy and hyperplasia. Diffuse drusen are associated with the development of a thin sub-RPE fibrovascular membrane, which may eventually lead to serous and/or haemorrhagic detachment of the RPE and/or neurosensory retina, exudates, haemorrhage and pigmentary abnormalities of the RPE. Fibrovascular membranes may also progress to disciform scarring with extensive exudation, tearing of the RPE and further neovascularization originating from the retinal vasculature (Fig. 4). The principle mechanism for severe visual loss is essentially CNV and subsequent exudation, haemorrhage, fibrovascular proliferation and ultimately disciform scarring. The current preferred treatment modality is laser photocoagulation, however submacular surgery is a newly evolving treatment alternative, now being studied in a

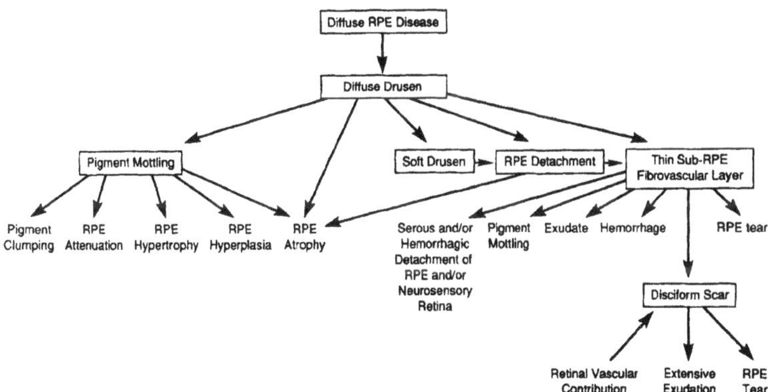

Fig. 4. Flow diagram shows the interrelationships of the various features of age-related macular degeneration.

randomized controlled clinical trial. Only a few submacular surgery cases have undergone detailed clinicopathological study. The value of surgical therapy compared with laser treatment remains to be elucidated.

Acknowledgements

Supported in part by the International Order of Odd Fellows, Winston-Salem, North Carolina and Core Grant EYO 01765-21 from the National Eye Institute, Bethesda, Maryland.

References

1. Kini, M.M., Leibowitz, H.M., Colton, T., Nickerson. R.J., Ganley, J., Dawber, T.R. Prevalence of senile cataract, diabetic retinopathy, senile macular degeneration, and open angle glaucoma in the Framingham Eye Study. Am J Ophthalmol. 1978; 85: 28–34.
2. Gass, J.D.M. Pathogenesis of disciform detachment of the neuroepithelium. III. Senile disciform macular degeneration. Am J Ophthalmol. 1967; 63: 617–44.
3. Sarks, S.H. New vessel formation beneath the retinal pigment epithelium in senile eyes. Br J Ophthalmol. 1973; 57: 951–965.
4. Green, W.R., Key, S.N. III. Senile macular degeneration: a histopathologic study. Trans Am Ophthalmol Soc. 1977; 75: 180–254.
5. Sarks, S.H. Ageing and degeneration in the macular region; a clinicopathological study. Br J Ophthalmol. 1976; 60: 324–331.
6. Sarks, S.H. Drusen and their relationship to senile macular degeneration. Aust J Ophthalmol. 1980; 8: 117–130.
7. Green, W.R., McDonnell, P.J., Yeo, J.H. Pathologic features of senile macular degeneration. Ophthalmology. 1985; 92: 615–627.
8. Bressler, N.M., Silva, J.C., Bressler, S.B., Fine, S.L., Green, W.R. Clinicopathologic correlation of drusen and retinal pigment epithelial abnormalities in age-related macular degeneration. Retina. 1994; 14: 130–142.
9. Green, W.R., Enger, C. Age-related macular degeneration histopathologic studies. Ophthalmology. 1993; 100: 1519–1535.
10. Kenyon, K.R., Maumenee, A.E., Ryan, S.J., Whitmore, P.V., Green, W.R. Diffuse drusen and associated complications. Am J Ophthalmol. 1985; 100: 119–128.
11. Burns, R.P., Feeney-Burns, L. Clinicopathologic correlations of drusen of Bruch's membrane. Trans Am Ophthalmol Soc. 1980; 78: 206.
12. El Baba, F., Green, W.R., Fleischmann, J., Finkelstein, D., de la Cruz, Z. Clinicopathologic correlation of lipidization and detachment of the retinal pigment epithelium. Am J Ophthalmol. 1986; 101: 576–583.
13. Green, W.R. Clinicopathologic studies of SMD. In: Nicholson, D.H. (ed): Ocular Pathology Update. New York, Masson, 1980: 115–144.
14. Fine, B.S., Kwapien, R.P. Pigment epithelial windows and drusen. An animal model. Invest Ophthalmol Vis Sci. 1978; 17: 1059.
15. Fine, B.S. Lipoidal degeneration of the retinal pigment epithelium. Am J Ophthalmol. 1981; 91: 469.
16. Dastgheib, K., Green, W.R. Granulomatous reaction to Bruch's membrane in age-related macular degeneration. Arch Ophthalmol. 1994; 112: 813–818.
17. Green, W.R., Wilson, D.J. Choroidal neovascularization. Ophthalmology. 1986; 93: 1169–1176.

18. Bressler, S.B., Silva, J.C., Bressler, N.B., Alexander, J., Green, W.R. Clinicopathologic correlation of occult choroidal neovascularization in age-related macular degeneration. Arch Ophthalmol. 1992; 110: 827–832.
19. Bressler, N.M., Bressler, S.B., Fine, S.L. Age-related macular degeneration. Surv Ophthalmol. 1988; 32: 375–413.
20. Bressler, N.M., Frost, L.A., Bressler, S.B., Murphy, R.P., Fine, S.L. Natural course of poorly defined choroidal neovascularization associated with macular degeneration. Arch Ophthalmol. 1988; 106: 1537–1542.
21. Bressler, N.M., Bressler, S.B., Gragoudas, E.S. Clinical characteristics of choroidal neovascular membranes. Arch Ophthalmol. 1987; 105: 209–213.
22. Freund, K.B., Yannuzzi, L.A., Sorenson, J.A. Age-related macular degeneration and choroidal neovascularization. Am J Ophthalmol. 1993; 115: 786–791.
23. Chang, T.S., Freund, K.B., de la Cruz, Z., Yannuzzi, L.A., Green, W.R. Clinicopathologic correlation of choroidal neovascularization demonstrated by indocyanine green angiography in a patient with retention of good vision for almost 4 years. Retina. 1994; 14: 114–124.
24. El Baba, F., Jarrett, W.H. II, Harbin, T.S. Jr. et al. Massive hemorrhage complicating age-related macular degeneration. Ophthalmology. 1986; 93: 1581–1592.
25. Macular Photocoagulation Study Group. Argon laser photocoagulation for neovascular maculopathy: five year results from randomized clinical trials. Arch Ophthalmol. 1991; 109: 1109–1114.
26. Macular Photocoagulation Study Group. Krypton laser photocoagulation for neovascular lesions of age-related macular degeneration: results of a randomized clinical trial. Arch Ophthalmol. 1990; 108: 816–824.
27. Macular Photocoagulation Study Group. Laser photocoagulation of subfoveal neovascular lesions in age-related macular degeneration: results of a randomized clinical trial. Arch Ophthalmol. 1991; 109: 1220–1231.
28. Glaser, B.M., Campochiaro, P.A., Davis, J.L., Sato, M. Retinal pigment epithelial cells release an inhibitor of neovascularization. Arch Ophthalmol. 1985; 103: 1870–1875.
29. Macular Photocoagulation Study Group. Evaluation of argon green vs krypton red laser for photocoagulation of subfoveal choroidal neovascularization in the macular photocoagulation study. Arch Ophthalmol. 1994; 112: 1176–1184.
30. Guyer, D.R., Fine, S.L., Murphy, R.P., Green, W.R. Clinicopathologic correlation of krypton and argon laser photocoagulation in a patient with a subfoveal choroidal neovascular membrane. Retina. 1986; 6: 157–163.
31. Green, W.R. Clinicopathologic studies of treated choroidal neovascular membranes. A review and report of two cases. Retina. 1991; 11: 328–356.
32. Macular Photocoagulation Study Group. Recurrent choroidal neovascularization after argon laser photocoagulation for neovascular maculopathy. Arch Ophthalmol. 1986; 104: 503–512.
33. Dastgheib, K., Bressler, S.B., Green, W.R. Clinicopathologic correlation of laser lesion expansion after treatment of choroidal neovascularization. Retina. 1993; 13: 345–352.
34. de Juan, E. Jr, Machemer, R. Vitreous surgery for hemorrhagic and fibrous complications of age-related macular degeneration. Am J Ophthalmol. 1988; 105: 25–29.
35. Blinder, K.J., Peyman, G.A., Paris, C.L., Gremillion, C.M. Jr. Submacular scar excision in age-related macular degeneration. Int Ophthalmol. 1991; 15: 215–222.
36. Lopez, P.F., Grossniklaus, H.E., Lambert, H.M. et al. Pathologic features of surgically excised subretinal neovascular membranes in age-related macular degeneration. Am J Ophthalmol. 1991; 112: 647–656.
37. Gehrs, K.M., Heriot, W.J., de Juan, E. Jr. Transmission electron microscopic study of a subretinal choroidal neovascular membrane due to age-related macular degeneration. Arch Ophthalmol. 1992; 110: 833–837.
38. Grossniklaus, H.E., Martinez, J.A., Brown, V.B. et al. Immunohistochemical properties of surgically excised subretinal neovascular membranes in age-related macular degeneration. Am J Ophthalmol. 1992; 114: 464–472.

39. Das, A., Puklin, J.E., Frank, R.N., Zhang, N.L. Ultrastructural immunocytochemistry of subretinal neovascular membranes in age-related macular degeneration. Ophthalmology. 1992; 99: 1368–1376.
40. Lopez, P.F., Lambert, H.M., Grossniklaus, H.E., Sternberg, P. Jr. Well defined subfoveal choroidal neovascular membranes in age-related macular degeneration. Ophthalmology. 1993; 100: 415–422.
41. Saxe, S.J., Grossniklaus, H.E., Lopez, P.F., Lambert, H.M., Sternberg, P. Jr, L'Hernault, M.A. Ultrastructural features of surgically excised subretinal neovascular membranes in the ocular histoplasmosis syndrome. Arch Ophthalmol. 1993; 111: 88–95.
42. Bynoe, L.A., Chang, T.S., Funata, M., Del Priore, L.V., Kaplan, H.J., Green, W.R. Histopathologic examination of vascular patterns in subfoveal neovascular membranes. Ophthalmology. 1994; 101: 1112–1117.
43. Grossniklaus, H.E., Hutchinson, A.K., Capone, A. Jr, Woolfson, J., Lambert, H.M. Clinicopathologic features of surgically excised choroidal neovascular membranes. Ophthalmology. 1994; 101: 1099–1111.
44. Amim, R., Puklin, J.E., Frank, R.N. Growth factor localization in choroidal neovascular membranes of age-related macular degeneration. Invest Ophthalmol Vis Sci. 1994; 35: 3178–3188.
45. Seregard, S., Algvere, P.V., Berglin, L. Immunohistochemical characterization of surgically removed subfoveal fibrovascular membranes. Graefe's Arch Clin Exp Ophthalmol. 1994; 232: 325–329.
46. Rosa, R.H., Thomas, M.A., Green, W.R. Clinicopathologic correlation of submacular membranectomy with retention of good vision in a patient with age-related macular degeneration. Arch Ophthalmol. 1996; 114: 480–487.
47. Hsu, J.K., Thomas, M.A., Ibanez, H., Green, W.R. Clinicopathologic studies of an eye after submacular membranectomy for choroidal neovascularization. Retina. 1995; 15: 43–52.
48. Young, R.W. Solar radiation and age-related macular degeneration. Surv Ophthalmol. 1988; 32: 252–269.

W. Richard Green
Eye Pathology Laboratory
Maumenee 427
Johns Hopkins Hospital
600 North Wolfe Street
Baltimore, MD 21287-9248, USA

53. Choroidal neovascularization prevention trial

A.J. BRUCKER

(Philadelphia, PA, USA)

Introduction

Severe visual loss in age related macular degeneration (ARMD) may be due to choroidal neovascularization (90%) or to geographic atrophy (10%). Drusen are the common precursor for the development of either of these forms of ARMD. Eyes with large drusen (also called soft drusen) have thickening of the basement membrane of the retinal pigment epithelium which predisposes to the development of choroidal neovascularization. Patients with small drusen (also called hard drusen) are at relatively low risk for the development of choroidal neovascularization. Patients aged over 65 with bilateral large (soft) drusen have an approximately 6% risk to either eye of developing choroidal neovascularization each year. Overall, patients with large drusen in one eye and choroidal neovascularization in the other eye are at a 30% risk of developing neovascularization in the second eye within 5 years. When large drusen are combined with pigmentation and choroidal neovascularization in the first eye, risk to the fellow eye approaches 60% over 5 years. Laser photocoagulation in eyes with drusen may result in the resolution or disappearance of drusen. The natural hope would be that the disappearance of drusen would be paralleled by a decrease in the risk of developing choroidal neovascularization. The purpose of this study was to determine whether laser photocoagulation of the periphery of the macula can reduce the risk of visual loss from choroidal neovascularization in eyes with high-risk drusen.

Materials and methods

Fellow eye

In patients with choroidal neovascularization or scarring in one eye and 10 or more high risk drusen in the fellow eye, the fellow eye was randomly assigned to photocoagulation or observation.

Bilateral drusen

Patients with high risk drusen in both eyes had the right eye assigned at random to photocoagulation or observation; the left eye received the opposite

G. Coscas and F. Cardillo Piccolino (eds.), Retinal Pigment Epithelium and Macular Diseases, pp. 323–324.
© *1998 Kluwer Academic Publishers.*

treatment. The first treatment tested comprised three rows of laser spots (20 laser burns) placed on the temporal side of the macula. The first row of spots will be placed 750 μm from the centre of the fovea with two additional rows approximately one burn width apart. If at 6 months there was not a reduction of at least 50% in the area of drusen, an additional 20 spots were applied to the nasal half of the macula in the same manner as designated for the temporal half. In the second treatment modality, eyes were treated with two rings of 12 evenly spaced laser spots surrounding the area of drusen and centred on the fovea. If at 6 months there were still 10 or more large drusen, a second double ring of laser burns was placed around the drusen. Eyes were examined at regular intervals for the development of geographic atrophy.

Results

Pilot clinical trials in 15 centres were initiated in October 1994 and 400 eyes of 245 patients were enrolled by October 1996. At 6 months a 50% reduction in drusen was achieved in one-quarter of the treated eyes. By one year, some reduction in drusen was achieved in 80% of eyes.

Conclusion

The National Eye Institute has awarded a planning grant to continue pilot studies and to prepare a grant for a multicentre clinical trial. The importance of the CNVPT is in the potential for widespread generalizability of this treatment to eyes with high risk drusen at risk of vision loss from complications of choroidal neovascularization. The possibility that a decrease in the number of drusen may also decrease the risk of atrophy associated with ARMD will also be measured in future studies.

Department of Ophthalmology
Scheie Eye Institute
Philadelphia, PA
USA

54. The one-year result of a prospective, randomized study of laser photocoagulation of eyes with soft drusen in early age-related maculopathy

C. FRENNESSON and S.E.G. NILSSON

(Linköping, Sweden)

Introduction

Age-related maculopathy (ARM) is the leading cause of visual loss among elderly people in Western countries[1]. Of all cases of severe visual loss due to ARM, the vast majority are caused by exudative/neovascular complications[2]. The Macular Photocoagulation Study Group (MPS) demonstrated that laser photocoagulation reduced or delayed severe visual loss in eyes with classic choroidal neovascularization secondary to ARM[3]. However, only a minority of the patients with exudative lesions are eligible for laser photocoagulation therapy[4], and recurrences are common[5].

Because of the limitations of laser treatment, attention has been directed towards preventing the development of choriodal neovascularization. Previous studies have consistently identified soft drusen as a risk factor for the development of choriodal neovascularization in ARM[6,7]: for patients with bilateral drusen, this risk is estimated to 13.5% at 3 years[7], while for patients with a disciform lesion in one eye, the risk for the fellow eye rises to 58% within 5 years[6]. Several studies reported laser photocoagulation to cause resolution not only of treated soft drusen but also of untreated drusen[8–10].

To investigate whether laser photocoagulation reduces the area of soft drusen and whether such a decrease in drusen area reduces the risk of progression to neovascular maculopathy we performed a prospective, randomized study[11,12]. Here we present the 12-month follow-up results.

Materials and methods

The prospective study included 38 patients with early ARM. All had soft drusen and mild pigmentary changes but no other pathology, i.e. no pigmentary clumping, no pigment epithelial detachment, no choroidal neovascularization or haemorrhage and no macular atrophy.

The patients were randomized into two groups, a treatment group and a control group. The treatment group consisted of 19 patients with a mean age of 72.2 ± 6.6 years. At study entry, mean visual acuity was 0.93 ± 0.1. The

G. Coscas and F. Cardillo Piccolino (eds.), Retinal Pigment Epithelium and Macular Diseases, pp. 325–327.
© *1998 Kluwer Academic Publishers. Printed in Great Britain.*

remaining 19 patients formed the control group, mean age 68.5 ± 6.2 years, with a mean visual acuity of 0.95 ± 0.1 at study entry. At study entry, there were no statistically significant differences in age or visual acuity between the two groups. Both cases and controls were seen at study entry, at 1 month after entry and then every 3 months. Each time the patient was examined for best corrected visual acuity, colour contrast sensitivity, central visual field and fundus condition.

Colour fundus photography and fluorescein angiography were performed at study entry and at 3, 6 and 12 months. Using a computer system, the area occupied by drusen was calculated in the colour fundus photographs and angiograms within a circle with a radius of 2500 μm and 1250 μm, respectively. At study entry, there were no statistically significant differences between the two groups regarding drusen area, nor regarding central visual field and colour contrast sensitivity.

Photocoagulation was performed using a green argon laser. The laser burns were placed on the drusen and scattered over drusen-free regions in a horse-shoe-shaped area temporal to the fovea. No laser burns were placed closer than approximately 500 μm to the centre of the fovea and the area of treatment extended to the vascular arcades. The spot size was 200 μm and the laser burns were mild (0.1–0.2 W, 0.05 s), just producing a greyish reaction in the retina.

Results

In the treatment group, the mean drusen area of the fundus photographs and the angiograms decreased significantly from 7.9% to 2.9% ($p < 0.001$) and from 19.2% to 7.2% ($p < 0.001$), respectively. In the control group, on the other hand, the mean drusen area tended to increase from 8.3% to 10.7% in the fundus photographs ($p = 0.060$) and from 17.4% to 22.1% in the angio-grams ($p = 0.076$). Comparing the change in mean drusen area from study entry to 12 months, there was a highly significant difference between the two groups ($p < 0.001$) for the fundus photographs as well as for the angiograms.

In the treatment group, visual acuity and colour contrast sensitivity did not change significantly from study entry to 12 months. In the control group, however, mean visual acuity decreased significantly from 0.95 ± 0.1 to 0.89 ± 0.1 ($p = 0.008$) as did the mean colour contrast sensitivity along the tritan axis ($p = 0.044$), indicating impairments in retinal function. No differ-ence was seen in either group regarding central visual field.

Furthermore, three patients in the control group advanced to an exudative/ neovascular stage of the disease. One patient developed a widespread macular haemorrhage due to choroidal neovascularization. Two other patients devel-oped a pigment epithelial detachment, one with occult choroidal neovasulari-zation and one with no signs of neovasularization. No patient in the treatment group developed exudative or neovascular lesions.

Conclusion

Perifoveal laser photocoagulation reduced the total drusen area significantly at 12 months, with no difference in visual acuity, colour contrast sensitivity or central visual field. In the control group, however, a significant decrease in visual acuity as well as in colour contrast sensitivity indicate an impairment of retinal function. In addition, three patients in the control group advanced to an exudative/neovascular stage of the disease. This did not occur in the treatment group. The long-term benefit of the treatment is yet to be determined but the outcome in the control group seems to indicate a prophylactic potential of the treatment.

References

1. Leibowitz, H.M., Kreuger, E., Maunder, L.R. The Framingham Eye Study Monograph. Surv Ophthalmol. 1980; 24: 335–607.
2. Ferris, F.L. III, Fine, S.L., Hymen, L. Age-related macular degeneration and blindness due to neovascular maculopathy. Arch Ophthalmol. 1984; 102: 1640–1642.
3. Macular Photocoagulation Study Group. Argon laser photocoagulation for neovascular maculopathy. Five-year results from randomized clinical trials. Arch Ophthalmol. 1991; 109: 1109-1114.
4. Moisseiev, J., Alhalel, A., Masuri, R., Treister, G. The impact of the Macular Photocoagulation Study results on the treatment of exudative age-related macular degeneration. Arch Ophthalmol. 1995; 113: 185–189.
5. Macular Photocoagulation Study Group. Recurrent choroidal neovascularisation after argon laser photocoagulation for neovascular maculopathy. Arch Ophthalmol. 1986; 104: 503–512.
6. Bressler, S.B., Maguire, M.G., Bressler, N.M., Fine, S.L. Macular Photocoagulation Study Group. Relationship of drusen and abnormalities of the retinal pigment epithelium to the prognosis of neovascular macular degeneration. Arch Ophthalmol. 1990; 108: 1442–1447.
7. Holz, F.G., Wolfensberger, T.J., Piguet, B. *et al.* Bilateral macular drusen in age-related macular degeneration. Ophthalmology. 1994; 101: 1522–1528.
8. Siegelman, J. Foveal drusen resorption one year after perifoveal laser photocoagulation. Ophthalmology. 1991; 98: 1379–1383.
9. Wetzig, P.C. Photocoagulation of drusen-related macular degeneration: a long-term outcome. Trans Am Ophthalmol Soc. 1994; 92: 299–306.
10. Figueroa, M.S., Regueras, A., Bertrand, J. Laser photocoagulation to treat soft drusen in age-related macular degeneration. Retina. 1994; 14: 391–396.
11. Frennesson, I.C., Nilsson, S.E.G. Effects of argon (green) laser treatment of soft drusen in early age-related maculopathy: a 6-month prospective study. Br J Ophthalmol. 1995; 79: 905–909.
12. Frennesson, I.C., Nilsson, S.E.G. Laser photocoagulation of soft drusen in early age-related maculopathy (ARM). The one-year results of a prospective, randomised trial. Eur J Ophthalmol. 1996; 6: 307–314

Department of Ophthalmology
Linköping University
S-581 85 Linköping, Sweden

55. ICG drusen-like alterations in the course of age-related macular degeneration

A. GIOVANNINI, G. AMATO, E. D'ALTOBRANDO, C. MARIOTTI
and B. SCASSELLATI-SFORZOLINI

(Ancona, Italy)

Introduction

Age-related macular degeneration (AMD) is the leading cause of blindness in patients older than 65 years of age in the industrialized countries and it ranks second after diabetic retinopathy in patients between 45 and 64[1-4]. Almost 30% of persons older than 75 years of age are affected by AMD[2,3]. The loss of vision can be caused by slow progressive geographic atrophy of the retinal pigment epithelium (in the atrophic form) or by the complications of a choroidal neovascularization (CNV) (in the exudative form). Drusen, especially large confluent soft drusen are common in eyes predisposed to the ingrowth of CNV.

The purpose of this chapter is to evaluate the prevalence, on a population of patients affected by AMD, of a new type of drusen-like hypofluorescent lesions detectable only with indocyanine green angiography (ICGA).

Materials and methods

We studied retrospectically with high definition videoangiography (Topcon IMAGEnet) 289 eyes (150 consecutive patients; 72 males and 78 females; age 56–88 years; mean age 71.5) affected by age-related macular degeneration (AMD).

All patients underwent a complete ophthalmic examination. Fundus photography, fluorescein angiography (FA) and ICGA were performed in both eyes. Indocyanine green (ICG) (Cardiogreen, Hynson, Westcott and Dunning, Inc, Baltimore, MD, USA) was reconstituted with the manufacturer-supplied aqueous solvent to a concentration of 5 mg/ml. ICGA was performed using 25 mg/patient of ICG injected into a peripheral arm vein and was followed immediately by 5 ml flush of sterile saline via a three-way stopcock.

Results

ICGA showed in 14 patients (23 eyes, 7.96%), small areas of blocked fluorescence (150–700 μm), clustered at the posterior pole in a ring or C shape

G. Coscas and F. Cardillo Piccolino (eds.), Retinal Pigment Epithelium and Macular Diseases, pp. 329–333.
© *1998 Kluwer Academic Publishers.*

(Figs 1–4). These alterations were never seen in the central macula. Although the pattern was similar to that of drusen or reticular pseudodrusen, these areas could not be visualized with neither FA or with red-free or blue light retinography and they did not correspond to blue light or reticular pseudo-drusen[5–8]. Hard or soft drusen where constantly observed, but located more centrally.

Conclusions

ICGA may allow identification of a new type of drusen, or at least Bruch's membrane alterations, in the course of AMD, which can not be visualized

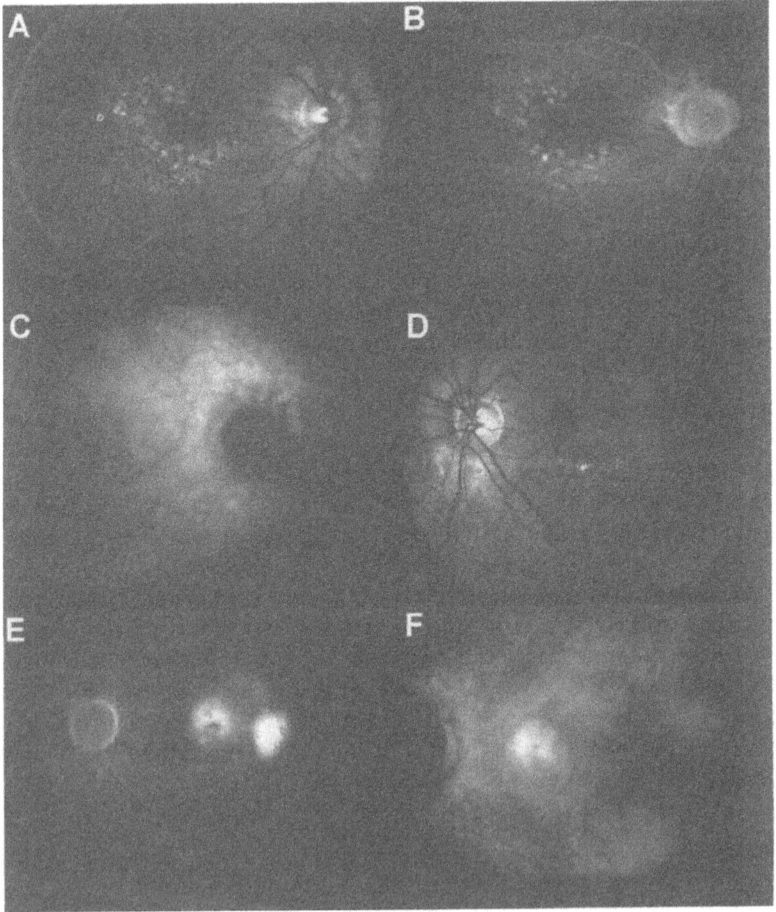

Fig. 1. 73-year-old woman. (a) Red-free image; (b) FA; (c) ICGA: late phase; (d) Red-free image; (e) FA; (f) ICGA: late phase.

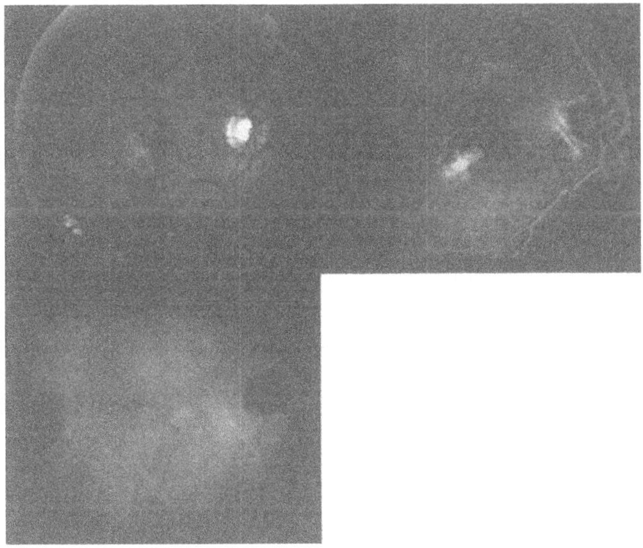

Fig. 2. 77-year-old woman. (a) Red-free image; (b) FA; (c) ICGA: late phase.

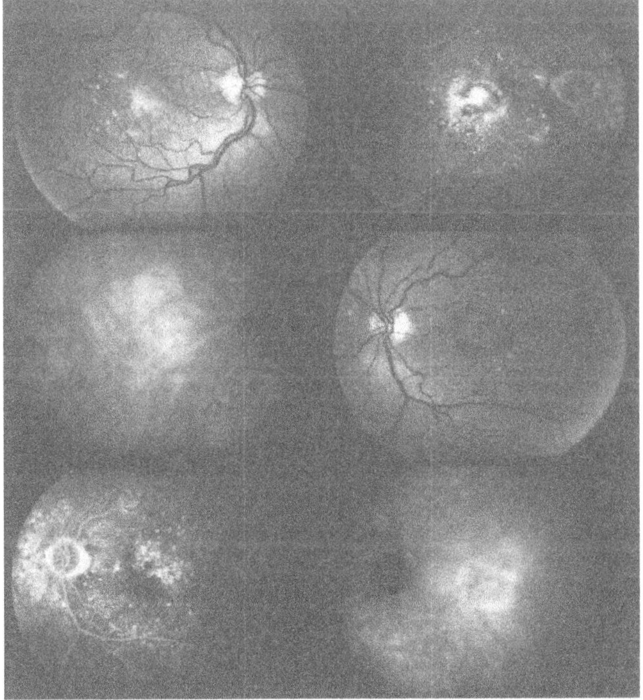

Fig. 3. 70-year-old man. (a) Red-free image; (b) FA; (c) ICGA: late phase; (d) Red-free image; (e) FA; (f) ICGA: late phase.

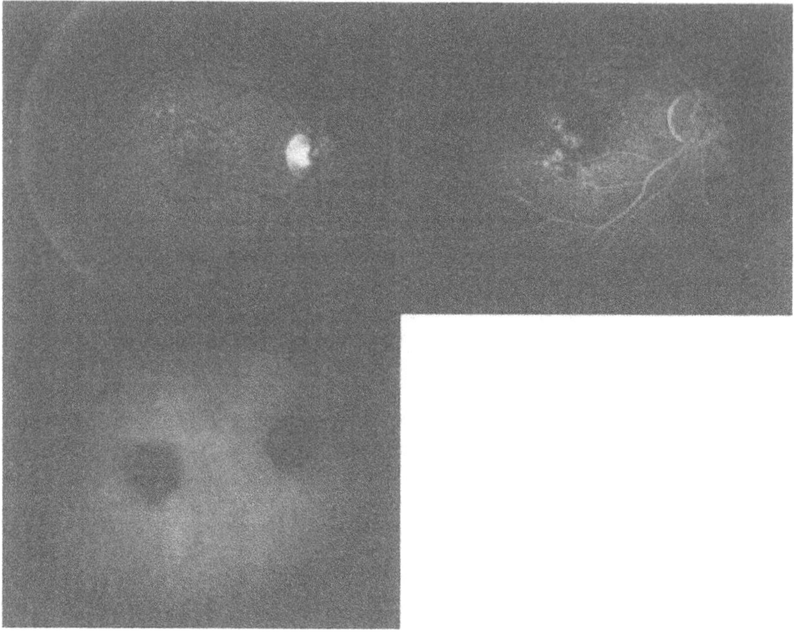

Fig. 4. 72-year-old woman. (a) Red-free image; (b) FA; (c) ICGA: late phase.

with FA, red-free or blue light retinography. The hypofluorescence observed in the late phases of ICGA could be the expression of the pre-choroidal deposits blocking the choroidal fluorescence or the staining of Bruch's membrane; the absence of block in the early phases would be in favour of the second hypothesis. These diffuse alterations of choroidal fluorescence could correspond to the 'basal laminar deposits or diffuse drusen' described in histopathological studies by Sarks[9,10], by Green *et al.*[11] and by Green and Enger[12]; ultrastructural examination showed that these deposits are composed of aggregates of collagen and abnormal basal membrane[9,11,13]. The significance of such ICG finding remains unknown, further studies and a follow-up are needed to establish whether these alterations may be a risk factor for the development of the complications of AMD.

References

1. Leibowitz, H.M., Krueger, D.E., Maunder, L.R. et al. The Framingham Eye Study monograph. An ophthalmological and epidemiological study of cataract, glaucoma, diabetic retinopathy, macular degeneration and visual acuity in a general population of 2631 adults, 1973–1975. Surv Ophthalmol. 1980; 24(suppl): 335–610.
2. Klein, B.E., Klein, R. Cataracts and macular degeneration in older Americans. Arch Ophthalmol. 1982; 100: 571–573.

3. Ferris, F.L. III. Senile macular degeneration: review of epidemiologic features. Am J Epidemiol. 1983; 118: 132–151.
4. Cullinan, T.M. The epidemiology of blindness. In Miller S, ed. Clinical Ophthalmology. Bristol, UK: Wright, 1987: 571–578.
5. Mimoun, G., Soubrane, G., Coscas, G. Macular drusen. J Fr Ophthalmol. 1990; 13: 511–530.
6. Coscas, G. Dégénérescences Maculaires Acquises Liées à l'Age et néovaisseaux Sous-retiniens. Masson, Paris 1991: 177.
7. Klein, R., Davis, M.D., Magli, Y.L., Segal, P., Klein, B.E.K., Hubbard, L. The Wisconsin age-related maculopathy grading system. Ophthalmology. 1991; 98: 1128–1134.
8. Arnold, J.J., Sarks, S.H., Killingsworth, M.C., Sarks, J.P. Reticular pseudodusen. A risk factor in age-related maculopathy. Retina. 1995; 15: 183–191.
9. Sarks, S.H. Ageing and degeneration in the macular region: a clinicopathological study. Br J Ophthalmol. 1976; 60: 324–341.
10. Sarks, S.H. Drusen and their relationship to senile macular degeneration. Aust J Ophthalmol. 1980; 8: 117–130.
11. Green, W.R., McDonnel, P.J., Yeo, J.H. Pathologic features of senile macular degeneration. Ophthalmology. 1985; 92: 615–627.
12. Green, W.R., Enger, C. Age-related macular degneration histopathologic studies. Ophthalmology. 1993; 100: 1519–1535.
13. Van der Schaft, T.L., De Bruijn, W.C., Mooy, C.M., Ketelaars, D.A.M., De Jong, P.T.V.M. Is basal laminar deposit unique for age-related macular degeneration? Arch Ophthalmol. 1991; 109: 420–425.

Department of Ophthalmology
University of Ancona
Ospedale di Torrette
60020 Ancona
Italy

56. Electrophysiological and neurophysiological symptoms of age-related macular dystrophy

A.M. SHAMSHINOVA, V.S. LISENKO, J.A. AREFIEVA and
A.P. DVORYANCHIKOVA

(Moscow, Russia)

Introduction

To date electrophysiological and psychophysiological research methods such as local electroretinography (LERG), light contrast and colour sensitivity have been used for evaluation of the functional state of the retinal macular region[1-5]. Taking into account anatomy and neurophysiology of the retina[6], and the presence of on/off channels of the cone system we suggest a new method of contrast sensitivity and topography of on/off channels of the cone system.

Materials and methods

Ninety patients with age related macular dystrophy (ARMD) were studied at different stages of the disease from drusen and pigmentation of macular region to choroidal neovascularization, fibrosis, detachment of pigment epithelium, exudative or exudative haemorrhage and pseudotumour. The original computerized methods of general and local ERG, topography of contrast and colour sensitivity, and activity of the on/off channels of the cone system of the retina, along with spatial contrast achromatic and chromatic sensitivity were used. The data were compared with the control group of normal subjects.

General ERG and local ERG were measured with a computer complex (MBN, Russia) using suction electrodes[3] with frosted front window for general ERG and with short-focus lens and red-green light emitting diode for local ERG. The size of the stimulating light for the local ERG was 15°, which always strike the macular region wherever the patient looked because the suction electrode moving with the eye.

The method of the contrast sensitivity was presented in an original mathematical program using sinusoidal achromatic and chromatic grating (red/black, green/black, blue/black, white/black) with 12 spatial frequencies from 0.5 to 22 cycle/degree.

The topography of on/off activity was studied with the original method using the registration of the motoresponse latency during equalization of the brightness of achromatic stimulus and the background. The moderately bright stimulus

G. Coscas and F. Cardillo Piccolino (eds.), Retinal Pigment Epithelium and Macular Diseases, pp. 335–339.
© *1998 Kluwer Academic Publishers.*

(2 mm) was presented on an achromatic background. The stimuli were darker than the background, and their brightness was gradually increased until the stimuli became brighter than the background in the central visual field.

The functional topography of colour vision was studied by maximization

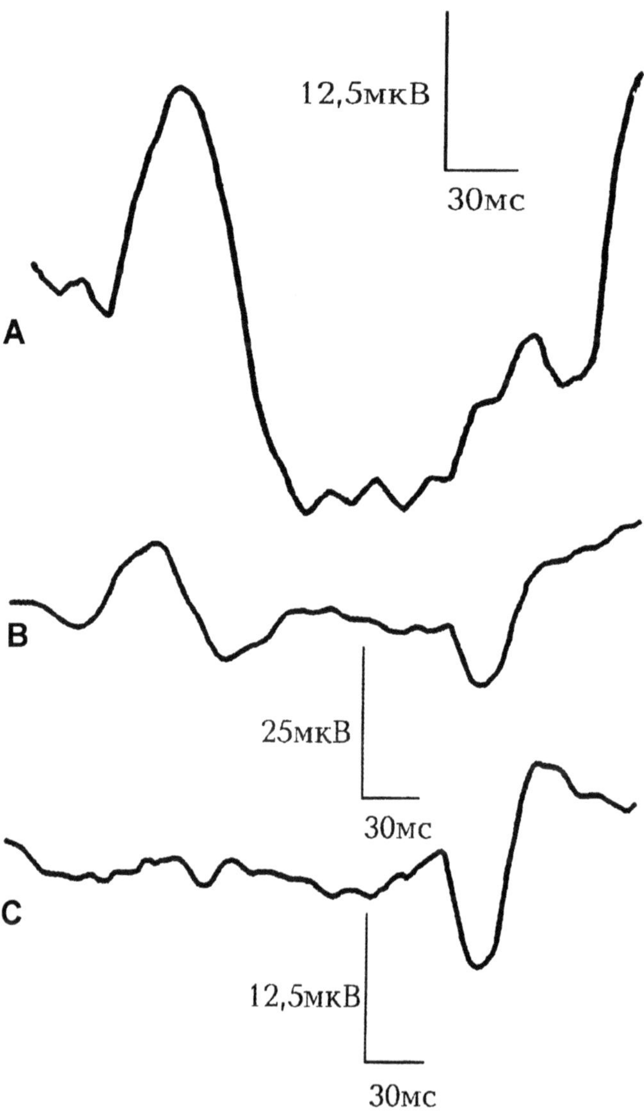

Fig. 1. Local ERG in different stages of ARMD. (a) normal; (b) OD (vision 0.6); and (c) LERG OS (vision 0.1). The asymmetry of the LERG was correlated with the visual aquity in the different stages of ARMD.

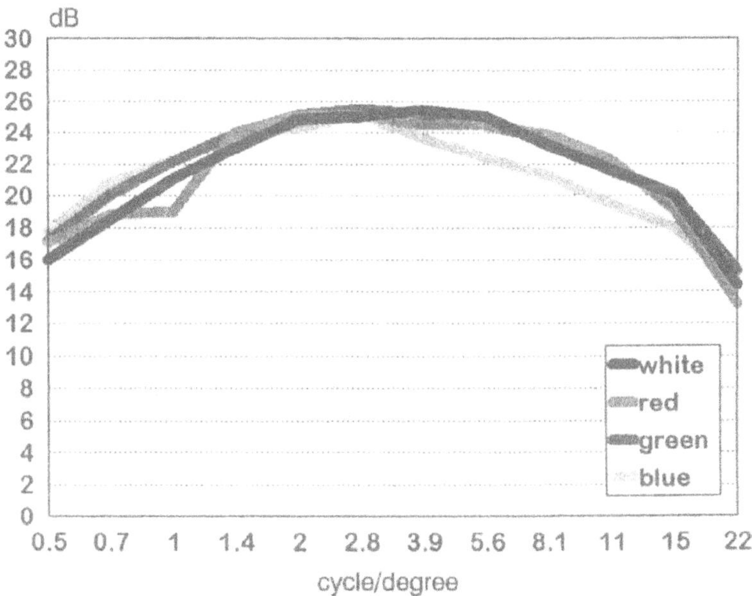

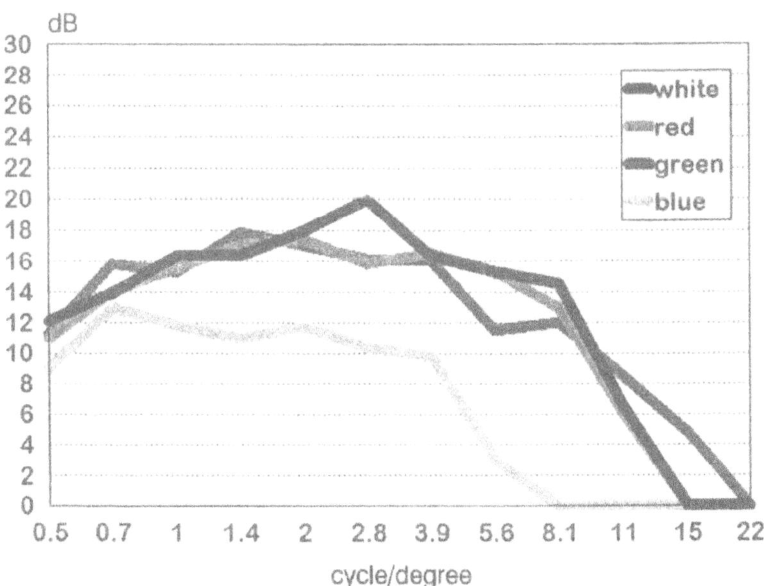

Fig. 2. Contrast sensitivity OD (vision OD 0.6) on the sinusoidal achromatic and chromatic grating (white/black, red/black, green/black, blue/black). *X*-axis: spatial frequencies of the gratings, *Y*-axis: contrast sensitivity (dB).

of the motoresponse latency during the equalization of brightness the colour stimulates and corresponding opponent colour background in each point of the central visual field, limited to 30°.

Results

Local ERG decreased progressively from normal to unrecordable with the evolution of the pathological process (Fig. 1). The bioelectrical activity of the macular region of patients with the different stages of ARMD demonstrated that electrogenesis disturbance mainly occurs in the late stages of the disease, correlating with the angiography data from patients with different stages of ARMD.

An unrecordable local ERG was always accompanied by hyperfluorescence in the central retinal region and pigment epithelium detachments. The general results were normal or subnormal.

The early stages of ARMD were characterized by depression of the contrast sensitivity in high spatial frequencies in both chromatic and achromatic grating (Fig. 2). Contrast and colour sensitivity were affected even in the early stages of the diseases.

Using the red, blue and green stimuli on the blue, yellow, red/blue, red/green background showed significant changes of the motoresponse latency corresponding to different disturbances of the red, green colour sensitivity during disease evolution in both central and paracentral regions. The RT were significantly higher at the presentation of the stimulus close to background in brightness than when there was a visible difference. In accordance with the increase in difference between the stimulus and the background in the direction of darker and lighter stimuli, the RT decreased symmetrically according to a conventional axis drawn through the point where the brightness of the stimulus and background were equal and RT were infinite (Fig. 3). These data showed a decreased sensitivity of on/off-channels of the cone system in ARMD. Asymmetry of the RT was an important diagnostic tag, because RT was higher when the stimulus was lighter than the background than when the stimulus was darker than the background. These data showed that the sensitivity of on-channels of the cone system were decreasing first and more rapidly in ARMD.

Conclusion

These data conform with current thinking on the pathogenesis of ARMD. Use of electrophysiological and psychophysiological investigations is necessary for determining the functions of different channels of the visual system (light, contrast and colour sensitivity, on/off-channels of the cone system), the localization of the pathological process and prognosis of the vision in ARMD.

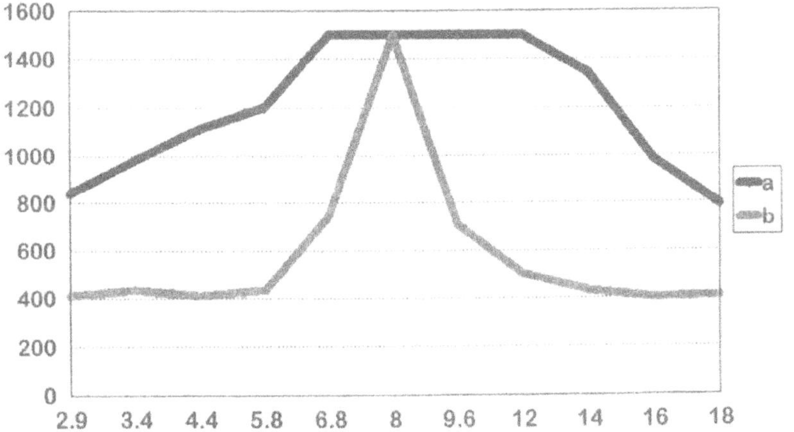

Fig. 3. On/off activity of cone system OD (vision 0.6). Dependence of reaction time during the equation the stimulus and the background by brightness in patient with ARMD. Right: reaction time for stimulus lighter than the background; left: for stimulus darker than the background.

It is necessary to compare the functional state of visual pathways with the results of modern indocyanine green angiography for definition of the mechanism of disturbance of visual acuity.

References

1. Campbell, R.W., Maffei, L. Electrophysiological evidence for the existence of orientation and size detectors in the human visual system. J Physiol. 1970; 207: 635–652.
2. Miyake, Y. Studies of local macular ERG. Acta Soc Ophthalmol. 1988; 92: 1419–1449.
3. Shamshinova, A.M. Local ERG for clinical examination of eye diseases. Doc Ophthalmol. 1990; 76: 1–11.
4. Folk, J.C. Aging macular degeneration: clinical features of treatable disease. Ophthalmology. 1985; 92: 594–602.
5. Heckenlively, J., Arden, G.B. Principles and Practice of Clinical Electrophysiology of Vision. Mosby Year Book 1991: 493.
6. Kolb, H., Fernandez, E., Ammermuller, J., Cuenca, N. Substance P: A neurotransmitter of amacrine and ganglion cells in the vertebrate retina. Histol Histopathol. 1995; 10: 947–968.

Helmholtz Research Institute of EYE Diseases
Sadovaya-Chernogriasskaya 14/19
Moscow 103064, Russia

57. Watershed filling in age-related macular degeneration: the implications of panretinal photocoagulation

J. BAROFSKY, R.D. ROSS, G. COHEN, W. BABER, S. PALAO
and K.A. GITTER

(New Orleans, USA)

Introduction

The previous literature describing choroidal vascular circulatory organization is highly controversial. *In vivo* indocyanine green (ICG) videoangiographic studies using dye subtraction algorithms confirm prior *in vitro* latex injection studies which demonstrated the choroidal vascular bed as one continuous, freely anastomotic system. In contrast, laser targeted fluorescein angiographic dye studies confirm previous conventional fluorescein angiographic studies which illustrated multiple choroidal vascular zones of watershed filling in the posterior pole. This latter type of choroidal watershed vascular physiology is consistent with clinical entities such as the triangular syndrome and Elschnig's spots. Overall, these findings may represent a normal spectrum of choroidal vascular physioanatomical heterogeneity, thereby explaining the variability found in the literature.

Watershed zones, the most distal end-arterial type segments, may be especially predisposed to ischemia in patients with age-related macular degeneration (ARMD), a condition associated with choroidal vascular circulatory compromise. The resultant ischaemia might portend to the development of associated choroidal neovascularization.

Peripheral panretinal photocoagulation (PPRP) has been shown previously to redirect choroidal blood flow centrally. It is then conceivable that PPRP could ameliorate central macular watershed zones. The subsequent improvement in macular choroidal blood flow might then minimize the development of choroidal neovascular disease.

Methods

In order to examine the potential relationship between choroidal watershed filling and choroidal neovascularization in ARMD, we retrospectively reviewed 100 consecutive ICG videoangiograms of 74 patients with ARMD and 26 age-matched normal control patients, looking for characteristic areas

G. Coscas and F. Cardillo Piccolino (eds.), Retinal Pigment Epithelium and Macular Diseases, pp. 341–342.
© *1998 Kluwer Academic Publishers.*

of early macular choroidal hypoperfusion assumed to represent watershed filling. We also prospectively studied pre- and post-PPRP ICG videoangiograms looking for attenuation of pre-existing watershed zones.

Results

Of the 60 ARMD patients with choroidal neovascularization, 35 (58.3%) exhibited watershed filling on ICG videoangiography vs. three of 26 (11.5%) age-matched normal control patients ($p < 0.01$). The watershed areas directly involved the fovea in more than 80% of cases with over 90% of associated choroidal neovascular membranes arising from these zones. Five of 14 (35.7%) dry ARMD patients had associated watershed filling on ICG videoangiography. These patients also exhibited large, soft, confluent drusen and focal retinal pigment epithelial hyperplasia on clinical examination. Additionally, a trend towards attenuation of pre-existing watershed zones in post-PPRP ICG videoangiograms was noted.

Conclusions

Our results suggest a possible predisposition for choroidal neovascularization in ARMD patients who manifest choroidal watershed vascular filling on ICG videoangiography. Prognostically, dry ARMD patients with watershed vascular filling may be at high risk for the eventual development of choroidal neovascular disease. This is supported by clinical examination which revealed associated large, soft, confluent drusen and focal retinal pigment epithelial hyperplasia, risk factors reported previously for the eventual development of choroidal neovascular disease. Finally, PPRP appears to redirect choroidal blood flow centrally, ameliorating potentially ischaemic central macular watershed zones. Thus, PPRP could be considered as a prophylactic treatment to minimize the risk of subsequent choroidal neovascular disease in high risk dry ARMD patients who exhibit ICG videoangiographic watershed vascular filling. This laser treatment could augment or replace prophylactic focal macular laser photocoagulation, a treatment approach which is now under multicentre clinical investigation. A large prospective controlled study should be carried out in order to assess the efficacy of this potential treatment modality.

Louisiana State University School of Medicine
Foundation for Retinal Research
New Orleans, USA

58. Isolated occult choroidal neovascularization: comparison between early and late phases of ICG angiography

G. SOUBRANE, G. COSCAS, D. KUHN and M. QUARANTA

(Créteil, France)

Introduction

Indocyanine (ICG) angiography is shown to be helpful in identifying choroidal new vessels when occult on fluorescein angiography[1-5]. Isolated occult choroidal neovascularization (CNV) or leakage of undetermined source (type II of the MPS classification) are not associated with serous haemorrhagic, or fibrovascular pigment epithelium detachment. On early phase ICG angiography, occult CNV may be converted into a well-defined net in about 40% of cases[6,7]. This conversion allows a good delination and definition of the limits of the neovascular complex. This early net is more often identified using scanning laser ophthalmoscope technology while using infrared fundus cameras. The identification of isolated occult CNV is based on the visualization in the late phases of hyperfluorescent plaque with hyperfluorescence. The signification of this late staining plaque is still controversial.

To approach and to analyse the meaning of the late staining plaque, an overlay of the early net on the late staining plaque was obtained on ICG angiograms.

Materials and methods

Thirty-four consecutive patients (34 eyes) with clinical and fluorescein angiographic features of isolated occult CNVs, related to age-related macular degeneration underwent a complete ophthalmological examination including ICG angiography performed with Heidelberg scanning laser ophthalmoscope (Germany). The early and late phases of ICG angiography were compared and overlaid after computer-assisted registration (OPH 1280, Medinfo France).

Results

In the early phase of ICG angiography, the macular area demonstrated delayed choroidal perfusion in all cases. Only large choroidal vessels were

G. Coscas and F. Cardillo Piccolino (eds.), Retinal Pigment Epithelium and Macular Diseases, pp. 343–346.
© *1998 Kluwer Academic Publishers.*

visible in this area. This subfoveal hypofluorescent zone was larger than on fluorescein angiography.

In the hypofluorescent macular zone, the neovascular complex was converted into a well-defined neovascular net in 28 eyes (82%). This complex had well defined limits and was partially surrounded by a hypofluorescent ring (Fig. 1a). In six other eyes (18%), small hyperfluorescent spots appeared within the early hypofluorescent zone.

In the late phase (10 min after injection), the fluorescence of the macular area persisted but its extent was partially reduced. The neovascular membrane was located within the initially hypofluorescent zone (Fig. 1b).

The overlay of the early and late phases of ICG angiograms showed that the late staining plaque corresponded exactly to the size of the early neovascular net in 12 out of 28 eyes (43%). In the remaining 16 eyes (57%), the initial hyperfluorescent net did not correspond to the same limits than the late staining plaque (Fig. 1). The early, multiple, hyperfluorescent spots either vanished or remained identical.

Discussion

The late staining plaque demonstrated to be larger than the net identified on the early frames of ICG angiography in more than half of the eyes. This difference suggests that there is a leakage of the ICG dye possibly into the associated fibrous tissue. Furthermore, the late staining plaques were also observed in normal controls[8] and in AMD eyes without evidence of CNV on

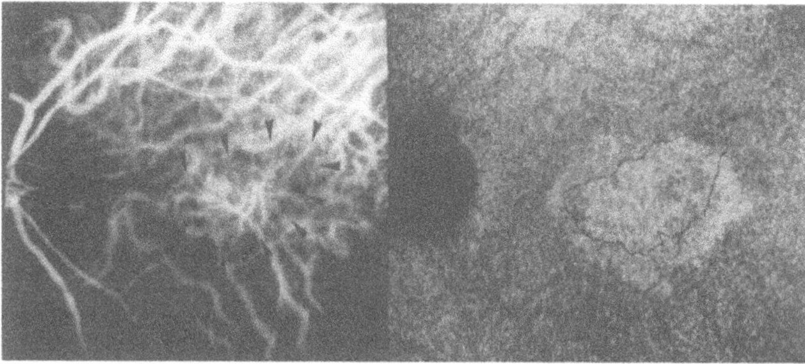

Fig. 1. Occult new vessels converted to a well defined network. (a) Early phase of ICG angiography. A hyperfluorescent network is well identified at this early venous phase (arrowheads). Central feeding vessels resolve in a capillary network. Note that the inferior macular area is darker than the superior area. (b) Late phase of ICG angiography. A large area in the macula is more hyperfluorescent that the choroidal background. This plaque has well defined borders. The limits of the early network is superimposed (black line). The difference in the two limits is obvious.

fluorescein angiography. Recent studies have suggested that the presence of this late staining plaque in AMD eyes is a risk factor for occurrence of active CNVs in a 1 year period[9].

The leakage of ICG dye into the associated fibrous tissue emphasizes that the early frames should be used when considering ICG-guided laser treatment[10], rather than the late staining plaques which are more extensive in half of the eyes.

The early hypofluorescent macular area[11] can be related to choroidal hypoperfusion. A histological analysis, by Pauleikhoff[12] has demonstrated a relationship between Bruch's membrane deposits (the histopathological hallmark of AMD) and choriocapillaris change. A choroidal hypoperfusion in AMD was suggested by Bird[13] on fluorescein angiography examinations. The similar aspect of Sorsby fundus dystrophy[14] provides support to this finding. The analysis of the choroidal macular perfusion on fluorescein angiography by Piguet[15] suggests that this delay is a risk factor for geographic atrophy.

An other possibility could be a masquage related to the deposited Bruch's membrane material. Green[16] has demonstrated on histopathological examinations that CNVs are associated with basal laminar or linear deposits. In addition, the alteration of the choriocapillaris perfusion could be a response to the modifications of the retinal pigment epithelium, as demonstrated in an experimental model by Korte[17]. Large drusen with indistinct margins are considered as marker of basal laminar deposits by Bressler[18] and to portend a high risk of occurrence of CNVs.

The observation of a macular choroidal hypofluorescence on ICG video angiography raises again the possibility of the involvement of the choriocapillaris in the pathogenesis of AMD. Moreover, the difference of size observed between early and late phase appearance of occult CNV, suggests that early frames should be used when considering ICG guided laser photocoagulation.

References

1. Flower, R.W. High-speed human choroidal angiography using indocyanine green dye and a continuous light source. Doc Ophthalmol Proc Ser. 1976; 9: 59–66.
2. Destro, M., Puliafito, C. Indocyanine green videoangiography of choroidal neovascularization. Ophthalmology. 1989; 96: 846–853.
3. Yannuzzi, L.A., Slakter, J.S., Sorenson, J.A., Guyer, D.R., Orlock, D.A. Digital indocyanine green video angiography and choroidal neovascularization. Retina. 1992; 12: 191–223.
4. Scheider, A., Kaboth, A., Neubauser, R. Detection of subretinal neovascular membranes with indocyanine green and an infrared scanning laser ophthalmoscope. Am J Ophthalmol. 1992; 113: 45–51.
5. Regillo, C.D., Benson, W.E., Maguire. J.F., Annesley, W.H. Indocyanine green angiography and occult choroidal neovascularization. Ophthalmology. 1994; 101: 280–288.
6. Lim, J.I., Sternberg, P., Capone, A., Aaberg, T.M., Gilman, J.P. Selective use of indocyanine green angiography for occult choroidal neovascularization. Am J Ophthalmol. 1995; 120: 75–82.

7. Wolf, S., Knabben, H., Krombech, H., Schaaf, A., Stolbach, U., Reim, M. Indocyanine green angiography in patients with occult choroidal neovascularization. Ger J Ophthalmol. 1996; 5: 251–256.

8. Soubrane, G., Coscas, G., Kuhn, D., Secretan, M., Herpe, C. Indocyanine green videoangiography in normal. 2nd International Symposium on indocyanine green angiography, Nara, Japan, 8/4/1995.

9. Guyer, D.R., Slakter, J.S., Hanutsaha, P. Indocyanine green videoangiography of drusen as a possible predictive indicator of exudative maculopathy. Annual Meeting of the American Academy of Ophthalmology. 1996, abstract book p. 125.

10. Slakter, J.S., Yannuzzi, L.A., Sorenson, J.A., Guyer, D.R., Hu, A.C., Orlock, D.A. A pilot study of indocyanine green videoangiography-guided laser photocoagulation of occult choroidal neovascularization in age-related macular degeneration. Arch Ophthalmol. 1994; 112: 465–472.

11. Quaranta, M., Krott, R., Soubrane, G., Coscas, G. Circulation choroïdienne et vidéoangiographie au vert d'indocyanine dans la néovascularisation choroïdienne occulte. Ophtalmologie. 1995; 9: 200–202.

12. Pauleikhoff, P., Chen, J.C., Chisholm, I.M., Bird, A.C. Choroidal perfusion abnormality with age-related Bruch's membrane change. Am J Ophthalmol. 1990; 109: 211–217.

13. Bird, A.C. Pathogenesis of retinal pigment epithelial detachment in the elderly: the relevance of Bruch's membrane change. Eye. 1991; 51: 1–12.

14. Polkinghorne, P., Capon, M.R., Berninger, T., Lyness, A.L., Sehmi, K., Bird, A.C. Sorsby's fundus dystrophy. A clinical study. Ophthalmology. 1989; 96: 1763–1768.

15. Piguet, B., Palmwang, I.B., Chisholm, I.M., Minassian, D., Bird, A.C. Evolution of age-related macular degeneration with choroidal perfusion abnormality. Am J Ophthalmol. 1992; 113: 657–663.

16. Green, W.R. Age-related macular degeneration histopatologic studies: the 1992 Lorenz E. Zimerman Lecture. Ophthalmology. 1993; 100: 1519–1535.

17. Korte, G.E., Repucci, V., Henkind, P. RPE destruction causes choriocapillary atrophy. Invest Ophthalmol Vis Sci. 1984; 25: 1135–1145.

18. Bressler, N.M., Silva, J.C., Bressler, S.B., Fine, S.L., Green, W.R. Clinicopathologic correlation of drusen and retinal pigment epithelial abnormalities in age-related macular degeneration. Retina. 1994; 14: 130–142.

Clinique Ophtalmologique Universitaire
Université Paris-XII
40, avenue de Verdun
94010 Créteil (France)

59. Indocyanine green angiography in age-related macular degeneration with fluorescein angiography occult neovascularization

A. PECE, U. INTROINI, G. BOLOGNESI, P. AVANZA, G. PACELLI
and R. BRANCATO

(Milan, Italy)

Introduction

Indocyanine green angiography (ICGA) has recently disclosed a new diagnostic approach to ARMD[1-15]. The characteristics of the dye, which is fluorescent in the near infrared and wholely bound to blood proteins, have already proved useful for investigating choroidal abnormalities, besides haemorrhages, turbid fluids and retinal pigment epithelium. The method, therefore, appears indicated in exudative ARMD when occult choroidal new vessels are suspected.

This study was designed to assess the ability of ICGA to detect CNV clearly, to study their angiographic characteristics and to establish the number of eyes eligible for laser treatment.

Patients and methods

We retrospectively reviewed the ICGA angiograms of 383 eyes of 355 consecutive patients with ARMD and occult new vessels, diagnosed on the basis of fluorescein angiography (FA); 117 were male (33%) and 238 female (67%); mean age was 73.4 (55–92 years). Inclusion criteria were age >55 years; presence of drusen and/or retinal pigment epithelium (RPE) changes in the affected or fellow eye; visual loss and/or metamorphopsia; exudative macular lesion with characteristics giving rise to a suspicion of occult CNV, haemorrhages, lipid exudates and FA evidence of late dye leakage or oozing. Eyes with evident CNV on FA, or with other associated chorioretinal diseases were excluded, as were eyes that had already undergone previous laser photocoagulation treatment.

Each patient underwent a complete ophthalmological examination, including best corrected visual acuity, slit-lamp examination and biomicroscopy.

FA were accepted only if recent (maximum 5 days before) and of good quality, otherwise they were repeated at the same time as ICGA, which was performed using the Topcon IMAGEnet System after IV injection of 25 mg indocyanine green. Each ICGA included color fundus stereo photographs, a

G. Coscas and F. Cardillo Piccolino (eds.), Retinal Pigment Epithelium and Macular Diseases, pp. 347–353.
© 1998 Kluwer Academic Publishers.

red-free photograph, early phases (from the choroidal filling to the retinal venous phase up to 5 min), mid-phases (10–15 min) and late phases (30–40 min).

Results

FA showed PED in 157 eyes (41%) of 143 patients; the remaining 226 eyes (59%) showed no FA evidence of a serous PED. On the basis of the ICGA images, we found focal CNV (less than 1 disc diameter (DD) and plaque CNV (larger than 1 DD). We compared these findings with the two groups of occult CNV: with PED or without PED.

Group with PED

In 35 of the eyes with PED (22.3%), ICGA did not show any hyperfluorescence ascribable to CNV. These PED were considered pure serous. Seventy-four eyes (47.1%) with PED presented focal CNV, with three different angiographic patterns according to their localization (beneath, marginal and parapapillary) with the following features:

(a) 30 eyes (40.5%) presented one or multiple focal hot-spots beneath the PED, frequently associated with large, confluent soft drusen (21/30) and small intraretinal haemorrhages, overlying the neovascularization (22/30). Their fluorescence appeared early as small bright roundish dots, clearly visible throughout all the angiographic phases, with a mid–late halo of leakage (Fig. 1);
(b) 35 eyes (47.3%) had a marginal focal CNV on the edge or contiguous with the boundaries of the PED, rarely combined with soft drusen (7/35). The discrete hyperfluorescent pattern frequently corresponded to the

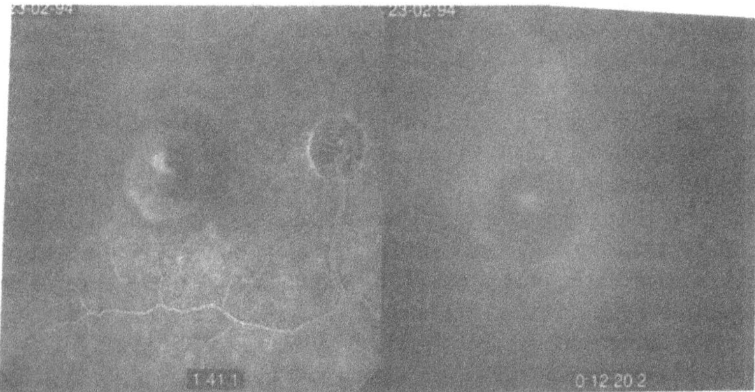

Fig. 1. FA (left) and ICGA (right). A ICGA CNV is present beneath the PED.

notch; these were generally larger than the previous type, with an irregular round/oval shape (Fig. 2);

(c) in nine eyes (12.2%) the CNV was near the optic disc; all these parapapillary neovascularizations showed a typical common pattern, consisting of multiple small hyperfluorescent dots, linked together (Fig. 1), and generally quite a distance from the PED boundaries. Their fluorescence usually appeared 3–5 min after the injection, when the layout of the vessels was extremely clear; during the examination the fluorescence increased with mild dye leakage 10–20 min after the injection (Fig. 3).

In the 35 eyes (22.3%) with a large hyperfluorescent area seen on ICGA, ascribable to a plaque CNV, this partially or completely involved the PED.

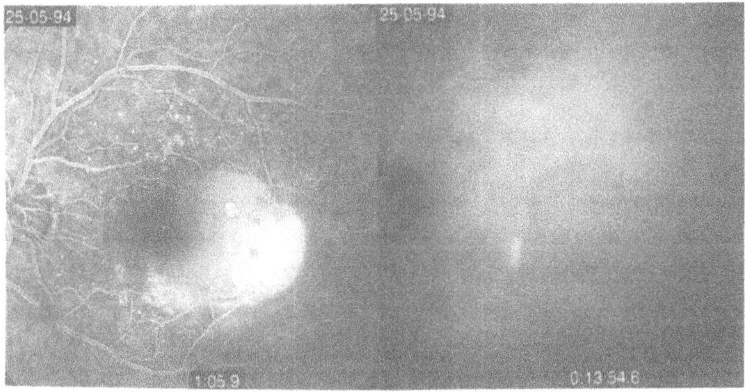

Fig. 2. FA (left) and ICGA (right). A ICGA well-evident CNV is present at the edge of the PED.

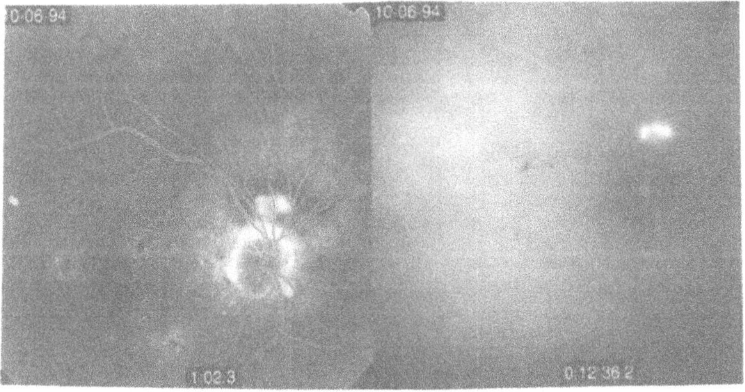

Fig. 3. FA (left) and ICGA (right). The parapapillary CNV is better delineated on ICGA.

Angiographically these large neovascularizations were usually characterized by a discrete hyperfluorescence of the CNV, much more visible after digitally enhancing the contrast (Fig. 4).

In 13 eyes (8.3%) with PED the CNV was barely visible or masked by massive haemorrhage.

Group without PED

Many cases in the group without PED (94 eyes, 41.6%) had plaque CNV while focal CNV was seen in 58 eyes (25.7%); five eyes of this group (8.6%) presented parapapillary CNV features. Among the focal macular CNV fluorescent patterns were largely similar: spots with variable degrees of fluorescence were seen (Fig. 5).

In the eyes with a large plaque CNV, two different hyperfluorescent figures could be identified. One type was not usually clearly detectable in the early phases; the complete new vessel extention was typically clear-cut in the late phases, appearing as a hyperfluorescent area with a granular pattern. The other plaque CNV showed irregular, more intense hyperfluorescence, frequently visible from the early phases, with dye leakage in the late phases. In 74 eyes (32.7%) in this group, ICGA did not show any detectable sign of neovascularization.

Well defined CNV was found in 261 eyes of the eyes examined by ICGA (68%). Excluding the eyes with subfoveal CNV and plaque CNV, we considered 103 of the total eyes (27%) eligible for laser treatment.

Discussion

In spite of many new therapeutic approaches to exudative ARMD, direct laser photocoagulation of well defined CNV remains the only effective therapy[16,17]. However only a small number of cases of exudative ARMD shows

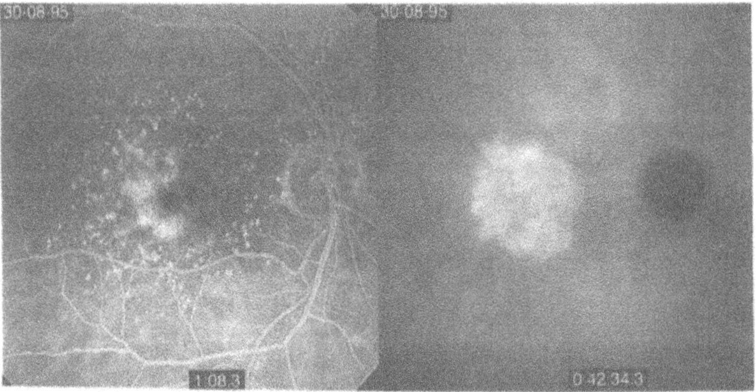

Fig. 4. FA (left) and ICGA (right). ICGA shows a well-evident plaque-CNV, not visible on FA.

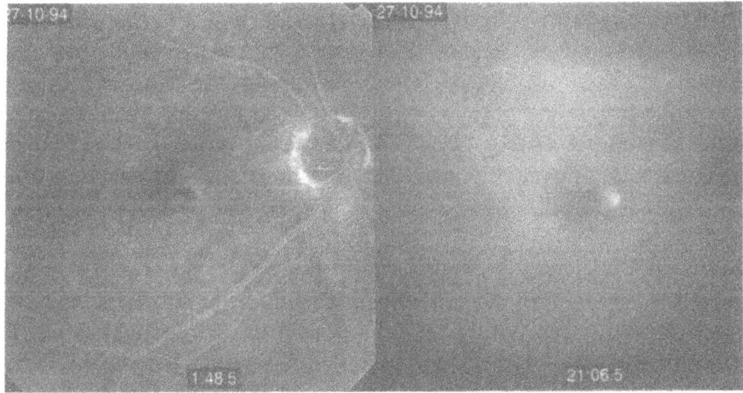

Fig. 5. FA (left) and ICGA (right). FA shows an occult CNV without PED. ICGA permits to evidence a focal well-defined CNV.

a well defined CNV. In fact most of CNV are undetectable by FA, being completely or partially occulted by turbid exudates, blood or simply by the retinal pigment epithelium; one report sustained that as much as 87% of the early diagnosed exudative ARMD were occult[18].

The introduction of infrared choroidal angiography made it possible to visualize CNV better which appear occult to FA. The utility of ICGA in identifying many CNV that appeared occult at FA has been largely confirmed[1-15]. However, when CNV become visible on ICGA, they present various angiographic patterns, probably related to their extent, location, age and activity.

In the present study, in fact, ICGA was not useful in about one-third of eyes with occult newvessels at FA. Considering all the eyes examined (with and without PED), ICGA failed to identify CNV in 122 eyes (32%). Such cases frequently present large, thick haemorrhages or turbid exudation that make it impossible to identify a CNV clearly. Moreover some CNV are only small, with a very poor blood flow, or are enveloped in an intense tissue reaction, such as pigmentation or fibrosis.

A focal CNV was detected in 35% of the eyes with well defined on ICGA CNV and a plaque CNV in 34%. As indicated by Yannuzzi[5,9,18], we considered two groups of CNV: with PED (41%) and without PED (59%), because of the different ICGA patterns and the different prognosis.

In the group with PED, a large number of pure serous PED was found (22.3%). This was strikingly more the 4% reported by Yannuzzi[5,18]. Different criteria for inclusion might explain the difference: in addition to PED larger than 2 DD associated with exudation or blood, we also included PED with a drusenoid aspect, or with pigment figures, but in any case accompanied by visual loss and metamorphopsia.

In the group of CNV with PED, we distinguished three types of focal CNV.

The CNV located beneath the PED usually appeared in the early phases as a small fluorescent point, its hyperfluorescence increasing during the examination, and showing late leakage; this pattern may correspond to a retino-choroidal anastomosis. Stereo photographs permit their spatial localization between the Bruchs' membrane and the detached RPE; sometimes a connection with a retinal vessel is seen[19]. In our series this CNV was frequently associated with an overlying intraretinal haemorrhage and with soft drusen. Their hyperfluorescence appeared more intense because of the surrounding hypofluorescent PED.

Marginal CNV, near the boundaries of the PED, showed different angiographic behaviour: their fluorescence, fainter than the previous type, sometimes had with edges, harder to distinguish from the contiguous flat RPE because of scant contrast around the lesion. A vascular net could be seen in the early phases but when this was present the shape was very similar to the CNV shown up well by FA.

Finally, parapapillary CNV were very close to the optic disc in a small proportion of patients; however all the eyes with parapapillary CNV presented the same pattern, which was different and clearly distinguishable from the other CNV arising in the macular area. We found parapapillary CNV in the groups with PED and without, though they were more frequent with PED (8 vs. 5). In eyes with PED, the boundaries of the detatchment may include the parapapillary CNV, or may be far from the new vessels, without any visible connection between the two lesions, in which case they are called 'remote'.

The special pattern of these vessels is clearly detectable from the early phases, when the more ectasic parts of the newvessels are seen as multiple focal fluorescent spots, close to each other. The subtle connections become visible 5–10 min after the injection, showing progressively stronger fluorescence with late dye leakage.

In the group of focal CNV without PED, the absence of a fluid beneath the retinal layer in the macular area the identification of different angiographic patterns; only the parapapillary CNV can be easily differentiated on account of their characteristic pattern and location,

Large plaques are differently distributed in the two groups. In the group with PED focal CNV was more frequent than the plaque type (47% vs. 22%); plaque CNV was found more often in CNV without PED (41% vs. 25%). This association, never reported before, was highly significant ($p < 0.001$).

In conclusion our findings confirms that, in ARMD complicated by the CNV occult to FA, ICGA helps considerably in the identification of the new vessels, making them well defined in 68% of the eyes examined here. We considered 103 eyes (27%) eligible for laser treatment.

References

1. Hayashi, K., de Laey, J.J. Indocyanine green angiography of choroidal neovascular membranes. Ophthalmologica. 1985: 190: 30–39.

2. Destro, M., Puliafito, C.A. Indocyanine green videoangiography of choroidal neovascularization Ophthalmology. 1989; 96: 846–853.
3. Scheider, A., Schroedel, C. High resolution indocyanine green angiography with scanning laser ophthalmoscope. Am J Ophthalmol. 1989; 108: 458–459
4. Guyer, D.R., Puliafito, C.A., Monés, J.M. *et al.* Digital indocyanine-green angiography in chorioretinal disorders. Ophthalmology. 1992; 99: 287–291.
5. Yannuzzi, L.A., Slakter, J.S., Sorenson, J.A. *et al.* Digital indocyanine green videoangiography and choroidal neovascularization. Retina. 1992; 12: 191–223.
6. Scheider, A., Kaboth, A., Neuhauser, L. Detection of subretinal neovascularization membranes with indocyanine green and infrared scanning laser ophthalmoscope. Am J Ophthalmol. 1992; 113: 45–51.
7. Kuck, H., Inhoffen, W., Schneider, U., Kreissig, I. Diagnosis of occult subretinal neovascularization in age-related macular degeneration by infrared scanning laser videoangiography. Retina. 1993; 13: 36–39.
8. Regillo, C.D., Benson, W.E., Maguire, J.I., Annesley, W.H. Indocyanine green angiography and occult choroidal neovascularization. Ophthalmology. 1994; 101: 280–288.
9. Guyer, D.R., Yannuzzi, L.A., Slakter, J.S., Sorenson, J.A., Hope-Ross, M., Orlock, D.R. Digital indocyanine-green videoangiography of occult choroidal neovascularization. Ophthalmology. 1994; 101: 1727–1737.
10. Chang, T., Freund, B., Green, W.R., Yannuzzi, L.A. Clinicopathologic correlation of indocyanine green angiography of occult choroidal neovascularization. Retina. 1994; 14: 114–124.
11. Yannuzzi, L.A., Sorenson, J.A., Guyer, D.R., Slakter, J.S., Chang, B., Orlock, D. Indocyanine green videoangiography: current status. Eur J Ophthalmol. 1994; 4: 69–81.
12. Yannuzzi, L.A., Hope-Ross, M., Slakter, J.S. *et al.* Analysis of vascularized pigment epithelium detachments using indocyanine greeen videoangiography. Retina. 1994; 14: 99–113.
13. Slakter, J.S., Yannuzzi, L.A., Sorenson, J.A. *et al.* A pilot study of indocyanine green videoangiography guided laser photocoagulation treatment of occult choroidal neovascularization. Arch Ophthalmol. 1994; 112: 465–472.
14. Reiche, E., Duker, J.S., Puliafito, C.A. Indocyanine green angiography and choroidal neovascularization obscured by hemorrhage. Ophthalmology. 1995; 102: 1871–1876.
15. Lim, J.I., Strerberg, P. Jr, Capone, A. Jr, Aaberg, T.M., Gilman, J.P. Selective use of indocyanine green angiography for occult choroidal neovascularization. Am J Ophthalmol. 1995; 120: 75–82.
16. Macular Photocoagulation Study Group. Argon laser photocoagulation for age-related macular degeneration. Arch Ophthalmol. 1982; 100: 912–918.
17. Macular Photocoagulation Study Group. Krypton laser photocoagulation for neovascularized lesions of age-related macular degeneration. Arch Ophthalmol. 1982; 108: 816–824.
18. Freund, K.B., Yannuzzi, L.A., Sorenson, J.A. Age-related macular degeneration and choroidal neovascularization. Am J Ophthalmol. 1993; 115: 786–791.
19. Khun, D., Meunier, I., Soubrane, G., Coscas, G. Imaging of chorioretinal anastomoses in vascularized retinal pigment epithelium detachments. Arch Ophthalmol. 1995; 113: 1392–1398.

Department of Ophthalmology and Visual Sciences
Scientific Institute S. Raffaele Hospital
University of Milano
Via Olgettina, 60
20132 Milano, Italy

60. Defined and occult choroidal neovessels in age-related macular degeneration by means of a scanning laser ophthalmoscope: a retrospective study of 100 cases

G. GIACOMELLI, M. SCRIVANTI, R. MENCUCCI, R. VOLPE
and G. SALVI

(Firenze, Italy)

Abstract

The authors examined 100 consecutive cases of exudative age-related macular degeneration (ARMD) from their own practice in a retrospective study to evaluate the ability of fluorangiography (FAG) and indocyanine green angiography (ICGA), performed with a scanning laser ophthalmoscope (SLO) to detect choroidal neovessels (CNVs). Sixteen percent of CNVs were imaged by FAG, 36% by ICGA, 2% of cases had a purely serous pigment epithelium detachment and 46% had occult CNVs. ICGA imaged 42.9% of occult CNVs after FAG. 27% of choroidal membranes were eligible for laser photocoagulation with central vision sparing: 13% detected by FAG and 14% by ICGA (extrafoveal or delineated feeder vessel). Among occult CNVs after FAG, ICGA detected 16.7% of cases eligible for laser photocoagulation. On the bases of FAG results, patients suffering from exudative ARMD can be eligible for laser photocoagulation only in a few cases. In our experience ICGA can enhance this number of over 100%. Nevertheless only 27% of our cases could be treated with foveal sparing. An early diagnosis and following fluorescein and indocyanine green angiography is important to stop evolution of CNV.

Introduction

Exudative age-related macular degeneration (ARMD) is the major cause of serious central poor vision in Western countries. Choroidal neovessels (CNVs) photocoagulation is the only sure treatment for these patients[1-3]. However, successful treatment requires a well-delineated neovascular membrane and, unfortunately, the great majority of cases has occult or poorly defined choroidal neovessels if studied with ophthalmoscopy and fluorescein angiography (FAG)[4]. Indocyanine green angiography (ICGA), performed with high

G. Coscas and F. Cardillo Piccolino (eds.), Retinal Pigment Epithelium and Macular Diseases, pp. 355–359.
© 1998 Kluwer Academic Publishers.

resolution digital systems or with a scanning laser ophthalmoscope (SLO) can image many occult CNV[5–14]. The aim of this study is to evaluate the ability of FAG and ICGA, performed with a SLO, to image CNV.

Patients and methods

We examined 100 cases of isolated exudative ARMD from 74 patients in a retrospective study (41 women, 33 men ranging in age from 57 to 91 years, median: 78.2 years). All patients underwent complete ophthalmologic examination including: visual acuity (Snellen), slit lamp examination, IOP (Goldmann), fundus biomicroscopy (90 dioptres lens). Fluorescein and indocyanine green angiography were performed consecutively with a SLO (Rodenstock SLO 101). Images were displayed on video-monitor in real time (25 frames/sec, 512 × 512 pixel) and recorded on videotape. Three different ophthalmologists analysed separately the angiographies before final diagnosis. CNVs were classified as occult and defined, focal spots, plaques and mixed forms (plaques with hot spots), extrafoveal and subfoveal, high, low, medium and no activity forms, mixed forms, (low activity plaques with 'hot spots'), imaged by FAG and by ICGA (early or late phases).

Results

The results are summarized in Fig. 1 and Table 1. We only discuss here results concerning the ability of FAG and ICGA to image CNVs (Fig. 1). In 100 cases of exudative ARMD 16% had imaged CNVs by FAG, 36% by ICGA, 2% cases had a purely serous pigment epithelium detachment and 46% had occult CNVs. ICGA delineated 42.9% of occult CNVs after FAG; 27% of choroidal membranes were eligible for laser photocoagulation with central vision sparing: 13% detected by FAG and 14% by ICGA (extrafoveal or delineated feeder vessel). Among occult CNVs after FAG, ICGA detected 16.7% cases eligible for laser photocoagulation.

Discussion

On the basis of FAG, only a few patients suffering from exudative ARMD can be treated by laser. Freund et al.[4], for example, found 13% among their cases and our results show 16% well-delineated and 13% treatable CNVs with foveal sparing. ICGA can increase this number by over 100% (from 13% to 27% in our study). Recent available literature shows some comparable results[5–7,10]. The scanning laser ophthalmoscope used for ICGA has some advantages and disadvantages, compared with high resolution digital systems, which have been widely studied by many authors. The main advantage of

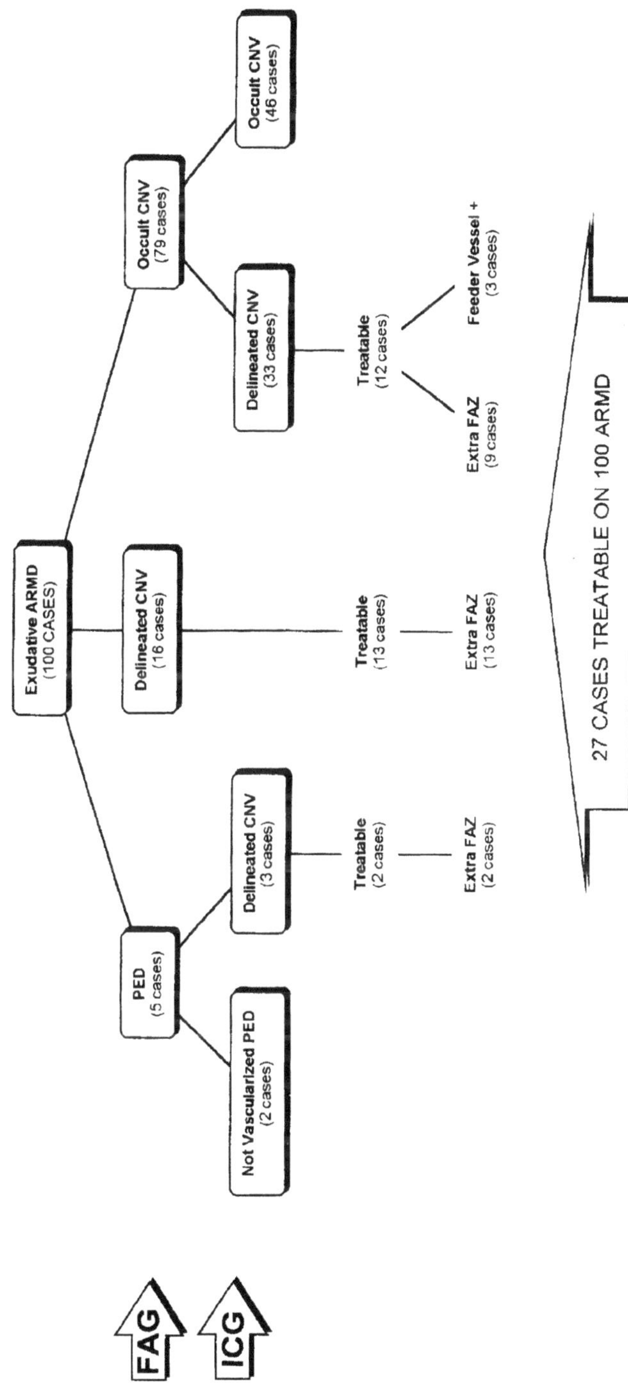

Fig. 1. Distribution of CNVs eligible for laser photocoagulation.

Table 1. CNV characteristics.

	Classic CNV	CNV with PED	CNV without PED

Morphologic classication	Focal CNV:
	  13 cases (12 treatable)
	Plaque CNV:
	  3 cases (1 treatable)
		Focal CNV:
		  3 cases (2 treatable)
		Plaque CNV:
		  no cases
			Focal CNV:
			  14 cases (8 treatable)
			Plaque CNV:
			  15 cases (4 treatable)
			Mixed CNV:
			  4 cases (no treatable)

CNV activity	High Activity:
	  5 cases (4 treatable)
	Medium Activity:
	  6 cases (5 treatable)
	Low Activity:
	  5 cases (4 treatable)
		High Activity:
		  1 case (1 treatable)
		Medium Activity:
		  2 cases (1 treatable)
		Low Activity:
		  no cases
			High Activity:
			  7 cases (3 treatable)
			Medium Activity:
			  14 cases (6 treatable)
			Low Activity:
			  7 cases (2 treatable)
			Zero Activity:
			  1 case (no treatable)
			Mixed Activity:
			  4 cases (1 treatable)

ICG phase of CNV detection	—	Early ICG +:
		  2 case (1 treatable)
		Early and Late ICG +:
		  1 case (1 treatable)
			Early ICG +:
			  5 cases (2 treatable)
			Late ICG +:
			  17 cases (3 treatable)
			Early and Late ICG +:
			  11 cases (7 treatable)

ICGA performed in exudative ARMD is its ability for dynamic recording in real time. This feature, associated with the tolerability of fundus illumination, allows a very good recording of early injection phases. Some CNVs with a low activity in late phases, and not well delineated in early phases because of choroidal capillaries quick filling, can be so detected. The main disadvantage is the low fluorescence in late images. Some CNVs with a low activity cannot be well imaged and their limits cannot be detected. However these neovascular membranes are plaques, often subfoveal, and rarely are eligible for laser treatment. Our ocular angiography service has been provided with a SLO recently and represents the only centre in Florence and near cities where ICGA is effected. We often perform ICGA in long-term exudative ARMD characterized by large plaques of subfoveal neovascularization that we can neither detect nor treat. We await results of examination of cases with a first or recent diagnosis. Finally, our data confirm the observation that for the majority of patients suffering from exudative ARMD our actual diagnostic and therapeutic interventions offer a little hope of recovery. Only one case in four can be treated with foveal avascular zone sparing and 50% of these will have a recurrence[2]. Nevertheless our data suggest that ICGA is helpful in these cases: ICGA enhances CNV detection by 200% and eligibility for photocoagulation by 100%. An early diagnosis and following FAG and ICGA is important to stop CNV evolution.

References

1. Macular Photocoagulation Study Group. Argon laser photocoagulation for senile macular degeneration. Results of a randomised clinical trial. Arch Ophthalmol. 1982; 100: 912–918.
2. Macular Photocoagulation Study Group. Persistent and recurrent neovascularization after krypton laser photocoagulation for neovascular lesion of age-related macular degeneration. Arch Ophthalmol. 1990; 108: 825–831.
3. Macular Photocoagulation Study Group. Laser photocoagulation of subfoveal neovascular lesions in age-related macular degeneration. Results of a randomized clinical trial. Arch Ophthalmol. 1991; 109: 1220–1231.
4. Freund, K.B., Yannuzzi, L.A., Sorenson, J.A. Age related macular degeneration and choroidal neovascularization. Am J Ophthalmol. 1993; 115: 786–791.
5. Regillo, C.D., Benson, W.E., Maguire, J.I., Annesley, W.H. Indocyanine green angiography and occult choroidal neovascularization. Ophthalmology. 1994; 101: 280–288.
6. Slatker, J.S., Yannuzzi, L.A., Sorenson, J.A. et al. A pilot study of indocyanine green video-angiography guided laser photocoagulation treatment of occult choroidal neovascularization. Arch Ophthalmol. 1994; 112: 465–472.
7. Bishoff, P., Speiser, P. Indocyanine green angiography and laser treatment of sub retinal membranes in age-related macular degeneration. Klin Monatsbl Augenheilkd. 1994; 204: 298–301.
8. Yannuzzi, L.A., Hope-Ross, M., Slatker, J.S. et al. Digital indocyanine green videoangiography and vascularized pigment epithelium detachment. Retina. 1994; 14: 99–113.
9. Wolf, S., Remky, A., Elsner, A.E. et al. Indocyanine green videoangiography in patients with age-related maculopathy-related retinal pigment epithelium detachments. Ger J Ophtalmol. 1994; 3: 224–227.
10. Guyer, D.R., Yannuzzi, L.A., Slatker, J.S. et al. Digital indocyanine green videoangiography of occult choroidal neovascularization. Ophthalmology. 1994; 101: 1727–1735.
11. Coscas, G., Soubrane, G. Indocyanine green videoangiography in laser photocoagulation for occult subretinal neovessels. Bull Soc Ophtalmol Fr. 1994; 94: 343–346.
12. Piermarocchi, S., Bertoja, E., Santin, G., Segato, T. Angiografia con SLO e verde di indo-cianina. Diagnosi delle membrane neovascolari sottoretiniche in corso di maculopatia degenerativa legata all'età. Boll Ocul. 1994; suppl. no. 3: 321–325.
13. Hayashi, K., De Laey, J.J. Indocyanine green angiography of choroidal neovascular membranes. Ophthalmologica. 1985; 190: 30–39.
14. Destro, M., Puliafito, C.A. Indocyanine green videoangiography of choroidal neovascularization. Ophthalmology. 1989; 96: 846–853.

University of Florence-1st Eye Clinic
viale Morgagni no. 85
50134-Firenze
Italy

61. Indocyanine green angiography follow-up of plaque choroidal neovascularization in age-related macular degeneration

A. PECE, G. BOLOGNESI, U. INTROINI, A. JANSEN
and R. BRANCATO

(Milan, Italy)

Introduction

In 1992 Yannuzzi and coworkers published the first report on digital indo-cyanine green angiography (ICGA) in age-related macular degeneration (ARMD), used to investigate occult choroidal neovascularization (CNV)[1]. That report identified a new ICGA pattern of CNV, referred to as plaque CNV. Four years later, there is still very little information about the natural course of plaque CNV, so this study was designed to cast some light on the question.

Materials and methods

A retrospective study was carried out on 19 consecutive eyes of 17 patients, seven males and 10 females. Fluorescein angiography (FA) showed occult CNV but ICGA indicated plaque CNV. A Topcon IMAGEnet 1024 System was used. Infracyanine dye was injected i.v. (25 mg) and pictures were taken in the early (5 min), middle (10–15 min) and late phases (after 30 min). Patients were followed up and two different observers (A and B) measured the plaque CNV area, using the Topcon Area Measurement System (Fig. 1).

Results

Mean follow-up was 7.78 ($\pm$4.8, range 3–19) months, initial and final mean visual acuity was 0.40 ($\pm$0.25, range 0.03–1) and 0.36 ($\pm$0.29, range 0.05–1). The initial mean size of plaque CNV, measured on ICGA was 5.458 mm^2 ($\pm$3.189) (observer A) and 5.742 mm^2 ($\pm$3.010) (B); the final mean size was 8.263 mm^2 ($\pm$5.507) (A) and 8.849 mm^2 ($\pm$5.434) (B) (Table 1). Mean size increased by 49% (A), and 56% (B).

G. Coscas and F. Cardillo Piccolino (eds.), Retinal Pigment Epithelium and Macular Diseases, pp. 361–364.
© 1998 Kluwer Academic Publishers.

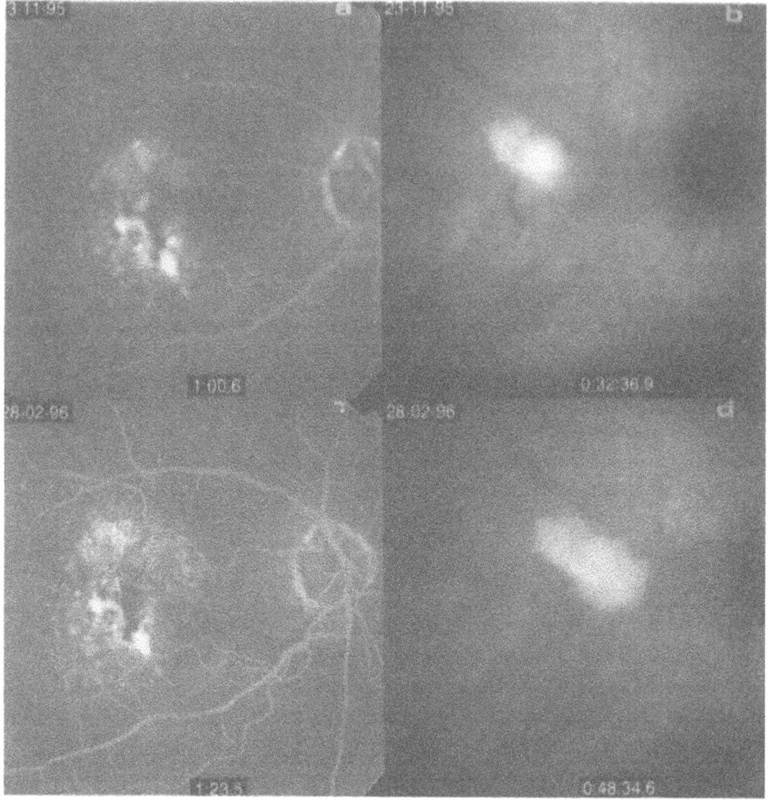

Fig. 1. Fluorescein angiography (a,c) and indocyanine green angiography (b,d) of a plaque CNV at the beginning and at the end of the study (V.E.). Initial size was 3.069 mm² (obs.A), final size was 6.149 mm². Follow-up period was 3 months.

Discussion

We considered a plaque CNV as a hyperfluorescent area larger than one disc diameter, with well defined borders, in the mid-late ICGA phases. Plaque CNV is believed to be a fairly inactive type of neovascularization[1] and in fact patients often have quite good visual acuity which tends to remain stable or decline only slowly. Sometimes, however, they complain of a sudden decrease in visual acuity with an evident CNV. Laser treatment is not normally indicated because plaque CNV is usually larger than one or two disc diameters and involves the subfoveal region.

The first question that arises is whether the ICGA plaque is really a CNV.

Table 1 Size of the lesion at the beginning and at the end of the study for observers A and B.

Patent	Size A 1	Size B 1	Size A 2	Size B 2
Z.L.	5.636	5.630	5.913	5.809
D.F	2.522	2.600	6.943	6.800
F.M.	4.241	3.201	6.874	6.220
L.F.	5.317	7.004	5.192	7.309
L.F.	1.966	2.246	1.771	2.251
V.T.	7.021	6.501	9.733	9.509
S.S.	4.054	4.511	6.214	5.954
R.P.	5.359	6.902	6.107	7.310
Z.F.	1.603	1.300	2.032	2.622
L.F.	2.043	4.439	2.041	4.653
L.E.	1.943	2.616	1.910	2.672
P.I.	6.174	6.232	17.738	18.466
A.E.	9.258	9.528	15.231	17.160
F.E.	9.833	9.152	17.050	17.916
I.V.	3.560	3.852	4.535	5.382
B.F.	7.310	8.012	9.656	10.880
V.E.	3.069	3.253	6.149	6.141
V.E.	11.564	11.305	14.913	15.510
S.F.	11.229	10.866	16.995	15.715

A 1, observer A beginning of study; B 1, observer B beginning of study; A 2, observer A end of study; B 2, observer B end of study.

These relatively inactive plaque CNV might be caused by the dye stain in the Bruch membrane-retinal pigment epithelium complex due to diffusion from the choriocapillaris altered by ARMD. Chang *et al.*[1] demonstrated histopathologically, however, that this ICGA hyperfluorescent area is due to a large amount of neovascular tissue. There is currently very little information about the plaque's natural progression.

Our study was only a preliminary investigation because both the number of patients and the follow up were limited. Nevertheless we found that the typical angiographic pattern may change, the plaque becoming bigger and fainter. The neovascularization became, on average, about 50% bigger. However visual acuity remained quite stable over time and there was no correlation with the size of the plaque CNV.

Conclusions

This study shows that the typical angiographic ICGA patterns of plaque CNV may change with time. These lesions often become bigger, though with minimal loss of visual acuity. This supports the current hypothesis that plaque CNV can be considered a type of CNV with little tendency to progression.

References

1. Yannuzzi, L.A., Slakter, J.S., Sorenson, J.A. et al. Digital indocyanine green videoangiography and choroidal neovascularization. Retina. 1992; 12: 191–223.
2. Chang, T., Freund, B., Green, W.R., Yannuzzi, L.A. Clinicopathologic correlation of indocyanine green angiography of occult choroidal neovascularization. Retina. 1994; 14: 114–124.

Department of Ophthalmology and Visual Sciences
Scientific Institute H S. Raffaele
University of Milano
Via Olgettina, 60
20132 Milano
Italy

62. Detection of recurrent choroidal neovascularization in age-related macular degeneration: comparison of clinical examination, fluorescein angiography and indocyanine green videoangiography

S. SAVIANO, M. BATTAGLIA PARODI, S. DA POZZO, D. IUSTULIN
and G. RAVALICO

(Trieste, Italy)

Introduction

Several reports and clinical trials have assessed the efficacy of laser treatment in selected cases of choroidal neovascularization (CNV) in age-related macular degeneration (AMD)[1-3]. However, in spite of laser photocoagulation, more than 50% of treated eyes develop persistent or recurrent CNV within 3 years after treatment[4,5]. Consequently, in order to identify as soon as possible the recurrence and to prevent a severe visual loss, there is a general agreement on the opportunity to perform frequent post-treatment clinical and instrumental examinations.

In recent years, indocyanine green videoangiography (ICG-V) has been usefully introduced in the imaging of recurrent CNV, particularly ill-defined lesions, thus giving an excellent support to fundus biomicroscopy and fluorescein angiography (FA); this fact has significantly increased the number of patients eligible for laser photocoagulation[6-9].

The purpose of this study was to evaluate the ability of ICG-V as a first choice investigation to detect the presence of recurrent CNV after krypton laser treatment in AMD.

Patients and methods

Forty-nine patients (64 eyes) were included in the study. All patients underwent krypton laser photocoagulation; post-treatment examinations were performed at the first, third and sixth month after laser treatment, in all 122 visits. The follow-up included clinical examination (fundus biomicroscopy using a 90 and 60-diopter lens). FA and ICG-V, all performed on the same day. The identification of recurrent CNV was based on FA as an early hyperfluorescent area along the edge of the laser scar with late dye leakage[4] and, on ICG-V, as an area of late staining[9]. Two of the authors (SS and

G. Coscas and F. Cardillo Piccolino (eds.), Retinal Pigment Epithelium and Macular Diseases, pp. 365–370.
© 1998 Kluwer Academic Publishers.

MBP) evaluated separately in a masked fashion each one of the three examinations and identified the presence of recurrent CNV, considering FA as the gold standard technique. All eyes were classified as having no recurrence, questionable or definite recurrence.

For purposes of calculating test accuracy parameters (sensitivity, specificity, positive and negative predictive value), the eyes classified as having definite and questionable recurrence were grouped together, on the assumption that a questionable recurrence is at high risk of becoming definite. If eligible for laser treatment, definite recurrences diagnosed during the follow-up were treated and the follow-up started again.

Of the 64 considered eyes, 37 had one treatment (no recurrence), nine had two treatments (one recurrence) and three had three treatments (two recurrences). Two patients had a bilateral treatment.

Results

At the first month clinical examination was slightly more sensitive than ICG-V whereas ICG-V is more specific, however without any statistical difference. Both examinations had high rate of false positives (15.6% and 10.9%, respectively) and false negatives (9.4%, 14.1%) (Figs 1, 2). A total of 28.5% of the false positives and 22% of the false negatives on ICG-V became true positive (on both angiographies) before next visit. At the third month ICG-V was completely sensitive but not so specific, with a high rate of false positives (18%). At the sixth month clinical examination had a very good sensitivity and specificity, while the same values were lower for ICG-V, but without any statistical difference. The questionable recurrences, indicating suspected but not certain lesions, were 30% on clinical examination, 19% on FA and 18% on ICG-V. Table 1 shows the calculated parameters by the comparison of clinical examination with FA are summarized. Comparison with ICG-V with FA is shown in Table 2. Table 3 shows the diagnostic accuracy values resulting from the comparison of clinical examination and of ICG-V with FA.

Discussion

The need to identify as early as possible the presence and the site of recurrent CNV is well documented to avoid further visual loss in patients with AMD. Since its introduction in the clinical use, ICG-V, combined with clinical examination and FA, has proved to be very useful to identify recurrent CNV, above all ill-defined CNV. This study compared separately both clinical examination and ICG-V with FA to evaluate their ability as a first choice investigation to detect the presence of recurrent CNV after krypton laser treatment in AMD. FA was considered as the gold standard examination because it has been used for longer and is more clearly understood than

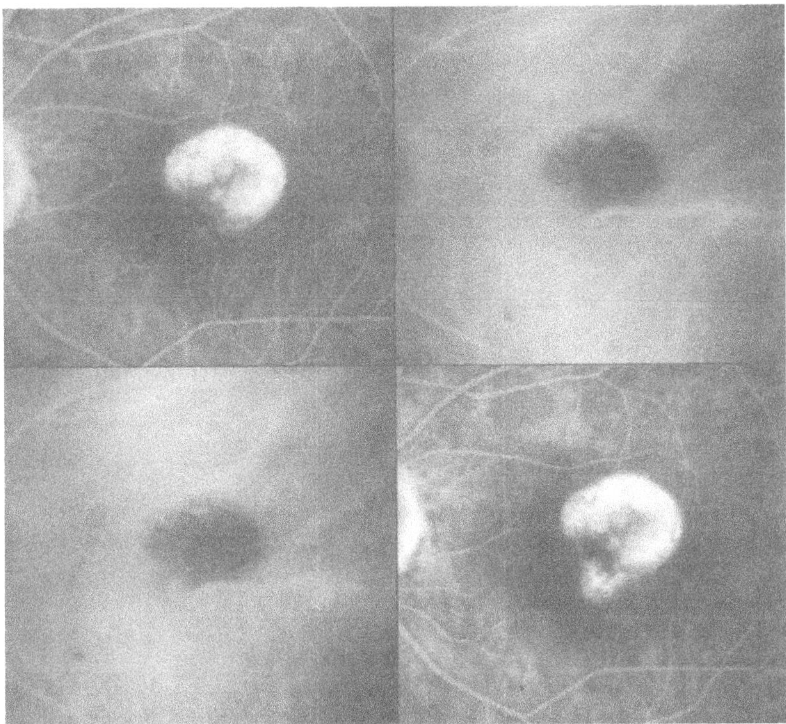

Fig. 1. Example of a false negative result (positive on FA, negative on ICG-V). FA shows a slight dye leakage at the foveal border of the laser scar (top left), suspect for a recurrent lesion. ICG-V (top right) shows no evidence of recurrent CNV. The presence of a recurrence is evident on both angiographs 1 month later (bottom left and right).

ICG-V. Although late hyperfluorescence and dye staining on FA can hide the location and the extension of recurrences, they are usually easily recognized, so revealing the presence of the lesion. Our results show that diagnostic accuracy, that combines sensitivity, specificity, positive and negative predictive value, improves during the follow-up with either clinical examination or ICG-V (Table 3). On the contrary, Sykes *et al.*[10] found clinical examination had a very good sensitivity and specificity at the sixth month. This probably arose because the longer the laser treatment, the greater is the resorption of lipid, haemorrhage and subretinal fluid and the better the demarcation between the laser scar and the surrounding retina. These confounding factors probably justify the high rate of questionable recurrences occurring at the first month control compared with a much lower rate at the sixth month (44 vs. 12%). These high sensitivity and specificity values at the sixth month could imply that retinal angiography should be performed on the basis of clinical examination.

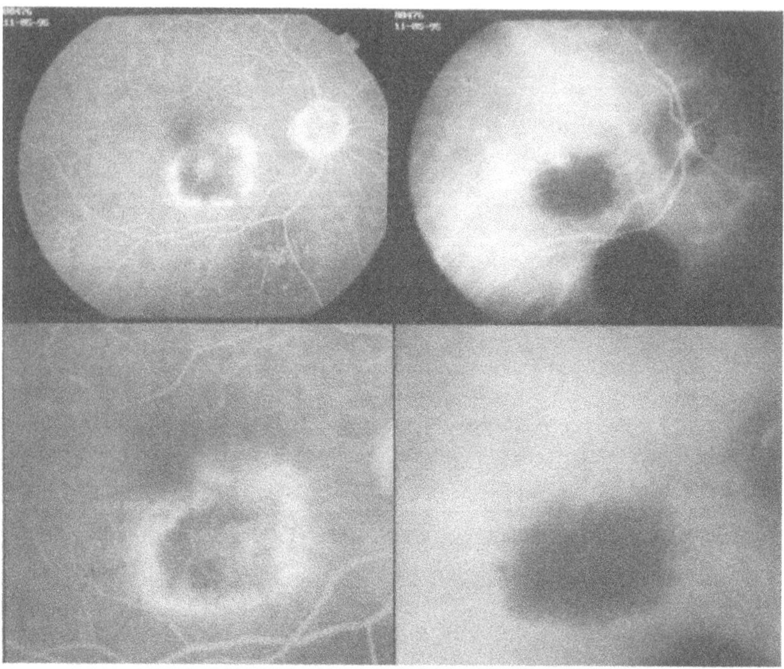

Fig. 2. Example of a false positive (negative on FA, positive on ICG-V). Biomicroscopy and FA (top left) do not demonstrate the presence of residual neovascularization 1 month after laser treatment. ICG-V (top right) shows a hyperfluorescent lesion at the foveal border of the laser scar. One month later, without any further laser photocoagulation, FA shows a slight dye leakage at the foveal border, whereas ICG-V does not show any lesion.

Table 1. Clinical examination vs. FA: test accuracy parameters values.

	First month (%)	*Third month* (%)	*Sixth month* (%)
Sensitivity	87.2	93.8	92.9
Specificity	41.2	82.4	90.9
Positive predictive value	80.4	83.3	92.9
Negative predictive values	53.8	93.3	90.9

ICG-V showed maximum of sensitivity at the third month and good specificity at the sixth month. That means, globally, high rate of false positive and false negative, above all at the first month. We do not know the reasons for these misdiagnosed cases. They could certainly depend on the difficulty in interpreting the images of angiographies. On one hand these results indicate that ICG-V cannot be considered as a first choice investigation in detecting the presence of recurrent CNV, have too high a false positive and negative rate, particularly in the first months after laser treatment. On the other hand

Table 2. ICG-V vs. FA: test accuracy parameters values.

	First month (%)	Third month (%)	Sixth month (%)
Sensitivity	80.9	100	85.7
Specificity	58.8		
		72.7	92.3
Negative predictive values	52.6	100	83.3

Table 3. Diagnostic accuracy values at first, third and sixth month.

	First month (%)	Third month (%)	Sixth month (%)
Clinical examination vs. FA	75	87.9	92
ICG-V vs. FA	75	81.8	88

the high rate of questionable recurrences, either out of FA or ICG-V, confirms the need of short follow-up intervals and suggests to use both retinal angiographies together to identify as early as possible a definite lesion.

In our opinion, and according to the results of this study, the best available protocol for recurrent CNV identification is the combination of the three techniques together. Further studies and longer follow-up are needed to improve and to better understand the imaging of retinal angiographies in patients treated for AMD. All variables, such as different angiographic patterns of recurrences or dye staining depending on laser-induced angiitis, should be considered to reduce as much as possible all doubts of interpretations.

References

1. Macular Photocoagulation Study Group. Argon laser photocoagulation for neovascular maculopathy: five-year results from randomized clinical trials. Arch Ophthalmol. 1991; 109: 1109–1114.
2. Macular Photocoagulation Study Group. Laser photocoagulation for juxtafoveal choroidal neovascularization: five-year results from randomized clinical trials. Arch Ophthalmol. 1994; 112: 500–509.
3. Macular Photocoagulation Study Group. Laser photocoagulation of subfoveal neovascular lesions of age-related macular degeneration: updated findings from two clinical trials. Arch Ophthalmol. 1993; 111: 1200–1209.
4. Macular Photocoagulation Study Group. Persistent and recurrent neovascularization after krypton laser photocoagulation for neovascular lesions of age-related macular degeneration. Arch Ophthalmol. 1990; 108: 825–831.
5. Macular Photocoagulation Study Group. Persistent and recurrent neovascularization after laser photocoagulation for subfoveal choroidal neovascularization of age-related macular degeneration. Arch Ophthalmol. 1994; 112: 489–499.

6. Yannuzzi, L.A., Slakter, J.S., Sorenson, J.A. *et al.* Digital indocyanine green videoangiography and choroidal neovascularization. Retina. 1992; 12: 191–223.
7. Regillo, C.D., Benson, W.E., Maguire, J.I. *et al.* Indocyanine green angiography and occult choroidal neovascularization. Ophthalmology. 1994; 101: 280–288.
8. Slakter, J.S., Yannuzzi, L.A., Sorenson, J.A. *et al.* A pilot study of indocyanine green video-angiography-guided laser photocoagulation of occult choroidal neovascularization in age-related macular degeneration. Arch Ophthalmol. 1994; 112: 465–472.
9. Sorenson, J.A., Yannuzzi, L.A., Slakter, J.S. *et al.* A pilot study of digital indocyanine green videoangiography for recurrent occult choroidal neovascularization in age-related macular degeneration. Arch Ophthalmol. 1994; 112: 473–479.
10. Sykes, S.O., Bressler, N.M., Maguire, M.G. *et al.* Detecting recurrent choroidal neovascularization. Comparison of clinical examination with and without fluorescein angiography. Arch Ophthalmol. 1994; 112: 1561–1566.
11. Dyer, D.S., Brant, A.M., Schachat, A.P. *et al.* Angiographic features and outcome of questionable recurrent choroidal neovascularization. Am J Ophthalmol. 1995; 120: 497–505.

Eye Clinic
University of Trieste
Italy

63. Massive subretinal haemorrhage in age-related macular degeneration

C. VEROUGSTRAETE, L. POSTELMANS and F. DIXSAUT

(Brussels, Belgium)

Introduction

A sudden and major visual loss may occur in age-related macular degeneration (AMD) after a massive macular subretinal haemorrhage[1-6]. The very poor prognosis of this complication led us to undertake a retrospective study in order to determine the characteristics of the eyes at risk, the type of neovascularization involved and their evolution before and after the haemorrhage.

Methods

Seventy-two eyes (69 patients) with AMD and subretinal haemorrhage of five disc areas or more were examined with fluorescein angiography (FA). When available, FA before the haemorrhage and during follow up after the haemorrhage were analysed, as well as FA of the fellow eye. The type of subretinal new vessels (SRNV) was determined with FA at the time of or just before the haemorrhage in 65 eyes. In four eyes it was determined after some resorption of the haemorrhage. In three eyes, it was based on the type of SRNV in the fellow eye.

Results

There were 66 subretinal and six vitreous haemorrhages. Seventy-one percent of patients were women and 29% were men, with a mean age for both groups of 77 years. Occult or mixed SRNV were responsible for 97% of haemorrhages (3/4 occult, 1/4 mixed; Fig. 1. Visual acuity (VA) before the haemorrhage was still $\geq 4/10$ in 34% of the cases (VA measured at a mean of 1.5 months before the haemorrhage). Mean time between the onset of SRNV and the haemorrhage was 30 months.

FA before the haemorrhage showed 65% occult SRNV, 21% mixed SRNV, 3% visible SRNV and 3% disciform scar with neovascular activity. In 9% SRNV had not been detected beforehand on FA but occult SRNV could be suspected retrospectively. Twenty-seven percent of eyes had a serous pigment

G. Coscas and F. Cardillo Piccolino (eds.), Retinal Pigment Epithelium and Macular Diseases, pp. 371–375.
© *1998 Kluwer Academic Publishers.*

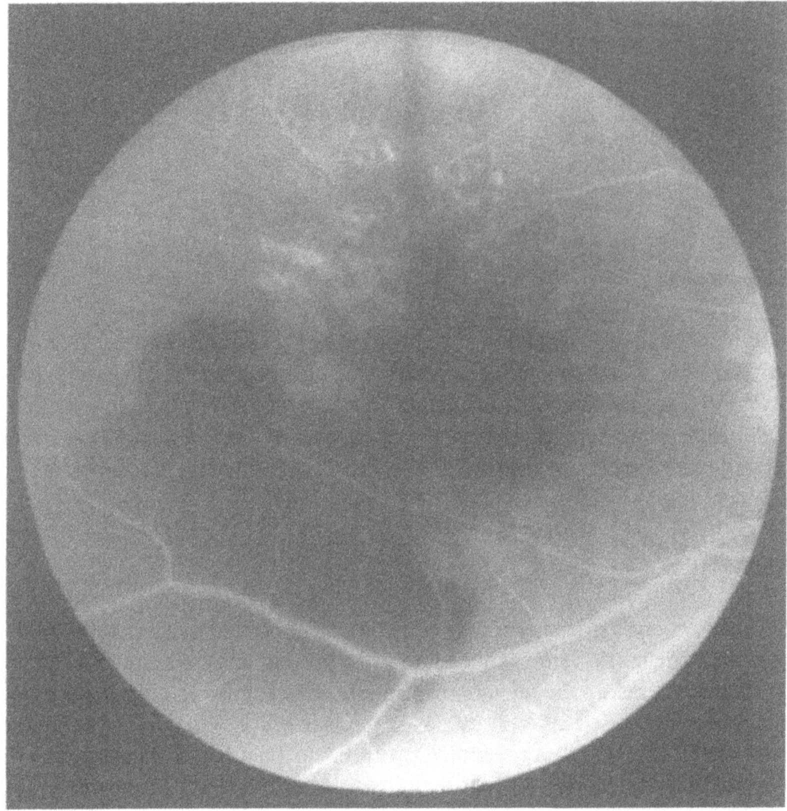

Fig. 1. Occult subretinal new vessels associated with a 10 disc area subretinal haemorrhage (visual acuity 7/10).

epithelium detachment (PED), of which two subsisted at the time of the haemorrhage. Three additional cases had a serous PED at the time of the haemorrhage.

Haemorrhagic recurrences occurred in 36% (Fig. 2) and were multiple in 15% of the eyes. They occurred most frequently within 7 months (32% of the eyes) and 38% invaded the vitreous. Hypertension and anticoagulant treatment were not more frequent than in the normal population. However, one patient with blood dyscrasia had a particularly severe haemorrhage with 360° retinal detachment and angle closure glaucoma.

In the fellow eye, 56% had a neovascular AMD, with 21% having early SRNV (10 eyes with occult SRNV and two with mixed SRNV) and 35% having a disciform scar (of which 1/4 still had occult or mixed neovascular activity). Four fellow eyes had a fresh massive subretinal macular haemorrhage during the follow up (6%).

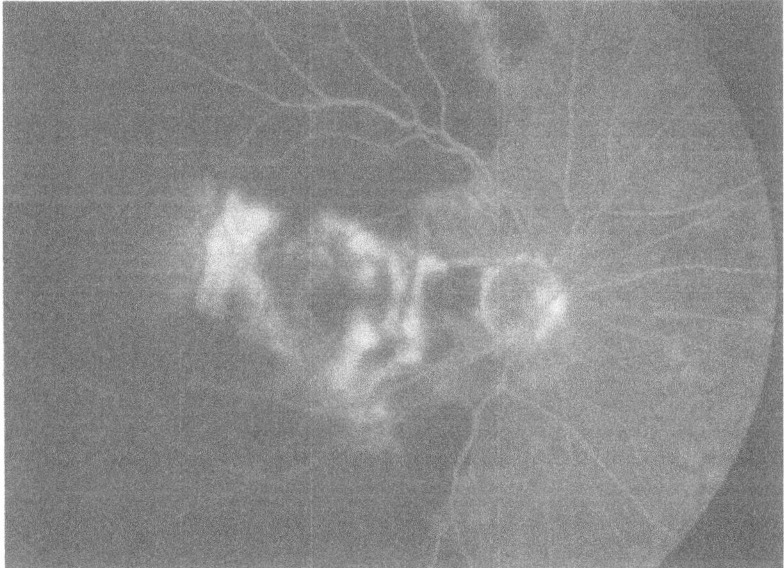

Fig. 2. Same patient 4 months later: massive subretinal haemorrhagic recurrence. Scar retraction and radial choroidal folds.

Final visual acuity was $<1/10$ in 88% of eyes, due to fibrous and atrophic central scars (Fig. 3).

Seven percent of eyes retained good vision $(>4/10)$; they had had an eccentric haemorrhage and a rather thin layer of blood at the level of the foveola.

Conclusions

Massive macular subretinal haemorrhages have a very poor visual prognosis. In our study they occurred mostly with occult or mixed SRNV, which explains why one-third of the eyes still had moderate to good vision before the haemorrhage, even though the SRNV had been longstanding[7], and also explains why 27% of the eyes had a PED before the haemorrhage[8-10].

We observed haemorrhagic recurrences in one-third of the eyes. However, some of the vitreous recurrences may have been delayed migration of subretinal blood. Hypertension, anti-agregant or anticoagulant medications had no major influence in causing the haemorrhage, but may have aggravated it. The fellow eye was at risk of massive macular subretinal haemorrhage. Occult SRNV may grow slowly, becoming quite large membranes in spite of minimal symptoms[7]. These membranes are connected to the choroid by capillaries passing through Bruchs membrane defects. These capillaries may, with time,

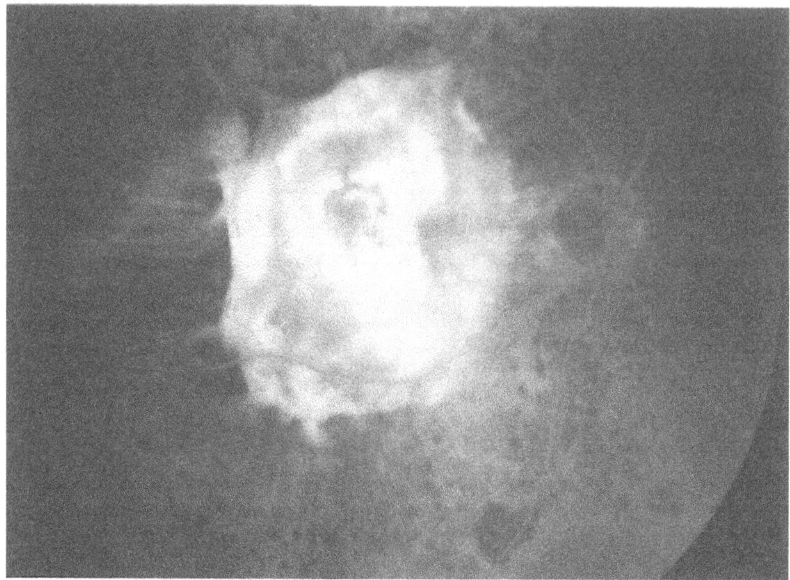

Fig. 3. Same patient 19 months later: large central fibrous scar and leopard spots due to haemorrhagic resorption (visual acuity < 1/10).

become large venous and arteriolar trunks[7,11-14]. We suggest that, either with natural evolution towards membrane fibrous retraction, or with treatment, traction stresses may cause mechanical tearing of large vessel walls, giving rise to vast haemorrhages of which the intensity will depend on the arterial, venous or capillary nature of the ruptured vessel. Another mechanism which could occur in advanced AMD with important serous detachment, is pressure necrosis of the artery wall, as suggested by El Baba *et al.*[2].

References

1. Bennett, S.R., Folk, J.C., Blodi, C.F., Klugman, M. Factors prognostic of visual outcome in patients with subretinal hemorrhage. Am J Ophthalmol. 1990; 109: 33–37.
2. El Baba, F., Jarrett, W.H. II, Harbin, T.S. Jr *et al.* Massive hemorrhage complicating age-related macular degeneration. Clinicopathologic correlation and role of anticoagulant. Ophthalmology. 1986; 93: 1581–1592.
3. Kreiger, A.E., Haidt, S.J. Vitreous hemorrhage in senile macular degeneration. Retina. 1983; 3: 318–321.
4. Smiddy, W.E., Isernhagen, R.D., Michels, R.G., Glaser, B.M., De Bustros, S.N. Vitrectomy for nondiabetic vitreous hemorrhage. Retinal and choroidal vascular disorders. Retina. 1988; 8: 88–95.
5. Tani, P.M., Buettner, H., Robertson, D.M. Massive vitreous hemorrhage and senile mcular choroidal degeneration. Am J Ophthalmol. 1980; 90: 525–533.

6. Wade, E.C., Flynn, H.W., Olsen, K.R., Blumenkranz, M.S., Nicholson, D.H. Subretinal hemorrhage management by pars plana vitrectomy and internal drainage. Arch Ophthalmol. 1990; 108: 973–978.

7. Chang, T.S., Freund, K.B., De La Cruz, Z., Yannuzzi, L.A., Green, W.R. Clinicopathologic correlation of choroidal neovascularization demonstrated by indocyanine green angiography in a patient with retention of good vision for almost four years. Retina. 1994; 14: 114–124.

8. Frederick, A.R. Jr, Morley, M.G., Topping, T.M., Peterson, T.J., Wilson, D.J. The appearance of stippled retinal pigment epithelial detachments. A sign of occult choroidal neovascularization in age-related macular degeneration. Retina. 1993; 13: 3–7.

9. Kuhn, D., Meunier, I., Soubrane, G., Coscas, G. Imaging of chorio-retinal anastomoses in vascularized retinal pigment epithelium detachments. Arch Ophthalmol. 1995; 113: 1392–1398.

10. Yannuzzi, L.A., Hope-Ross, M., Slakter, J.S. *et al.* Analysis of vascularized pigment epithelial detachments using indocyanine green videoangiography. Retina. 1994; 14: 99–113.

11. Googe, J.M., Hirose, T., Apple, D.J., Melgen, S. Vitreous hemorrhage secondary to age-related macular degeneration. Surv Ophthalmol. 1987; 32: 123–130.

12. Green, W.R., Enger, C. Age-related macular degeneration. Histopathologic studies. Ophthalmology. 1993; 100: 1519–1535.

13. MacCumber, M.W., Dastgheib, K., Bressler, N.M. *et al.* Clinicopathologic correlation of the multiple recurrent serosanguineous retinal pigment epithelial detachments syndrome. Retina. 1994; 14: 143–152.

14. Wolter, J.R., McWilliams, J.R. Rupture of disciform macular degeneration causing massive retroretinal hemorrhage. Am J Ophthalmol. 1965; 59: 1044–1047.

Brugmann University Hospital
4, Place Van Gehuchten
1020 Brussels, Belgium

64. Choroidal neovascular membrane in age-related macular degeneration, histopathological and clinical correlation

N. ORZALESI, L. MIGLIAVACCA and G. STAURENGHI

(Milan, Italy)

Purpose

Indocyanine green angiography (ICGA) has been recently introduced in the clinical practice for better visualization of choroidal neovascular membranes (CNM). In particular, ICGA helps in identifying occult membranes or small feeder vessels in subfoveal CNM. There is just one report describing clinico-pathological correlation, with an interval of 15 months between the dye study and the histopathology. We report the first case of neovascular ARMD in which a complete clinical examination, including infrared imaging, ICGA and scotometry was correlated with pathology assessed after 12 h in the intact eye enucleated for an untreatable melanosarcoma.

Methods

A 65-year-old woman with an untreatable choroidal melanosarcoma and a subfoveal choroidal neovascular membrane was studied with infrared imaging (IR), scotometry, FA and ICGA using a scanning laser ophthalmoscope (SLO; Rodenstock GmbH). The eye was enucleated 12 h later and embedded in epoxy resin for histology and transmission electron microscopy (TEM). A computerized three dimensional (3D) reconstruction of the membrane, based on 1300 serial sections (1 micron thick), was used to correlate pathology with clinical retinal imaging and scotometry.

Results

FA revealed a classic neovascular membrane with ill-defined borders due to the presence of blood. A feeder vessel (FV) was clearly evident in the early phase of ICGA. IR imaging with the SLO showed very clearly the sharp boundaries of the membrane. The 3D reconstruction of the membrane showed a close correlation between histological size and shape of the membrane and the boundary indicated by IR imaging. The FV shown by ICGA was the

G. Coscas and F. Cardillo Piccolino (eds.), Retinal Pigment Epithelium and Macular Diseases, pp. 377–378.
© *1998 Kluwer Academic Publishers.*

only feeder shown also by histological examination and was located in the centre of the membrane. Histology revealed two components of the membrane, the main one located beneath the RPE and the other in the intraretinal space. Only few feeder vessels of the intraretinal portion of the membrane arising from the sub-epitelial net were seen crossing the RPE. Remarkable TEM features of the membrane are also presented. These included many fibroblasts and fibrils connected with the newly formed vessels which were of the mature and immature type with relatively few fenestrations. The vessels were concentrated in the middle of the membrane whereas the periphery was almost entirely fibrous. These results are compared with previous data available in the literature on the structure and clinical-pathological correlation of CNM.

Conclusion

Information of this kind, which may be available only exceptionally, appears useful for a better understanding of neovascularization in ARMD and its correlation to new clinical data based on infrared imaging, ICGA and scotometry.

University Eye Clinic
Institute of Biomedical Science
San Paolo Hospital
Milan, Italy

65. Indocyanine green angiography-guided laser photocoagulation of choroidal neovascularization in age-related macular degeneration

U. INTROINI, A. PECE, G. PACELLI, G. BOLOGNESI,
G. TRABUCCHI, P. AVANZA and R. BRANCATO

(Milan, Italy)

Purpose

Indocyanine green angiography (ICGA) is an important diagnostic tool in the management of age-related macular degeneration (ARMD), enabling ophthalmologists to convert fluorescein-occult choroidal neovascularization (CNV) to ICGA well-defined CNV in 40–50% of cases[1-3]. About 30% of these can be treated with laser photocoagulation, which is the only proven therapy for exudative ARMD[4,5]. The aim of this study was to evaluate the effectiveness of ICGA-guided laser treatment in eyes with ICGA well-defined focal CNV.

Methods

We retrospectively reviewed 86 eyes of 84 consecutive patients with ARMD and well defined extrafoveal focal CNV on ICGA, either associated or not with pigment epithelium detachment (PED). We distinguished four groups. In group 1 (21 eyes), all had hot-spots beneath the PED. Fluorescence showed early bright small dots, well visible during all angiographic phases, which were considered to be chorio-retinal anastomoses (CRA)[6]. Group 2 (27 eyes) had PED with a marginal focal CNV, on the edge of or close to the boundaries of the PED. This CNV frequently lies over the 'notch' of the PED. Group 3 (11 eyes) had macular PED and CNV near the optic disc area; a typical pattern showed multiple small hyperfluorescent dots, linked together and generally far from the PED boundaries. Group 4 (27 eyes) had an ICGA well defined focal CNV with no fluorescein angiography (FA) evidence of PED. In this last group no distinct fluorescent patterns of CNV were detectable.

Results

Group 1 showed an initial mean visual acuity of 20/80, and mean follow-up was 9 months. At final examination, 18/21 (86%) eyes had a subfoveal

G. Coscas and F. Cardillo Piccolino (eds.), Retinal Pigment Epithelium and Macular Diseases, pp. 379–381.
© *1998 Kluwer Academic Publishers.*

involvement with huge CNV recurrences. Final visual acuity (mean 20/300) was stable in two eyes (10%) and worsened in the remaining 19 eyes (90%). No eyes showed an improvement.

In group 2 (27 eyes) initial mean visual acuity was 20/40. After a mean follow-up of 10 months, nine eyes (33%) attained obliteration of the CNV, while 18 (67%) had untreatable recurrences. Final visual acuity (mean 20/80) increased in two eyes (8%), was stable in six (22%) and was worse in 19 (70%).

Group 3 (11 eyes) showed a mean initial visual acuity of 20/50. Only one eye (9%) needed a second successful laser treatment. After a mean follow-up of 13 months nine eyes (82%) showed complete obliteration of the CNV. After more than 1 year only two eyes (18%) had a recurrence. Final visual acuity (mean 20/32) was improved in six eyes (55%), stable in four (36%) and worse in one (9%).

Group 4 (27 eyes) had an initial visual acuity of 20/63. After a mean follow-up of 12 months 11 eyes (41%) achieved obliteration of the CNV, and 16 (59%) had a subfoveal recurrence. Final visual acuity (mean 20/80) had improved in six eyes (22%), was stable in four (15%) and worse in 17 (63%).

Discussion

Direct laser photocoagulation is the only effective therapy for exudative ARMD, when CNV are well defined by FA[4,5]. However in 85% of the cases CNV are occult to FA[7]. These CNV can be seen well with ICGA though this has widened the indication for angiography-guided laser treatment of CNV in the last few years[1-3].

Using Yannuzzi's classification of occult CNV, we divided CNV as focal (bright fluorescent points called 'hot-spots' smaller than 1 DD) or plaque CNV (bigger than 1 DD)[1]. In our pilot study we only considered the laser treatment of focal CNV, and investigated how the presence of a serous PED influenced the prognosis in the laser treatment of a focal CNV. In our innovative study, we detected three different patterns of focal CNV among ARMD with PED. In the first group, CRA with PED, we obtained the worst results. The diagnosis of CRA is made by clinical and dynamic observation of the lesion. FA and ICGA both confirm the presence of an abnormal retinal vessel connected to the hyperfluorescent spot[6]. Most of the frequent persistencies occurred in the first 6 weeks of follow-up.

In the second group the PED was complicated by a marginal CNV, partially or completely covered by the detachment itself. The microvascular net of new vessels is visible in early ICGA phases. Laser treatment gave better results, than in the first group. After 6 months 45% of the eyes maintained obliteration of the CNV, and 33% after 1 year.

The third group, with parapapillary CNV, achieved the best results (82% of final CNV obliteration). The particular pattern of these new vessels or their location seem to be the reason for the success photocoagulation. In all but two, CNV were far from the PED, but even in the eyes with the PED overlying the CNV, a successful result was attained, with obliteration of the CNV and flattening of the PED.

In the fourth group, which included eyes without PED, laser treatment had a success rate of 56% within the first 6 months. After 1 year, 41% of the eyes maintained obliteration of the CNV, this final result almost confirming the outcome in the second group (33%). These findings disagree with the theory, put forward in an earlier pilot study, that the presence of PED strongly worsens the prognosis of laser treatment. That study reported that CNV obliteration was obtained in 43% of the eyes with PED and in 66% without PED, after 6 months. However, it comprised only one group of focal CNV and PED, including all types of focal spots[8].

Our initial classification of the various patterns was virtually guesswork, but it was then supported by the differences found between the four groups. The results of laser treatment in the different groups demonstrate the prognostic importance of our classification. Our findings confirm that the presence of a PED with a suspected CRA can badly influence ICGA-guided laser treatment[6]. However the outcome after 1 year of patients with and without PED (groups 2 and 4) were similar; the exceptions are eyes with PED associated with a parapapillary CNV, which achieved good functional and anatomical results.

Our retrospective pilot study only deals with preliminary results, very different for the four groups considered, but not backed by case-control groups. A randomized multicentre trial in which all new patients are enrolled is now needed to give guidelines about ICGA laser-guided eligibility.

References

1. Yannuzzi, L.A., Slakter, J.S., Sorenson, J.A. *et al.* Digital indocyanine green videoangiography and choroidal neovascularization. Retina. 1992; 12: 191–223.
2. Guyer, D.R., Yannuzzi, L.A., Slakter, J.S. *et al.* Digital indocyanine-green videoangiography of occult choroidal neovascularization. Ophthalmology. 1994; 101: 1727–1737.
3. Yannuzzi, L.A., Hope-Ross, M., Slakter, J.S. *et al.* Digital indocyanine greeen video angiography and vascularized pigment epithelium detachment. Retina. 1994; 14: 99–113.
4. Macular Photocoagulation Study Group. Argon laser photocoagulation for age-related macular degeneration. Arch Ophthalmol. 1982; 100: 912–918.
5. Macular Photocoagulation Study Group. Krypton laser photocoagulation for neovascularized lesions of age-related macular degeneration. Arch Ophthalmol. 1990; 108: 816–824.
6. Khun, D., Meunier, I., Soubrane, G., Coscas, G. Imaging of chorioretinal anastomoses in vascularized retinal pigment epithelium detachments. Arch Ophthalmol. 1995; 113: 1392–1398.
7. Freund, K.B., Yannuzzi, L.A., Sorenson, J.A. Age-related macular degeneration and choroidal neovascularization. Am J Ophthalmol. 1993; 115: 786–791.
8. Slakter, J.S., Yannuzzi, L.A., Sorenson, J.A. *et al.* A pilot study of indocyanine green videoangiography guided laser photocoagulation treatment of occult choroidal neovascularization. Arch Ophthalmol. 1994; 112: 465–472

Department of Ophthalmology and Visual Sciences
Scientific Institute H. S. Raffaele
University of Milano
20132 Milano, Italy

66. Photocoagulation of choroidal neovascular membrane (CNV) with diode laser (805 nm)

P. LANZETTA, U. MENCHINI and G. VIRGILI

(Udine, Italy)

Introduction

Laser photocoagulation of CNV was introduced in the early 1970s[1-3]. Several multicentre studies have demonstrated that argon or krypton laser treatment reduces the incidence of severe visual loss[4,5]. Recently a semiconductor diode laser that emits in the near-infrared wavelength at 805–810 nm was introduced in ophthalmology. This photocoagulator has many operating benefits such as its compact dimensions, efficient electric-optical conversion (over 50%), the absence of cooling requirements and a long useful life with minimal maintenance[6-10]. This wavelength has good transmission through dioptric media, an almost total absence of absorption by the foveal pigment and lower absorption by the retinal pigment epithelium (RPE) with respect to argon and krypton laser[11-13]. We verified its efficacy in the treatment of CNV.

Patients and methods

Twenty-four eyes with a well-defined parafoveal CNV were selected for laser photocoagulation. The eyes were treated with a near infrared diode laser (Visulas diode by Zeiss, 807 nm; diode laser by IRIS Medical, 805 nm). Seventeen of the eyes presented age related macular degeneration, five were affected with myopic macular degeneration, one had angioid streaks and one had idiopathic CNV.

Direct treatment on the lesion was carried out. Photocoagulation produced a whitening of the zone treated. All eyes underwent colour retinography of the fundus and fluorescein angiography no more than 72 h prior to treatment. The efficacy of the treatment was verified by an independent specialist. Visual acuity was evaluated (a variation of at least 2 lines on the Snellen chart) at 1 week, 2 weeks, 1 month and 2 months, and then every 3 months with an average follow-up of 9.9 months (range 2–30 months; SD 8.4). The success of laser treatment was evaluated by fluorescein angiogram evaluating the presence of any recurrence at the end of follow-up time.

G. Coscas and F. Cardillo Piccolino (eds.), Retinal Pigment Epithelium and Macular Diseases, pp. 383–385.
© 1998 Kluwer Academic Publishers.

Results

Treatment parameters were a 160–200 µm spot with a power of 400–800 mW. Exposure time varied from 0.5 to 1 s in both groups. None of the patients had undesirable eye movements or complained of pain during treatment. Fluorescein angiography soon after photocoagulation appeared totally hypofluorescent in the zone treated. Visual acuity after treatment improved in eight eyes (33.3%), unchanged in 11 (45.8%) and worsened in five (20.9%). Mean visual acuity was 0.37 before treatment and 0.35 after treatment. The success of laser photocoagulation was angiographically assessed in 19 eyes (79.2%) while five eyes (21.8%) presented recurrent CNV.

Discussion

Laser photocoagulation is still the only available therapy during CNV. Semiconductor diode lasers emit in the near-infrared. This wavelength has good transmission characteristics through the dioptric media even in presence of lens opacities (cataract) or vitreous haemorrhages. Diode transmission through transparent dioptric media exceeds 95%. RPE wavelength absorption is of the order of 30–35%. The absorption is lower than for red krypton (about 65%) and substantially higher than that for the CW Nd:YAG infrared laser (7–8%)[14]. Absorption by the RPE is therefore lower than is the case with shorter wavelengths, such as green argon. Radiation is blocked to a lesser degree by the RPE so that there is greater penetration of the radiation into the choriocapillaris and an increased level of energy is required to produce the whitening effect typical of retinal photocoagulation. In the patients that we treated, the effective power (400–800 mW) was on average three times higher than that generally needed with krypton laser (150–250 mW).

Near-infrared radiation is also capable of passing through thin layers of preretinal blood[15]. Moreover near-infrared radiation does not cause an unpleasant sensation of haze. The closure of the neovascular membrane could depend upon an acute occlusion which may derive from the transmission of heat absorbed by the RPE and choroidal melanocytes to the CNV vessels. Definitive closure of the CNV may be a consequence of atrophy and the cicatricial phenomena that lead to its constriction. Some authors have found that photocoagulated human RPE cells secrete inhibitors of proliferation[16]. Diode laser treatment of CNVs may have some difficulties related to the epiphenomena accompanying neovascularization. The presence of detachment of the neuroepithelium, subretinal liquid or detachment of the RPE make retinal whitening more difficult. Greater energy is required to obtain whitening, which may cause the occlusion of sections of the choriocapillaris and abnormal tissue atrophy. However we did not identify any occlusion of large vessels of the choroid or of sections of the choriocapillaris adjacent to the area treated. This aspect requires further investigation on a larger scale.

In conclusion although long-term efficacy should naturally be verified on a large number of patients, the results that we recorded favourably encourage CNV photocoagulation with near infrared diode laser wavelength.

References

1. Gass, J.D.M. Photocoagulation of macular lesions. Trans Am Acad Ophthalmol Otolaryngol. 1971; 75: 581–608.
2. Schatz, H., Patz, A. Exudative senile maculopathy: 1. Results of argon laser treatment. Arch Ophthalmol. 1973; 90: 183–196.
3. Bird, A.C. Recent advantages in the treatment of senile disciform macular degeneration by photocoagulation. Br J Ophthalmol. 1974; 58: 367–76.
4. Macular Photocoagualtion Study Group. Argon laser photocoagulation for neovascular maculopathy: five year results from randomized clinical trials. Arch Ophthalmol. 1991; 109: 1109–1114.
5. Macular Photocoagualtion Study Group. Krypton laser photocoagulation for neovascular lesions of age-related macular degeneration: results of a randomized clinical trial. Arch Ophthalmol. 1990; 108: 816–824.
6. Brancato, R., Pratesi, R., Leoni, G. *et al.* Retinal photocoagulation with diode laser operating from a slitlamp microscope. Lasers Light Ophthalmol. 1988; 2: 73–78.
7. McHugh, J.D.A., Marshall, J., Capon, M. *et al.* Transpupillary retinal photocoagulation in the eyes of rabbit and human using a diode laser. Lasers Light Ophthalmol. 1988; 2: 125–43.
8. McHugh, J.D.A., Marshall, J., ffytche, T.J. *et al.* Initial clinical experience using a diode laser in the treatment of retinal vascular disease. Eye. 1989; 3: 516–527.
9. Puliafito, C.A., Deutsch, T.F., Boll, J., To, K. Semiconductor laser endophotocoagulation of the retina. Arch Ophthalmol. 1987; 105: 424–427.
10. Brancato, R., Pratesi, R., Leoni, G. *et al.* Histopathology of diode and argon laser lesions in rabbit retina. Invest Ophthalmol Vis Sci. 1989; 30: 1504–1510.
11. Gabel, V.P., Birngruber, R., Hillenkamp, F. Visible and near infrared light absorption in pigment epithelium and choroid. In: Shimizu, K. (ed.), International Congress Series nr 450, XXIII Concilium Ophthalmol Kyoto. Amsterdam: Excerpta Medica, 1978; 658–662.
12. Fankhauser, F., Van Der Zypen, E., Kwasniewska, S., Loertscher, H. The effect of thermal mode Nd:YAG laser radiation on vessels and ocular tissues. Ophthalmology. 1985; 3: 419–426.
13. Brancato, R., Menchini, U. Microchirurgia Laser in Oftalmologia. Milano: Ghedini editore, 1989: 605–635.
14. Menchini, U., Lanzetta, P., Soldano, F., Ferrari, E., Virgili, G. CW Nd:YAG laser photocoagulation in proliferative diabetic retinopathy. Br J Ophthalmol. 1995; 79: 642–645.
15. Cohen, S.M., Weishaar, P.D., Murray, T.G. Effect of photocoagulation on laser power transmission through human retina. Invest Ophthalmol Vis Sci. 1995; 36(4, suppl): 833.
16. Yoshimura, N., Matsumoto, M., Shimizu, H. *et al.* Photocoagulated human retinal pigment epithelial cells produce an inhibitor of vascular endothelial cell proliferation. Invest Ophthalmol Vis Sci. 1995; 36: 1686–1691.

Department of Ophthalmology
University of Udine
Viale Venezia 410
33100 Udine, Italy

67. Radiation therapy for age-related subfoveal neovascular membranes

B. SNYDERS, L. RENARD, C. KONINCKX and M. CIOFFI

(Brussels, Belgium)

Introduction

Age-related macular degeneration is the leading cause of blindness in patients older than 50 years of age in the Western world. The natural visual course for patients with subfoveal membranes is poor. Retrospective studies have shown that about 60–70% of affected have final acuity of 0.1 or worse within 12–18 months[1–4]. Although previous studies have shown some long-term benefit of laser treatment for subfoveal CNV, the patient has to be prepared for a large decrease in visual acuity immediately following therapy[5–7].

Recent pilot studies have shown favourable responses after low dose of radiation therapy, which selectively damages proliferating new vessels. The potential advantage of radiation is the preservation of intact retinal and choroidal tissue[8–12].

In this study, we examined the clinical course of 26 patients treated by radiation therapy with a follow-up longer than 9 months.

Material and methods

Since June 1994, 60 patients with subfoveal CNV have been treated in our hospital by low dose radiation therapy delivered by a 8 MV photon beam. All the patients received a total dose of 20 Gy given in 10 fractions of 2 Gy, 5 days a week. The 95% isodose curve encompassed the macula and optic disc. Less than 10% encompassed the lens. The eyes were irradiated through a single lateral port (slightly oblique anterior).

Our study concerns 26 patients with a mean follow-up of 13 months. In 21 patients, the follow-up was longer than 1 year and in five patients, 9–12 months. Twelve (46%) patients are males, and 14 (54%) females. The mean age at the initial time was 77 years (63–87). There was no control group.

The first inclusion criterion was the presence of angiographically proven classic or occult subfoveal CNV. Fifteen patients had well defined CNV. Eleven patients had the occult type with or without pigment epithelium detachment (PED). Twelve cases in the series had a subfoveal recurrence after previous laser treatment. Other inclusion criteria included recent onset of

G. Coscas and F. Cardillo Piccolino (eds.), Retinal Pigment Epithelium and Macular Diseases, pp. 387–392.
© 1998 Kluwer Academic Publishers.

symptoms with a vision better than 0.05 in all except one, poor vision in the other eye, the age of more than 60 years and the patient's consent. We excluded patients with other concomitant retinal disease and patients with a previous history of eyes or brain radiotherapy. The interval between the baseline examination and the treatment by radiation varied from 1 to 5 weeks (mean 2 weeks).

Results

A complete ophthalmological examination undertaken at (1), 3, 6, (9), 12 and 18 months, included best corrected visual acuity, Amsler grid test, slit lamp examination, ophthalmoscopy, colour photographs and fluorescein angiography. The two studied parameters were the visual outcome and the CNV evolution. The CNV size and leakage were observed from photographs and fluorescein angiograms.

Visual acuity

The mean visual acuity before RTH (radiation therapy) and 1, 3, 6 and 12 months after is shown in Fig. 1. For the total series, the mean initial vision was 0.2 and the final 0.11. There was a similar decrease for each subgroup. The most significant visual loss occured during the first weeks after the initial examination. Figure 2 shows the number of patients for each level of vision,

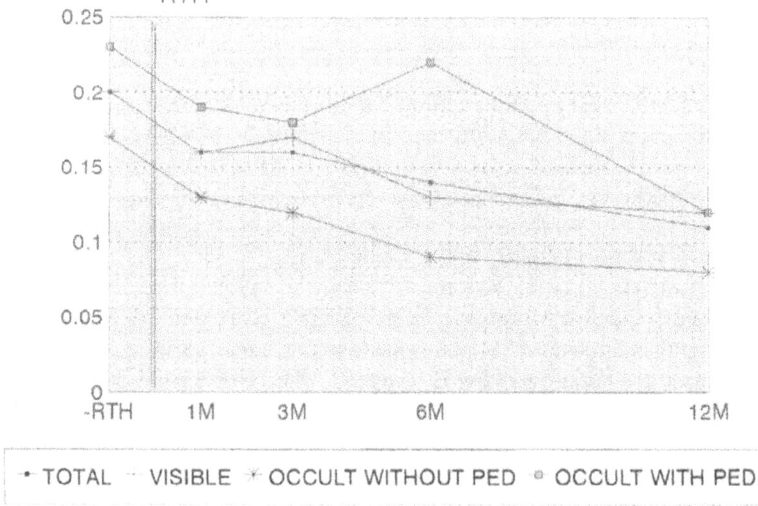

Fig. 1. Visual outcome: mean visual acuity before radiation therapy and 1, 3, 6, and 12 months after.

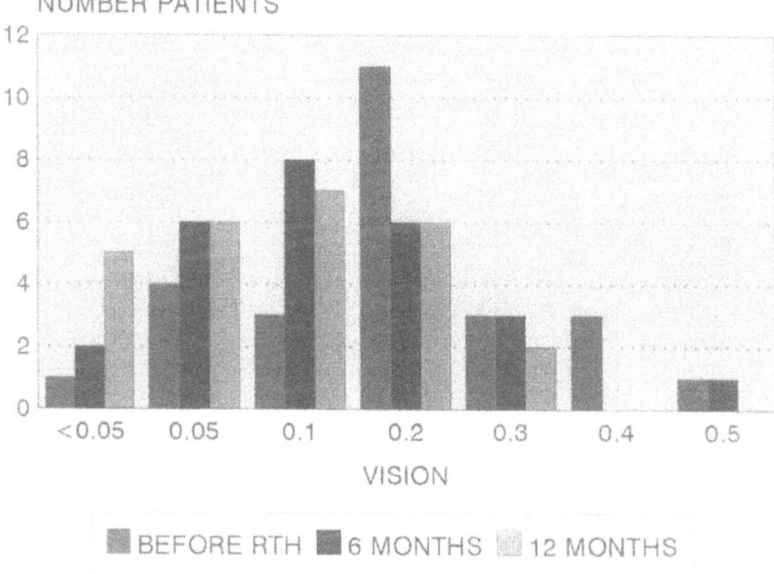

Fig. 2. Visual outcome: number of patients at each level of vision before radiation therapy and after 6 and 12 months.

before RTH and after 6 and 12 months. Before RTH, a visual acuity of ≥ 0.1 was found for 81% of the patients, after 6 months for 69% and after 12 months for 58%. In 11 patients (42%) there was no change between the initial and final visual acuity, although in some the fluorescein angiogram showed a deterioration of the ocular fundus.

Angiographic changes

The second studied parameter was CNV evolution. This was evaluated at each control by comparing the photographs and the fluorescein angiograms to the previous one, assessing four possible situations: no change, regression of the CNV, progression of the CNV or undetermined status. The last situation comes from the presence of occult membranes which sometimes makes difficult to compare the fluorescein angiograms or from the absence of well performed angiograms.

Regression of the membrane was seen in 19% at 3 months, 35% at 6 months and 46% at 12 months. Progression of the membrane was predominant in the first 3 months (46%), but was also documented later in the follow-up (Table 1, Fig. 3). The total macular scar size, combining active and atrophic lesions, is obviously enlarged in 17 cases (65%) between the initial and the final time. One case of vascularized PED developed a retinal tear several

Table 1. Funduscopic evolution: number of patients with no change, regression, progression or dubious/indeterminate status of the CNV complex between each control (1–3 months, 6 months, 9–12 months, 18 months).

	1–3 months	6 months	9–12 months	18 months
No change	4 (15%)	3 (11%)	5 (19%)	1 (14%)
Regression	5 (19%)	9 (35%)	12 (46%)*	4 (57%)
Progression	12 (46%)	7 (27%)	9 (35%)	2 (28%)
Dubious/ind**	5 (19%)	7 (27%)		
Total cases	26	26	26	7

* At 9–12 months regression was complete in 7 cases (27%) partial in 5 cases (19%).
** Sometimes difficult to compare FA with occult CNV.

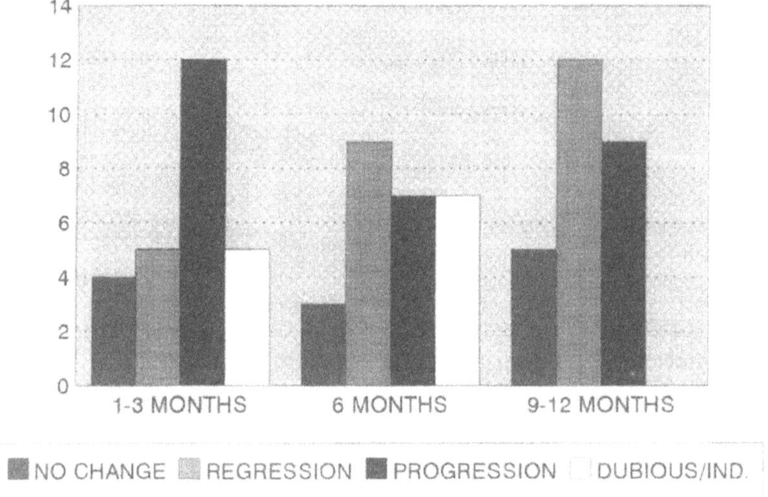

Fig. 3. Funduscopic evolution: illustration of CNV evolution in the series (see Table 1).

months after the treatment. No negative side effects, including dry eye syndrome, cataract, radiation optic neuropathy and radiation retinopathy, have been observed in this series.

Discussion

In this study, the visual outcome and CNV evolution were evaluated in 26 patients who underwent radiation therapy for subfoveal CNV and whose follow-up was at least 9 months (mean 13 months). Previous pilot studies indeed suggest a beneficial effect of radiation therapy on the natural course of age-related subfoveal neovascularization[8-12].

The Belfast group found a stable or improved visual acuity of 63% at 12 months[8]. In the Nijmegen group, with the use of 12, 18 and 24 Gy, the results were similar[9,10]. In our study, only 42% of the patients maintained the same visual acuity during the follow-up. There was a significant mean decrease in the vision during the first weeks after the initial examination followed by a stabilization or a slight decrease between 3 and 12 months. Corresponding to the significant decrease of the vision observed in the first weeks, we noted the largest rate of progression of the CNV (46%) in the interval of the first 3 months after the treatment. The hypothesis to explain this initial deterioration in the vision and the CNV evolution short after the treatment may be the delay between the baseline examination and angiogram, and the beginning of the treatment. Another hypothesis could be the delay necessary for low dose radiation to be effective.

The Belfast group noticed significant angiographically proven neovascular membrane regression in 77% of the treated patients at 12 months[8]. The Nijmegen group could only note an inhibition of the expansion of the CNV membrane after radiation therapy[9,10]. In our study, after 12 months, we found an angiographically proven complete CNV regression in seven cases only. Four of these had occult CNV, two with and two without PED. In the two cases with neovascularized PED, we found a discordance between the dry aspect of the fluorescein angiogram after 12 months and the persistance of well visible PED at biomicroscopic observation. In our study, an obvious enlargement of the total scar size was observed between 0 and 12 months in 65% of the cases. There was no significant difference in the results between each subgroups.

Conclusion

Although this study is limited to a small number of patients without control series and to a quite short follow-up time, it shows that low dose radiation can, in some cases, improve the natural history of age-related subfoveal membrane. In our series, the benefits however seemed not to be as optimistic as those reported in other pilot studies. The results of prospective and randomized studies are expected before approving radiation therapy as the appropriate treatment in subfoveal membranes.

References

1. Bressler, N.M., Bressler, S.B., Fine, S.L. Age-related macular degeneration. Surv Ophthalmol. 1988; 32: 375–412.
2. Bressler, N.M., Frost, L.A., Bressler, S.B., Murphy, R.P., Fine, S.L. Natural course of poorly defined choroidal neovascularisation associated with macular degeneration. Arch Ophthalmol. 1988; 106: 1537–1542.

3. Guyer, D.R., Fine, S.L., Maguire, M.G., Hawkins, B.S., Owens, S.L., Murphy, R.P. Subfoveal choroidal neovascular membranes in age-related macular degeneration. Visual prognosis in eyes with relative good visual acuity. Arch Ophthalmol. 1986; 104: 702–705.

4. Singerman, L.J., Stockfish, J.H. Natural history of subfoveal pigment epithelial detachments associated with subfoveal or unindentifiable choroidal neovascularisation complicating age-related macular degeneration. Graefe's Arch Clin Exp Ophthalmol. 1989; 227: 501–507.

5. Coscas, G., Soubrane, G., Ramahefasolo, C., Fardeau, C. Perifoveal laser treatment for subfoveal choroidal new vessels in age-related macular degeneration: results of a randomized clinical trial. Arch Ophthalmol. 1991; 109: 1258–1265.

6. Macular Photocoagulation Study Group. Laser photocoagulation of subfoveal neovascular lesions in age-related macular degeneration. Arch Ophthalmol. 1991; 109: 1220–1231.

7. Macular Photocoagulation Study Group. Subfoveal neovascular lesions in age-related macular degeneration: guidelines for evaluation and treatment in the macular photocoagulation study. Arch Ophthalmol. 1991; 109: 1242–1257.

8. Chakravarthy, U., Houston, R.F., Archer, D.B. Treatment of age-related subfoveal neovascular membranes by teletherapy: a pilot study. Br J Ophthalmol. 1993; 77: 265–273.

9. Bergink, G.J., Deutman, A.F., van den Broek, J.F., van Daal, W.A., van der Maazen, R.W. Radiation therapy for subfoveal choroidal neovascular membranes in age-related macular degeneration. A pilot study. Graefes Arch Clin Exp Ophthalmol. 1994; 232: 591–598.

10. Bergink, G.J., Deutman, A.F., van den Broek, J.F., van Daal, W.A., van der Maazen, R.W. Radiation therapy for age-related subfoveal choroidal membranes. A pilot study. Doc Ophthalmol. 1995; 90: 67–74.

11. Hart, P.M., Archer, D.B., Chakravarthy, U. Asymmetry of disciform scarring in bilateral disease when one eye is treated with radiotherapy. Br J Ophthalmol. 1995; 70: 562–568.

12. Valmaggia, C., Bischoff, P., Ries, G. Niedrig dosierte Radiotherapie der subfoveolären Neovaskularisationen bei altersabhängiger Makuladegeneration. Vorläufige Resultate. Klin Monatsbl Augenheilkd. 1995; 206: 343–346.

Department of Ophthalmology
St-Luc Hospital
Av. Hippocrate
10-B-1200 Brussels
Belgium

68. The disc-to-macula circulation time in diabetic retinopathy

T. OKANO

(Ibaraki, Japan)

This study was performed to determine the retardation of retinal circulation in diabetic eye. The velocity of retinal circulation in diabetes was evaluated by means of rapid serial fluorescein angiography, employing a scanning laser ophthalmoscope (SLO).

Method and materials

Fluorescein angiography was conducted at the rate of 30 frames/s with a SLO (Rodenstock) in videotape following injection of 5 ml of 10% fluorescein sodium into the antecubital vein. Disc-to-macula circulation time (DMCT) was defined as the time interval between the initial appearance of the dye bolus in the central retinal artery and the moment of maximum dye filling in the parafoveal capillaries[1-3] (Fig. 1A–C).

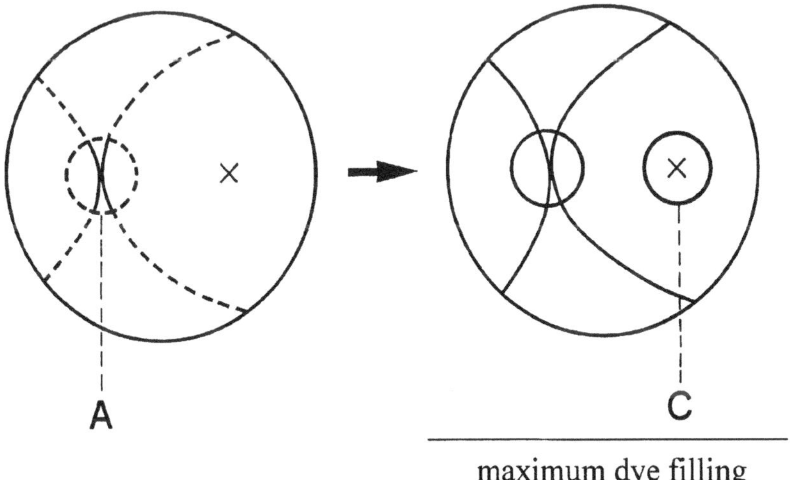

Fig. 1. Disc-to-macula circulation time.

G. Coscas and F. Cardillo Piccolino (eds.), Retinal Pigment Epithelium and Macular Diseases, pp. 393–395.
© *1998 Kluwer Academic Publishers.*

Thirty normal eyes were used as control, and 70 diabetic eyes with (simple, 30; pre- or proliferative 15) or without (15) retinopathy were examined in order to measure DMCT.

Results

The distribution of DMCT by SLO is shown in Fig. 2. The average values in these groups are shown in Table 1. The DMCT in 70 diabetic subjects, with or without retinopathy, averaged 6.9 ± 1.6 s. This value was significantly longer than that in normal eyes (4.9 ± 0.6 s). A significant tendency present for the DMCT to prolong along with the presence and severity of retinopathy.

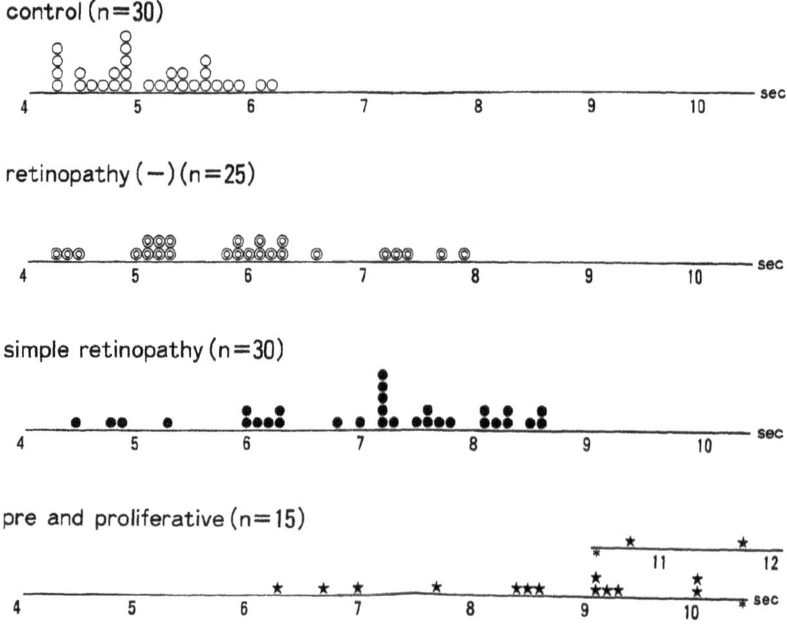

Fig. 2. Distribution of DMCT.

Table 1. Disc-to-macula circulation time (DMCT).

Group	Seconds
Control ($n = 30$)	4.9 ± 0.6
Diabetes ($n = 70$)	
No retinopathy ($n = 25$)	5.8 ± 1.0
Simple retinopathy ($n = 30$)	7.0 ± 1.2
Pre- and proliferative retinopathy ($n = 15$)	8.8 ± 1.5
Mean of diabetics	6.9 ± 1.6

These findings indicate that retinal circulation is retarded in diabetics even before the onset of diabetic retinopathy. In cases with retinopathy, the retardation is correlated with the degree of retinopathy: control $<$ DM without retinopathy ($p < 0.01$); without retinopathy $<$ simple retinopathy ($p < 0.05$); simple retinopathy $<$ pre- and proliferative retinopathy ($p < 0.05$).

Discussion

My present method (DMCT) is of certain practical value. It may be used as a routine clinical procedure[1-3], is not too disturbing to either the examiner or patient and may be applied to long-term follow-up studies[2]. While it may be more ideal to study the earliest dye filling in one of the capillaries nearest to the fovea instead of the maximum dye filling as the end point, because the former is more closely correlated to the velocity of retinal circulation, the latter still serves as a parameter for flow velocity, is less dependent upon technical skill of the observer and, therefore, gives more reproductible results. The former may be possible to be measured by means of SLO.

Conclusion

The retinal circulation is retarded in diabetic eye even before the onset of diabetic retinopathy. In cases with retinopathy, the retardation is correlated with degree of retinopathy. The DMCT, a concept proposed by the present authors, is a useful clinical indicator for the velocity of retinal circulation in diabetes and in pathological fundus conditions in general.

References

1. Okano, T., Horiuchi, T., Saruya, S., Sukegawa, Y. Circulation times in diabetic retinopathy, Part 2, Disc-to-macula circulation time. Acta Soc Ophthalmol Jpn. 1993; 77: 1476–1485.
2. Okano, T., Horiuchi, T., Saruya, S., Sukegawa, Y. Effect of photocoagulation in diabetic retinopathy. Acta Soc Ophthalmol Jpn. 1974; 78: 926–938.
3. Shimizu, K., Okano, T. Retinal circulation times in diabetic subjects. In: Acta XXII Concilium Ophthalmologicum, 1974. Paris, Masson, 1976, v. 1: 345–347.

Deptartment of Ophthalmology
Tokyo Medical College Kasumigaura
3-20-1 Chuo, Ami, Inashiki
Ibaraki, 300-3, Japan

69. Non-proliferative diabetic retinopathy – new findings in indocyanine green angiography

Y. YASSUR, D. WEINBERGER, M. KREMER, D. GATON,
R. AXER-SIEGAL and E.R. PRIEL

(Petah-Tikva, Israel)

Introduction

Diabetic retinopathy, as the term implies, has long been considered to be a disease of the retina alone, afflicting the retinal vasculature and thus the retina surrounding the damaged vessels. Fluorescein angiography (FA), by delineating the fine retinal vessels at the various stages of the disease, greatly increased our understanding of the processes underlying the nature and progression of the vasculopathy, leading to the implementation of retinal laser photocoagulation as the treatment of choice. The possible involvement of the choroidal vasculature in diabetic retinopathy has been explored in only a few studies, including light and electron microscopy[1–5]. Indocyanine green angiography (ICGA) is used to study the choroid, primarily in age-related macular degeneration in order to pin-point the location of choroidal neo-vascular membranes.

In the present study we examined the involvement of the choroid in diabetic retinopathy using ICGA in patients with non-proliferative diabetic retinopathy NPDR and then correlating the findings with FA.

Patients and methods

Thirty patients with NPDR were evaluated. Digital ICGA and FA were performed using the Topcon IMAGENet 1024 system. The two images were compared and evaluated, and superimposed using the image comparison option in the software. Patients with opaque media, who had undergone laser treatment and/or suffered from any other retinal or choroidal disease were not assigned to this study. Thus we were able to identify the various fluorescent findings as originating in either the FA (involving the retina) or the ICGA (implying primarily choroidal involvement).

The three major findings related to the choroid arising from this study (using ICGA to evaluate NPDR patients) are:

1. Late-phase hyperfluorescent areas under areas of retinal edema and thickening.

G. Coscas and F. Cardillo Piccolino (eds.), Retinal Pigment Epithelium and Macular Diseases, pp. 397–399.
© *1998 Kluwer Academic Publishers.*

2. A unique pattern of spotted hypo- and hyperfluorescence in mild NPDR patients which appeared in the late phase of ICGA.
3. Microaneurysms which appeared on either ICGA or FA or both.

Indications as to the existence of diabetic choroidopathy are clearly present in histological studies. Light and electron microscopy study of the choroid in diabetic patients revealed noticeable thickening of the choriocapillaris basement membrane as well as in other small choroidal vessels. Scanning electron microscopy of the choroid[2,3] of Type I diabetic patients revealed significant involvement of the uvea, including increased tortuosity of blood vessels, focal vascular dilatation and narrowing, hypercellularity, vascular loops and microaneurisms, areas of non-perfusion and sinus-like formations between the choroidal lobules.

Bischoff and Flower[6] describe their preliminary findings from the ICGA diabetic patients as including choroidal vessel abnormalities, delayed and irregular filling of the choroidal vessels in most of the patients with proliferative diabetic retinopathy and in about half of those with NPDR. The areas of diffuse hyperfluorescence we noted in the ICGA, which appeared under areas of retinal thickening and edema can be explained as stemming from dye leakage in areas of diabetic choroidopathy and as both fluorescing through the retina and affecting it. The increased vascular permeability present in the more advanced stages of NPDR can account for the ability of the larger ICG molecule to leak and create areas of apparent diffuse hyperfluorescence.

The unique spotted 'salt and pepper' appearance noted in the late-phase images of the ICGA's in the mild NPDR patients, as opposed to the more common ground glass pattern seen in most late-phase images in normal individual[7], can be explained as arising from the selective filling of the choriocapillaris in these patients. This pattern appeared mainly in the milder cases of NPDR and may indicate the earlier involvement of the choroid in the diabetic retinopathy process.

The study of the various types of microaneurysms as demonstrated in the two different angiographies yielded the conclusion that not all microaneurysms are retinal in origin, as until now has been suggested by FA.

The various factors determining the orientation and appearance of the various microaneurysms include their size, structure, origin (retina or choroid) and the different properties of the to dyes, specifically their molecular weight and protein-binding properties.

The microaneurysms which appeared only on ICGA may represent larger fenestrations in the choroidal vessels wall or the existence of small buds of choroidal neovascularization, but further electron microscopy data are needed in this area. On routine FA these microaneurysms would not be noted, since they would be obscured by the intense flush of the fluorescein during most of the study. The microaneurysms which appeared only on FA and not on ICGA may pinpoint the known microaneurysms which develop in the retinal blood vessels in patients with NPDR, but which are not large enough to admit the indocyanine green dye. These microaneurysms are naturally filled by fluorescein and often leak, but are not visible during ICGA. Conversely, microaneurysms which were visible on both angiographies may be larger up to 50 µm in diameter[2], and would thus allow entry of the protein-bound indocyanine green molecule. Such microaneurysms, although situated in the retina, would thus be imaged in both types of angiographies.

These ICGA findings strongly imply that the degree of diabetic retinopathy as judged routinely by FA may reveal only part of the pathological events which occur in the vascular system of the fundus of diabetic patients. As ICGA, applied to diabetic retinopathy seems to provide additional information and insight into our understanding of the disease, its role in earlier diagnosis, and its possible application to additional or different treatment modalities should be further investigated.

References

1. Hiyadat, A.A., Fine, B.S. Diabetic choroidopathy. Light and electron microscopic observations of seven cases. Ophthalmology. 1985; 92: 512–522.
2. Fryczkowsky, A.W., Sato, E., Hodes, B.L. Changes in diabetic choroidal vasculature: Scanning electron microscopy findings. Ann Ophthalmol. 1988; 20: 299–305.
3. Fryczkowsky, A.W., Chambers, D.O., Crag, E.J., Walker, J., Davidoff, F.H. Scanning electron microscopic study of microaneurysms in diabetic retina. Ann Ophthalmol. 1991; 23: 130–136.
4. Weinberger, D., Fink-Cohen, S., Gaton, D., Priel, E., Yassur, Y. Nonretinovascular leakage in diabetic retinopathy. Br J Ophthalmol. 1995; 79: 728–731.
5. Freyler, H., Prskavec, F., Stelzer, N. Diabetic choroidopathy – a retrospective fluorescein angiography study. Preliminary report. Klin Montabsbl Augenhelikd. 1986; 189: 144–147.
6. Bischoff, P.M., Flower, R.W. Ten-year experience with choroidal angiography using indocyanine green dye: a new routine examination or an epilogue? Doc Ophthalmol. 1985; 60: 235–292.
7. Yannuzzi, L.A., Slakter, J.S., Sorenson, J.A., Guyer, D.R. Orlock, D.A. Digital indocyanine green videoangiography and choroidal neovascularization. Retina. 1992; 12: 191–223.

Department of Ophthalmology
Rabin Medical Center - Beilinson Campus
Petah-Tikva, 49100
Israel

70. The use of pentoxifylline (Trental) in diabetic retinopathy

G.M. GOMBOS and D.S. GOMBOS

(New York and Philadelphia, USA)

Introduction

Pentoxifylline represents a new class of medications used to treat peripheral vascular disease. Its mechanism of action is to decrease blood viscosity by increasing red blood cell flexibility and reducing serum fibrinogen levels[1]. This drug corrects impaired erythrocyte deformability and exerts a beneficial effect on the clinical symptoms of vascular diseases. The expected rheological properties of pentoxifylline mainly affect blood flow in small vessels and capillaries. Available evidence suggests that diabetic haemorrheological changes may be important in the pathogenesis and progression of diabetic microangiopathy[2].

Pentoxifylline increases the intracellular ATP content and affects erythrocyte membrane functions, including electrolyte exchange; moreover, pentoxifylline depresses platelet aggregation[3] and reduces plasma fibrinogen levels[4].

The aim of the present study was to determine the therapeutic effectiveness of pentoxifylline on the ocular microcirculation and the preservation of visual acuity of patients with diabetic retinopathy.

Patients and methods

Thirty diabetic patients (26 males and 4 females), age 39–70 years were selected. The mean duration of diabetes mellitus in these patients was 12.4 years (range 10–20 years). Diabetic retinopathy, exudative type, was observed in 24 patients (microaneurysm, haemorrhages and exudates). Six patients had no clinical evidence of diabetic retinal changes observed by ophthalmoscopy. However microaneurysms, capillary drop-out areas and intraretinal microvascular abnormalities were found on fluorescein angiography. There were no cases of proliferative diabetic retinopathy. Patients having other eye pathologies than exudative diabetic changes were excluded from the study. The visual acuity of all participants was documented at the beginning and at the end of this research work. At the beginning and at the end of the study fluorescein angiography was performed, and the results were analysed and compared.

G. Coscas and F. Cardillo Piccolino (eds.), Retinal Pigment Epithelium and Macular Diseases, pp. 401–403.
© *1998 Kluwer Academic Publishers.*

Results

No change in visual acuity was observed among the patients enrolled in this study, vision remaining in the range 20/20 – 20/40 with best correction. Fluorescein angiography studies of each patient were compared before and after therapy. The capillary phase was lengthened significantly in 25 cases (80%). Avascular areas had decreased in six eyes (50% of all avascular areas found in this study). Better tissue perfusion was observed in all post treatment angiography studies.

Discussion

Pentoxifylline is the best known of a new group of haemorrheologic agents. Several investigators have shown that pentoxifylline therapy improves haemorrheologic abnormalities associated with diabetes and atherosclerosis[5]. In ophthalmology Iwafune and Yoshimoto found pentoxifylline to be effective in preventing retinal and intravitreal neovascularization caused by retinal ischaemia[6]. Subsequently Solerte and Ferrari found pentoxifylline administration to be an effective drug for treatment of diabetic vascular complications[7].

Our study relied on fluorescein angiography interpretation and the maintenance of visual acuity. Better capillary blood flow and improved tissue perfusion of the retina were demonstrated in 80% of the patients.

In conclusion, long-term treatment with pentoxifylline improved haemorrheological paramenters in diabetic patients. Pentoxifylline was found to be an useful therapeutic agent in the treatment of diabetic vascular disorders in general and in diabetic retinopathy in particular. Pentoxifylline should be considered as an excellent, beneficial adjunct in the global effort to prevent the progress of diabetic retinopathy.

References

1. DiPerri, T., Guerrini, M. Placebo controlled double blind study with pentoxifylline of walking performance in patients with intermittent claudication. Angiology. 1983; 34: 40–45.
2. Barnes, A.J., Locke, P., Scudder, P.R., Dormandy, T.L., Dorsmandy, J.A., Slack, J. Is hyperviscosity a treatable component of diabetic microcirculatory disease? Lancet. 1977; 2: 789–791.
3. Muller, R., Lehrach, F. Haemorrheological role of platelet aggregation and hypercoagulability in microcirculation: therapeutical approach with pentoxifylline. Pharmatherapeutica. 1980; 2: 372–379.
4. Muggeo, M., Calabro, A., Businaro, V. et al. Blood clotting, fibrinolytic and haemorrheological parameters in ischemic vascular disease: The effects of pentoxifylline in the treatment of acute cerebral vascular disease. Pharmatherapeutica. 1983; 3 (Suppl. 1): 74–90.
5. Ehrly, A.M. The effect of pentoxifylline on the deformability of erythrocytes and on muscular oxigen pressure in patients with chronic arterial disease. J Med. 1979; 10: 331–334.
6. Iwafune, Y., Yoshimoto, H. Clinical use of pentoxifylline in haemorrhagic disorders of the retina. Pharmatherapeutica. 1980; 2: 429–438.

7. Solente, S.B., Ferrari, E. Diabetic retinal vascular complications and erythrocyte filtrability: Result of a 2 year follow up study with pentoxifylline. Pharmatherapeutica. 1985; 4: 341–350.

Department of veterans affairs
Brooklyn
New York

Scheie Eye Institute
University of Pennsylvania

71. Laser treatment of diabetic cystoid macular oedema with a grid extended to the foveal avascular zone

E. GANDOLFO, F. MORESCALCHI, E. ZINZINI, L. ROSA,
P. CAMARDI and E. SCURI

(Brescia, Italy)

Introduction

Cystoid macular oedema (CME) is an important cause of visual impairment in diabetic patients and its treatment is an unsolved problem for ophthalmologists.The typical polycystic aspect of the diabetic CME may be caused either by extramacular exudation or by a leakage from the perifoveal capillaries. Generally, it is reported that grid or focal laser photocoagulation is able to improve the fluorangiographic aspect of CME but this often fails to improve the visual acuity significantly[1-6]. On the other hand it is reported that CME may resolve spontaneously or fluctuate for months or years before causing severe loss of vision[7]. When the visual acuity tends to decrease to less than 0.5 a perifoveal grid photocoagulation should be performed[8,9]. here we present our experience about the use of a perifoveolar laser grid extended to the edge of the foveal avascular zone (FAZ) in reducing CME.

Patients and methods

The studied sample consisted of 50 eyes in 34 patients (22 women and 12 men), aged 32–73 years (mean 65.5); 25 were NIDDM (10 were on insulin, 15 were controlled with oral hypoglycemic agents) and nine were IDDM. Diabetes lasted for an average of 6 years (± 20, range 3–30). All these eyes had CME as indicated by the biomicroscopy and by late-phase fluorangiographic features. At the beginning of this study all patients had a good glycaemic compensation (glycaemia < 170 mg/dl at the last two examinations) and glycosylated haemoglobin < 10 mg/ml; diastolic blood pressure was well controlled (< 100 mmHg); patients with renal failure requiring dialysis were excluded from the study: the influence of these systemic factors on evolution of macular oedema is well known[10-13]. Thirty-eight eyes had CME unchanged despite a focal laser treatment or a grid performed avoiding the FAZ; most of these patients had already been treated with a panretinal photocoagulation ended at least 6 months before. Twelve eyes were affected by a CME primarily arising from a diffuse oedema of the posterior pole; this caused a rapid

G. Coscas and F. Cardillo Piccolino (eds.), Retinal Pigment Epithelium and Macular Diseases, pp. 405–411.
© 1998 Kluwer Academic Publishers.

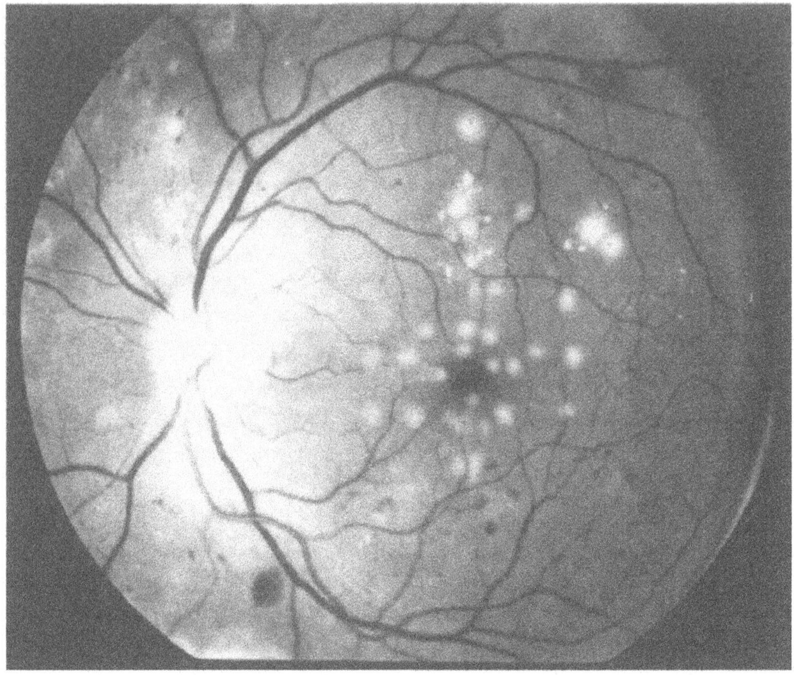

Fig. 1. Typical example of perifoveal laser grid.

decrease in visual acuity (more than two lines in 4 months). These eyes had never had previous laser treatment. The baseline examination included the following parameters: best corrected distance and near visual acuity; a fluor-angiographic examination, using 5 ml of 10% sodium fluorescein intravenously, taking late phase (500 s) frames; static threshold testing of the visual field, performed with the Octopus 2000-R perimeter, using the M1 program in which central and paracentral sensitivity is tested using a pattern of 59 locations distributed in the 24° with an increasing resolution toward the centre. This grid is capable of detecting defects of 1.4°, within the central 5°. The threshold in every location is tested twice. All eyes were treated using a coherent argon dye laser (514 nm), handling a Mainster or a Volk area centralis lens focusing the image to obtain the smallest diameter of the spots. All treatments were performed by the same ophthalmologist (E.S.) who used 50–150 μm spots, with exposure time of 0.2 s and 200–250 mW power. Argon laser therapy consisted of focal photocoagulation of the microaneurysms and dilated capillaries that displayed focal fluorescein leakage near the macula on angiography and of a grid regularly applied around the area of CME and extended over the edge of the foveal avascular zone. Light burns were performed in order to create a mild fading of the retina; an average of 41.3 (±14.5) spots per eye were used applying 4–8 spots inside the FAZ, 200 μm away from the fovea. The first follow-up visit was 1 month after the treatment, then every 4–6 months; during each examination the distance and the near visual acuity were tested and fluorangiography was used to take pictures of the late phases. Visual field examination was performed after 4 months from the treatment, then after every 6 months. The mean follow up was 24 ± 8 months (range 12–36 months). In order to obtain a homogeneous group of samples we divided thetreated eyes into two subgroups depending on their visual acuity; Group A: 16 eyes having a visual acuity <0.3; Group B: ≥ 34 eyes having a visual acuity 0.3, in this group 28 eyes (82%) had CME lasting less than 6 months. Statistical analysis was performed using the two sample Student *t*-test to show differences between the visual acuity before and after the treatment and using the Wilcoxon matched-pair signed ranks test to evidence the statistical differences between the perimetric data.

Results

Fluorescein angiograms, on the whole, showed that CME cleared up or decreased in 29 eyes (58%) while it remained stable in 21 eyes (42%). In 12 eyes (24%) the typical polycystic aspect of the CME was substituted by a light late hyperfluorescence.

After a single laser treatment exudates resolution occurred almost completely in 42 eyes (84%) after an average period of 4–8 months. Results are summarized in Table 1. On the whole, visual acuity improved in 16 eyes (32%, two eyes of Group A and in 14 eyes of Group B) in 9 eyes by 2 or more lines; in 27 eyes (54%) visual acuity was stable and in seven eyes (14%) it was decreased by one line. All the 12 eyes with primary developed CME improved their visual outcome. It was worthy of note that 41.2% of cyes belonging to Group B improved their visual performance, while stabilization

*Table 1.*Ocular findings and results

CME fluorangiographic aspect 12 months after treatment

	Resolved	Decreased	Unchanged
Group A ($n = 16$)	0	7 (43%)	9 (56.2%)
Group B) ($n = 34$)	17 (50%)	5 (11.7%)	12 (35.2%)

Visual acuity (v.a.) changement 12 months after treatment

	Improvement		Unchanged v.a.	Worsening	
	2 lines	1 line		1 line	2 lines
Group A	0	2 (12.5%)	10 (62.5%)	3 (18.7%)	1 (6.25%)
Group B*	9 (26.4%)	5 (14.7%)	17 (50%)	3 (8.8%)	0

$p = 0.037$.

of visual acuity was generally the most evident result (62.5% in Group A, 50% in Group B). There was a significant improvement of the subjective (assessed by the patient) and objective ability to read fluently, despite their distance acuity remaining unchanged.

The two sample t-test showed no significant change in group A visual acuity: pretreatment mean value was 0.16 ± 0.09, 1 year post-treatment mean value was 0.19 ± 0.12 ($t = -0.995$; $p = 0.336$). In Group B mean visual acuity before treatment was 0.63 ± 0.26; 1 year after treatment it improved to 0.71 ± 0.25 ($t = -2.175$, $p = 0.037$).

The typical visual field of patients with CME was characterized by a relative central scotoma with clusters, more or less deep and large, scattered all over the paracentral area, corresponding to thickned retina, exudates or haemorrhages. Perimetric data generally showed a depression of the foveal threshold, with pathological values of the mean sensitivity and of the corrected loss variance. Usually, 30° of visual field corresponded to the retinal area photographed by the fundus camera centred on the macula[14]. In some cases, the visual fields were inverted and superimposed to the retinal area, but it was not possible to correlate the scotomas to the laser scars. The pattern of the scotomas did not change even though the overal field appeared slightly worsened after each laser treatment. The effects of grid treatment on the sensitivity of the central 24° of the visual field was relevant only in patients of Group B: they are summarized in Table 2. Wilcoxon matched-pair signed ranks test did not reveal, in Group A, any significant change of the perimetric indices. In Group B it showed both a mild improvement of the foveal threshold (average $+ 0.72$ dB; $p < 0.06$),and a slight worsening of the mean sensitivity (average $+ 0.9$ dB; $p < 0.06$) and of the corrected loss variance (average $+ 2.0$ dB; $p < 0.06$). The average sensitivity variation was less than the long term fluctuation value (mean normal value $= 1.16$ dB).

Table 2. Static perimetry findings (dB)

	Before treatment	*After treatment*	*Wilcoxon-T*	*p*	
Visual field in Group A					
MS	14.2 ± 8	14.0 ± 5.1	$W = -35$	>0.06	
MD	14 ± 6	14.85 ± 4.8	$W = -20$	>0.06	
CLV	41.9 ± 22.3	42.25 ± 20.7	$W = -34$	>0.06	
SF	2.38 ± 0.3	2.47 ± 0.29	$W = -26$	>0.06	
Foveal threshold	14.9 ± 6.2	15.17 ± 5.8	$W = -35$	>0.06	
Visual field modification in Group B					
MS	17.11 ± 8	16.2 ± 5	$W = -80$	<0.06	$\Delta -0.9$ dB
MD	11.13 ± 8.5	12.09 ± 7.32	$W = -78$	<0.06	$\Delta +0.9$ dB
CLV	16.0 ± 11	17.98 ± 10.2	$W = -90$	<0.06	$\Delta +2$ dB
SF	2.3 ± 0.6	2.2 ± 0.42	$W = -21$	>0.06	
Foveal threshold	25 ± 0.5	25.7 ± 7.5	$W = -91$	<0.06	$\Delta +0.7$ dB

Discussion

CME is the major cause of poor vision in diabetic subjects. It usually appears after a long-lasting non-cystoid macular oedema, and its development reflects an increase in macular oedema. Visual acuity begins to deteriorate when CME appears, especially when a large central foveal cyst occurs, due to polycystic expansion of the external granular and plexiform layer filled by serous exudate. Spontaneous resolution of the CME is referred to be possible, but uncommon after a significant decrease in visual acuity. Treatment of CME is difficult and remains a major problem for the ophthalmologists. The hypothetical laser effect could be due to the closure of leaking intraretinal microvascular anomalies, to the stimulation of the RPE metabolism and to the mechanical elimination of the oedema by scars. The regeneration of the RPE or the release by these cells of a diffusable factor inducing endothelial reparation may promote the intraretinal fluid absorbtion[16,18]. A mechanical effect could also be present, since multiple regular scars may thin the retina, reducing the space available for fluid accumulation. Several treatments have been used for a number of years with variable success. At first, a laser grid not extending over 500 µm from the fovea was performed with uncertain results. In recent studies, some authors showed good visual results in performing very crowded laser grids (200–500 spots per treatment) to the edge of the FAZ[6,17]. This was followed by a significant drop of the mean sensitivity of the visual field after every treatment (average -3.4 dB per treatment). Other papers reported the possibility, after many years, of an enlargement of the laser scars that can involve the fovea with a severe visual loss[19]. This phenomenon was particularly evident for the strong laser photocoagulations of neovascularizations and has not been documented for mild laser grids. Several authors emphasize the opportunity to perform at first a focal treatment of the lesions which leak fluorescein before treating the CME with a laser grid[7]. The visual outcome, however, was not grossly improved. In our study treatment consisted of a focal photocoagulation of all the microvascular anomalies which caused exudation and were located at the centre of circinates, combined with a mild laser grid extended up to the foveal avascular zone. This caused a trend toward a visual improvement in those patients whose visual loss was not yet severe (generally >0.6); the same patients had a relatively short duration of CME (less than 6 months). An interesting finding was the general improvement of the reading ability reported subjectively in 60% of our patients, although their distance visual acuity remained unchanged. The same phenomenon has already been noted by other authors[20]. This treatment caused only a mild drop of the mean sensitivity, without changing the pattern of the scotomas; this visual field worsening was not significant if compared with the normal values of the long term fluctuation. The improvement of the foveal threshold in Group B was well correlated with the better visual acuity of these subjects after the treatment. In conclusion, from these results, the perifoveal laser grid is a reasonable therapy not to be delayed in patients whose visual acuity is not yet compromised, especially if CME is recent. This treatment should be performed only by expert and well trained ophthalmologists to lower the risks of a perifoveal laser treatment, including the occurrence of paracentral laser scotomas, subretinal neovascularization and progressive enlargement of laser scars.

Reference

1. British Multicentre Study Group. Photocoagulation for diabetic maculopathy: a randomized controlled clinical trial using xenon. Diabetes. 1983; 32: 1010–1016.
2. Blankenship, G.W. Diabetic macular edema and argon laser photocoagulation: a prospective randomized study. Ophthalmology. 1979: 86: 69–78.
3. Townsend, C., Bailey, J., Kohner, E. Xenon arc photocoagulation for treatment of diabetic maculopathy; interim report of a multicentre controlled clinical study. Br J Ophthalmol. 1980; 64: 385–391.
4. Early Treatment Diabetic Retinopathy Study Research Group. Photocoagulation for diabetic macular edema: ETDRS report number 1. Arch Ophthalmol. 1985; 103: 1796–1806.
5. ETDRS Research Group. Treatment techniques and clinical guidelines for photocoagulation of diabetic macular edema: report number 2. Ophthalmology. 1987; 94: 761–774.
6. Olk, J. Modified grid argon (blue-green) laser photocoagulation for diffuse diabetic macular edema. Ophthalmology. 1986; 93: 938–950.
7. Massin-Korobelnik, P., Gaudric, A., Coscas, G. Spontaneous evolution and photocoagulationof diabetic cystoid macular edema. Graefe's Arch Clin Exp Ophthalmol. 1994; 232: 279–289.
8. Schatz, H., Patz, A. Cystoid maculopathy in diabetes. Arch Ophthalmol. 1976; 94: 761–768.
9. McDonald, R.H., Schatz, H. Grid photocoagulation for diffuse macular edema. Retina. 1985; 5: 65–72.
10. Bresnick, G.H. Systemic factors affecting diabetic macular edema. Am J Ophthalmol. 1988; 105: 211–220.
11. Aiello, L.M., Rand, L.I., Briones, J.C., Weiss, J.N., Wafai, M.Z. Nonocular clinical risk factors in the progression of diabetic retinopathy. In: Little, H.L., Jack, R.L., Patz, A., Forsham, P.H. (eds). Diabetic Retinopathy. New York: Thieme Stratton, 1983: 21–32.
12. Klein, R., Klein, B.E.K., Moss, S.E., Davis, M.D., De Melts, D.L. The Wisconsin Epidemiologic Study of diabetic retinopathhy IV. Diabetic macular edema. Ophthalmology. 1984; 91: 1464–1474.
13. Perkovich, B.T., Meyers, S.M. Systemic factors affecting diabetic macular edema. Am J Ophthalmol. 1988; 105: 211–212.
14. Henricsson, M. and Hejil, A. Visual fields at different stages of diabetic retinopathy. Acta Ophthalmol. 1994; 72: 560–569.
15. Flammer, J., Drance, S.M., Schulzer, M. The estimation and testing of the components of long-term fluctuation or the differential light threshold. Doc Ophthamol Proc Series 1983; 35: 383–389.
16. Marshall, J., Clover, G., Rothery, S. Some new findings on retinal irradiation by krypton and argon lasers. Doc Ophthalmol Proc Ser. 1984; 36: 21–37.
17. Strip, G.G., Hart, W.M., Olk, J. Modified grid laser photocoagulation for diabetic macular edema. The effect on the central visual field. Ophthalmology. 1988; 95: 1673–1679.
18. Wallow, J.H. Repair of the pigment epithelial barrier following photocoagulation. Arch Ophthalmol. 1984; 102: 126–135.

19. Schatz, H., Madeira, D., McDonald, R., Jhonson, R.N. Progressive enlargement of laser scars following grid laser photocoagulation for diffuse diabetic macular edema. Arch Ophthalmol. 1991; 109: 1549–1551.
20. McNaught, E.I., Foldus, W.S., Allan, D. Grid photocoagulation improves reading ability in diffuse diabetic macular edema. Ophthalmology. 1988; 93: 938–950.

Clinica Oculistica
Spedali Civili
Pad. Satellite
Brescia
PC 25123
Italy

72. Idiopathic retinal occlusive vasculitis and the macula

P. SUMMANEN and L. LAATIKAINEN

(Helsinki, Finland)

Introduction

Retinal vasculitis is an inflammatory disease which may result in visual loss[1-3]. It is characterized by intraocular inflammation and abnormalities in any or all types of retinal vessels[1]. Vasculitis may be paraneoplastic or associated with infection or chronic inflammatory systemic disease[1,4]. Permanent loss of vision occurs due to vascular leakage, occlusion or both[1,2]. The vaso-occlusion in the macular area has been recognized only quite recently[5]. In the following two patients, retinal vasculitis seemed to be idiopathic and of ischaemic type in both, but differed in the macular involvement and thus in the visual outcome.

Case reports

Case 1

A 40-year-old female visited a local ophthalmologist, in November 1987, because of a chalazion. She had coeliac disease and lactose-intolerance, which remained controlled on an approriate diet. She used no systemic medication. Unexpectedly, retinal vascular changes were noted, and she was referred to the Helsinki University Eye Hospital. On examination, visual acuity (VA) was full in the right eye, and mildly impaired in the left eye at 0.9. The anterior chamber was quiet, but some cells in the vitreous were seen in both eyes. Ophthalmoscopy showed calibre variation in the main retinal vessels, with occasional macroaneurysm-like dilatations in arterioles, surrounded by local lipid exudation. Fluorescein angiograms revealed extensive peripheral vascular occlusion in both eyes (Fig. 1a,b).

The aetiology of the vasculitis remained unknown despite thorough examination (chest X-ray, complete blood count, erythrocyte sedimentation rate (ESR), angiotensin converting enzyme (ACE), lysozyme, antistreptolysin titre (AST), rheumatoid factor (RF), serum electrophoresis, immunoglobulins, complement count, *Yersinia* antibodies and urinalysis were all within normal limits. Four parabulbar corticosteroid injections were given in 2 months. Due to vascular leakage and widespread vaso-occlusion panphotocoagulation of 2000 burns was given in both eyes during the next 2 years.

G. Coscas and F. Cardillo Piccolino (eds.), Retinal Pigment Epithelium and Macular Diseases, pp. 413–420.
© 1998 Kluwer Academic Publishers.

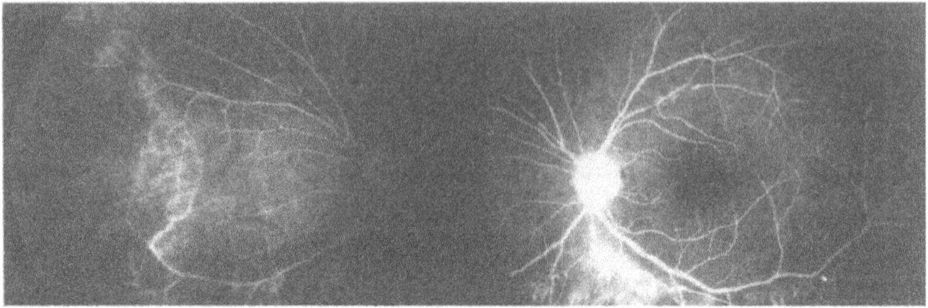

Fig. 1. Patient 1 in August 1988, left eye (a,b). Changes both in the main arterioles and venules. The peripheral retina totally non-perfused (b).

In May 1996, 8.5 years later, the patient is symptomless and her vision is full in both eyes. The fundi are quiet with panphotocoagulation scars. Fluorescein angiography reveals mild leakage from some of the macro-aneurysms still present but the macular vessels are normal (Fig. 2a,b).

Case 2

A 23-year-old female experienced floaters in the right eye in January 1991. A few days after an ordinary winter flu, she lost the vision in the right eye. Except for acne, she was well. She used hormonal contraception, and had changed the pills recently. She smoked. She was referred to the Helsinki University Eye Hospital by a local ophthalmologist. On examination, her visual acuity was 0.1 in the right eye and 0.6 in the left. There were no signs of intraocular inflammation in either eye, but there was a dense vitreous haemorrhage in the right eye, and disc neovascularization as well as occluded, dilated and tortuous vessels in the retina in the left eye. No cotton wool spots or lipid exudation were seen. On fluorescein angiogram, leakage of the dye was seen at both discs indicating neovascularization (Fig. 3a,b) and peripheral

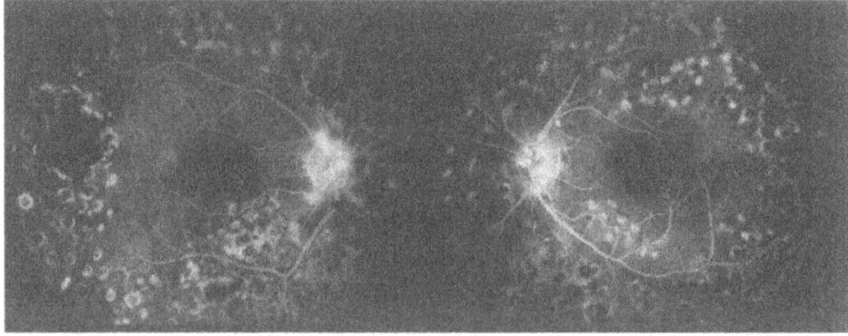

Fig. 2. Patient 1 in May 1996, 8 years after panphotocoagulation. Some macroaneurysm-like changes in the arterioles (arrows) in both eyes (a,b) and dilated capillaries temporal to the macula in the left eye (b). The centre of the macula unaffected.

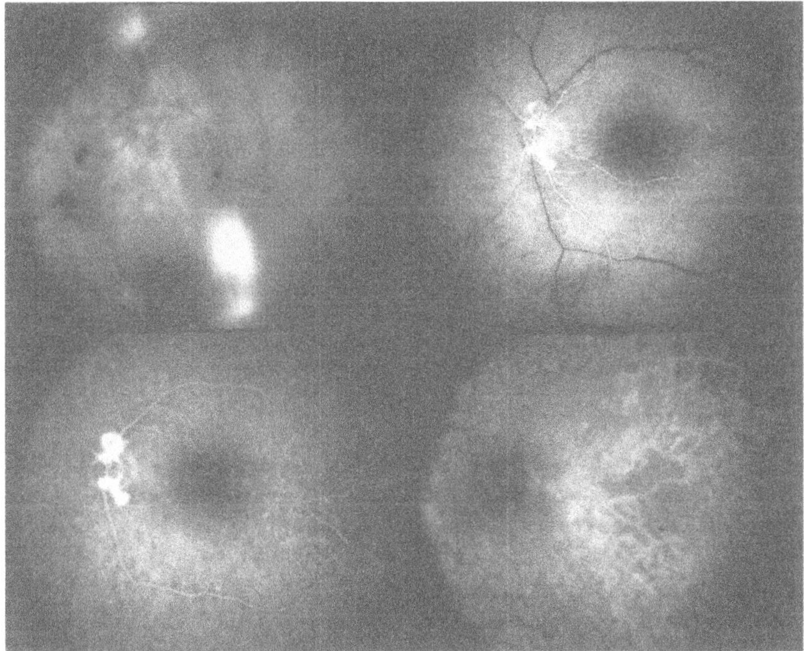

Fig. 3. Patient 2 in January 1991. Massive fluorescein leakage from the neovascular vessels on the disc and midperiphery in the right eye, otherwise the view obscured by vitreous haemorrhage (a). In the left eye, leakage from the disc neovascularization and enlarged foveal avascular zone and capillary abnormalities and closure temporal to the macula (b,c). At the late stage, leakage of the macular capillaries and staining of the vessel walls in the nonperfused temporal periphery (d).

vascular occlusion temporal to the macula was seen in the left eye (Fig. 3c,d). Furthermore, the foveal avascular zone was somewhat irregular indicating capillary closure.

Thorough diagnostic investigation revealed only a slightly elevated lysozyme enzyme (10.3, the normal upper limit being 9). Chest and sinus X-rays were normal, as were the results of complete blood count, ESR, ACE, rheumatoid factor, immunoglobulins, serum electrophoresis, complement system, viral antibodies and urinalysis. She was HLA B27-negative.

Oral contraception was stopped. Parabulbar corticosteroid injection was given once for both eyes. Panphotocoagulation was given for occluded areas; 3000 burns to the right, and 2200 burns to the left eye within 1 year. When the vitreous cleared, the vision in the right eye improved to 0.7 and has remained at that level. Visual acuity in the left eye was full, and neovascularization in the left optic disc disappeared and became fibrotic (Fig. 4a,b). The foveal avascular zone was enlarged, but leakage from the vessels in and around the macular area had diminished (Fig. 4a,b).

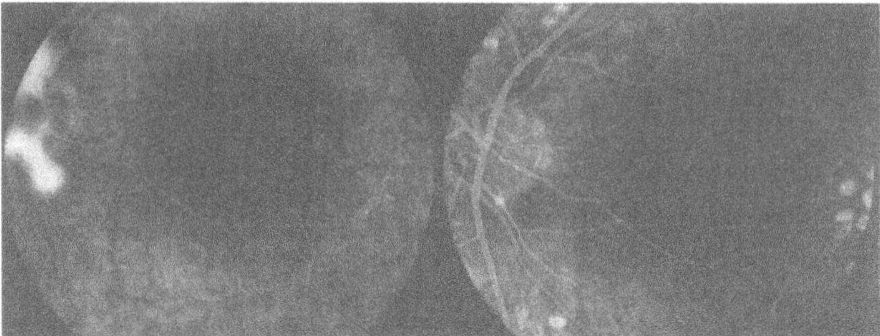

Fig. 4. Patient 2. Active neovascularization on the disc (a) regressed soon after the completion of panphotocoagulation (b). Leakage in the macular area diminished, foveal avascular zone enlarged (a,b).

Three and a half years from diagnosis, she developed herpes zoster of the face: local and systemic acyclovir therapy was given and the keratitis healed. A year later, her local ophthalmologist noticed dilated capillaries in the left macular region and referred her for further evaluation to the Helsinki University Eye Hospital suspecting activation of the retinal vasculitis. On examination, the overall appearance of the fundi was quiet. Fluorescein angiogram, however, revealed that vascular occlusion had progressed especially temporal to and in the centre of the macula; the foveal avascular zones had enlarged and now coalesced with the peripheral non-perfused areas in both eyes (Fig. 5a–d).

Detailed examinations did not reveal any definite cause of the retinal vasculitis. Assessment of antinuclear antibodies (ANA-Ab, ENA-Ab, ANC-Ab), complement levels (C3, C4), RF and DNA antibodies did not show any abnormalities, and no thrombotic abnormalities were found. A gynacologist and dermatologist were also consulted. She was advised to use acetylsalicylic acid (ASA) 100 mg per day, and tetracyclin therapy was started for acne (tetracycline 500 mg ×3 for a week, ×2 for 3 months).

In spite of slow progression of the vaso-occlusive process 5.5 years from the diagnosis of occlusive vasculopathy, the VA was 0.6 in the right eye, and 1.0 in the left in May 1996. There was no active neovascularization in the disc or in the retina in the left eye, but some small new vessels in the right disc are open. The remaining capillaries along the border of the avascular area in the macula are dilated and tortuous in both eyes, but no cotton wool spots or exudation are present in either eye.

Discussion

The aetiology of retinal vasculitis often remains unknown, although patients with this disorder have been said to be over-investigated[2], and thus at present,

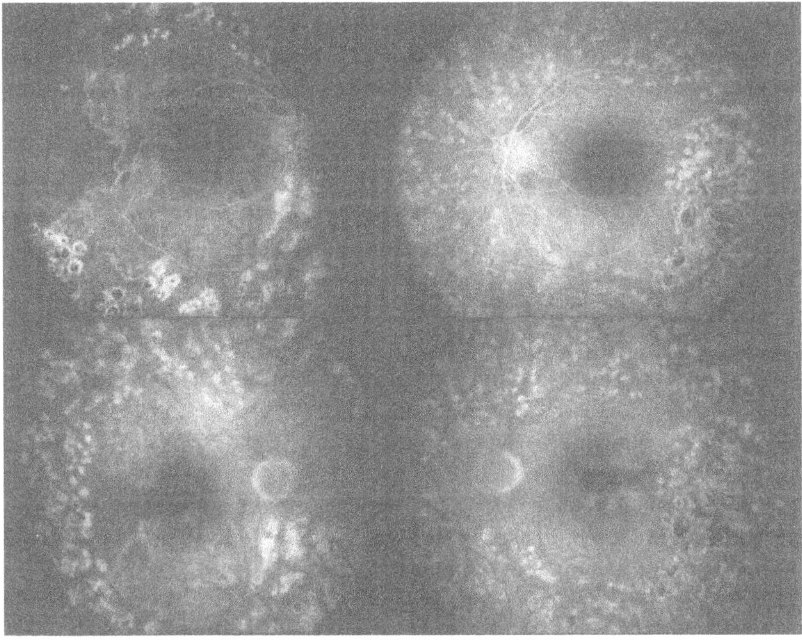

Fig. 5. Patient 2 in December 1991, neovascularization on the disc regressed in both eyes (a,b). Some leakage of the dye from the abnormal vasculature in the macula in the right eye (a). Four years later in December 1995, vaso-occlusion has progressed in both eyes (c,d); the markedly enlarged foveal avascular zones now coalescence with the peripheral nonperfused area (c,d).

systemic evaluation is advised to be tailored according to symptoms[2,6]. In our patients the aetiology of retinal vascular occlusion remained unknown inspite of thorough examinations. Patient 1 has coeliac disease and mild lactose intolerance, and Patient 2 has acne vulgaris, all relatively common disorders which are not generally known to cause retinal vasculitis. The term idiopathic or isolated retinal vasculitis may thus be used. Idiopathic retinal vasculitis/arteritis is suspected to be an autoimmune disease in which antibodies towards leucocytes, endothelial cells or thrombocytes cause endothelial damage, coagulation disturbances and thrombosis[1]. Nothing in our patients pointed towards autoimmune process, however.

The type of retinal vasculitis was found to be ischaemic by fluorescein angiograms in both of our patients. The clinical picture and the outcome showed, however, some dissimilarities. Patient 2 resembles so called Eales' disease, named after Henry Eales who first reported the disease in 1880[7]. Similar to Eales' patient our patient presented with vitreous haemorrhage as the first sign of the advanced vaso-occlusive process in the retina. She did, however, not have epistaxis, constipation or impaired hearing, and was not of male sex. Tuberculin hypersensitivity has not been studied in her, but nothing has been pointing towards cerebral infarctions which were reported by Renie and co-workers[8] to be typical for Eales' disease. In Eales' disease, venules are said to be mainly affected[8]. In Patient 2 the primary changes seemed to be in capillaries causing secondary occlusion of both arterioles and venules.

The clinical picture of Patient 1 shared features of a recently described clinical entity IRVAN (idiopathic retinal vasculitis, aneurysms and neuroretinitis)[2] described by Kincaid and Schatz[9]. Arteriolar changes at and near the optic nerve head distinguish this entity from Eales' disease[2]. In Patient 1, arterioles seemed to be mainly affected, and in addition to peripheral vascular nonperfusion she had peripapillary exudative retinopathy related to macroaneurysm-like retinal arteriolar changes. In Patient 2 corresponding arteriolar changes were not seen, and the exudative reaction was lacking. Instead, she developed capillary occlusion in the macula.

The visual outcome in patients with Eales' disease has been reported as good[10,11]. In eyes with ischaemic retinal vasculitis the visual prognosis was, however, significantly less favourable than in eyes with non-ischaemic vasculitis[3]. After a minimum follow-up of 5 years (range 5–20 years), 34% of eyes in the ischaemic group had a final vision of 6/60 or less, compared with 6% of eyes with non-ischaemic retinal vasculitis[3].

In our patients, more than 5 years after the detection of ischaemic retinal vasculitis, the visual function is still good, although in Patient 2 the progressing vascular closure in the centre of the macula may eventually threaten the central vision. Macular ischaemia is not common in retinal vasculitis, and has been appreciated only recently[5]: it was reported to occur in two out of 20 patients with ischaemic retinal vasculitis compared with two of 33 patients with non-ischaemic retinal vasculitis[3]. Macular ischaemia was not a major cause of poor vision but rather, when present, a contributing factor, and the main causes of poor visual outcome were optic atrophy, and cystoid maculopathy or macular epiretinal membrane[3]. Altogether, after a follow-up of minimun 5 years only 10% of patients with ischaemic retinal vasculitis had bilateral visual loss, which, however, compares with none of the patients with non-ischaemic retinal vasculitis[3]. As seen in Patient 2, the progression in vaso-occlusion in the idiopathic occlusive vasculopathy may be very slow and it may remain symptomless for years.

Of the possible risk factors, smoking has been shown to be more prevalent in patients with the ischaemic retinal vasculitis than in those with the non-ischaemic vasculitis[3,14]. In the smoking group, Palmer and co-workers[14] showed von Willebrand's factor and fibrinogen levels to be significantly higher than in their non-smoking counterparts. Increased levels may be due to endothelial damage caused by smoking and therefore represent an epiphenomenon[15,16] or they may have a real causative role[14]. In spite of thorough examination we did not find any coagulation disturbances in our patients.

Unfortunately, no systemic therapy is known to be effective in ischaemic retinal vasculitis[2,3,6]. Howe and his co-workers[12] have suggested that high-dose oral steroids should be used as the initial management before contemplating other more complicated regimes. It should also be kept in mind that retinal ischaemia may be made worse by the potentially procoagulant effects of immunosuppressants[13]. We have not given systemic corticosteroids or second-line immunosuppressants to our patients. The need for concomitant anticoagulant therapy to patients with ischaemic retinal vasculitis receiving procoagulant immunosuppressive treatment has been raised[3], or the use of anticoagulants alone for vascular diseases due to antiphospholipid antibodies has been advised[6].

Laser coagulation is commonly used for the treatment of leaking and occluded areas in retinal vasculitis[2,3], as was used in Patient 1, and for neovascular complications[2,3] as used in Patient 2. It proved to be effective in both patients, and most probably it also prevented neovascularization in Patient 1.

References

1. Sanders, M.D. Retinal arteritis, retinal vasculitis and autoimmune retinal vasculitis. Eye. 1987; 1: 441–465.
2. Chang, T.S., Aylward, W., Davis, J.L. et al. Idiopathic retinal vasculitis, aneurysms, and neuroretinitis. Ophthalmology. 1995; 102: 1089–1097.
3. Palmer, H.E., Stanford, M.R., Sanders, M.D., Graham, E.M. Visual outcome of patients with idiopathic ischaemic and non-ischaemic retinal vasculitis. Eye. 1996; 10: 343–348.
4. Graham, E.M., Stanford, M.R., Sanders, M.D., Kasp, E., Dumonde, D.C. A point prevalence study of 150 patients with idiopathic retinal vasculitis: 1. Diagnostic value of ophthalmological features. Br J Ophthalmol. 1989; 73: 714–721.
5. Bentley, C.R., Stanford, R.M., Shilling, J.S., Sanders, M.D., Graham, E.M. Macular ischaemia in posterior uveitis. Eye. 1993; 7: 411–414.
6. Rosenbaum, J.T., Robertson, J.E., Watzke, R.C. Retinal vasculitis – a primer. West J Med. 1991; 154: 182–185.
7. Eales, H. Cases of retinal haemorrhage associated with epistaxis and constipation. Birmingham Med Rev. 1880; 9: 262.
8. Renie, W.A., Murphy, R.P., Anderson, K.C. et al. The evaluation of patients with Eales' disease. Retina. 1983; 3: 243–248.
9. Kincaid, J., Schatz, H. Bilateral retinal arteritis with multiple aneurysmal dilatations. Retina. 1983; 3: 171–178.
10. Elliot, A.J. Thirty year observation of patients with Eales' disease. Am J Ophthalmol. 1975; 80: 404–408.
11. Atmaca, L.S., Idil, A., Gunduz, K. Visualisation of retinal vasculitis in Eales' disease. Ocul Immunol Inflamm. 1993; 1: 41–48.
12. Howe, L.J., Stanford, M.R., Edelsten, C., Graham, E.M. The efficiency of systemic corticosteroids in sight-threatening retinal vasculitis. Eye 1994; 8: 443–7.
13. Vanrenterghem, Y., Roels, L., Lerut, T., Gruwez, J. et al. Thromboembolic complications and haemostatic changes in cyclosporin-treated cadaveric kidney allograft recipients. Lancet. 1985; 8436: 999–1002.
14. Palmer, H.E., Jurd, K.M., Hunt, B.J., Zaman, A.G., Stanford, M.R., Sanders, M.D., Graham, E.M. Thrombophilic factors in ischaemic and non-ischaemic retinal vasculitis. Eye. 1995; 9: 507–512.

15. Blann, A.D., McCollum, C.N. Adverse influence of cigarette smoking on the endothelium. Thromb Haemost. 1993; 70: 707–711.
16. Ernst, E. Fibrinogen: an independent risk factor for cardiovascular disease. BMJ. 1991; 303: 596–597.

Department of Ophthalmology
University of Helsinki
Helsinki University Central Hospital
Haartmaninkatu 4 C,
FIN-00290 Helsinki
Finland

73. Macroaneurysms secondary to branch retinal vein occlusion

M. BATTAGLIA PARODI, S. DA POZZO, S. SAVIANO
and G. RAVALICO

(Trieste, Italy)

Introduction

Common consequences of branch retinal vein occlusion (BRVO) include microaneurysms, teleangiectatic and non-perfused capillaries, collateral vessels and macroaneurysms. Only few reports had described the development of macroaneurysms following retinal vein occlusions[1-4], until 1990, when Cousins and co-workers emphasized the occurrence, and the clinical and angiographic features of macroaneurysms secondary to BRVO[5]. The authors, reviewing the clinical and angiographic records of 147 patients enrolled in the Branch Vein Occlusion Study, distinguished four types of lesions: arterial, venous, capillary and collateral, pointing out the association with capillary non-perfusion.

Our research describes the clinical and angiographic aspects of 22 cases of BRVO, in which retinal macroaneurysms developed, in an attempt to analyse the pathogenetical features.

Patients and methods

The study considered 133 patients, referred to our fluorescein angiography centre with a clinical diagnosis of BRVO. Each patient underwent complete ophthalmologic examination, including biomicroscopic evaluation, fundus photography and fluorescein angiography.

BRVO diagnosis was based on the ophthalmoscopic appearance (superficial and/or deep retinal hemorrhages in just one quadrant, congestion and tortuosity of venous vessel, with or without presence of surrounding exudates) and the fluorescein angiography finding of delayed venous filling. The criteria previously proposed by Cousins[5] were used in the identification of macroaneurysms and for the evaluation of their size and type. Fluorescein angiography was performed at an average interval of 2 months (range: 1–4 months) from the onset of the disease with a mean follow-up of 40 months (range: 30–55 months). A careful examination was made in order to determine the presence of capillary non-perfusion and the amount of retinal venous collaterals. As suggested by the Branch Vein Occlusion Study Group[6], capillary non-

G. Coscas and F. Cardillo Piccolino (eds.), Retinal Pigment Epithelium and Macular Diseases, pp. 421–426.
© *1998 Kluwer Academic Publishers.*

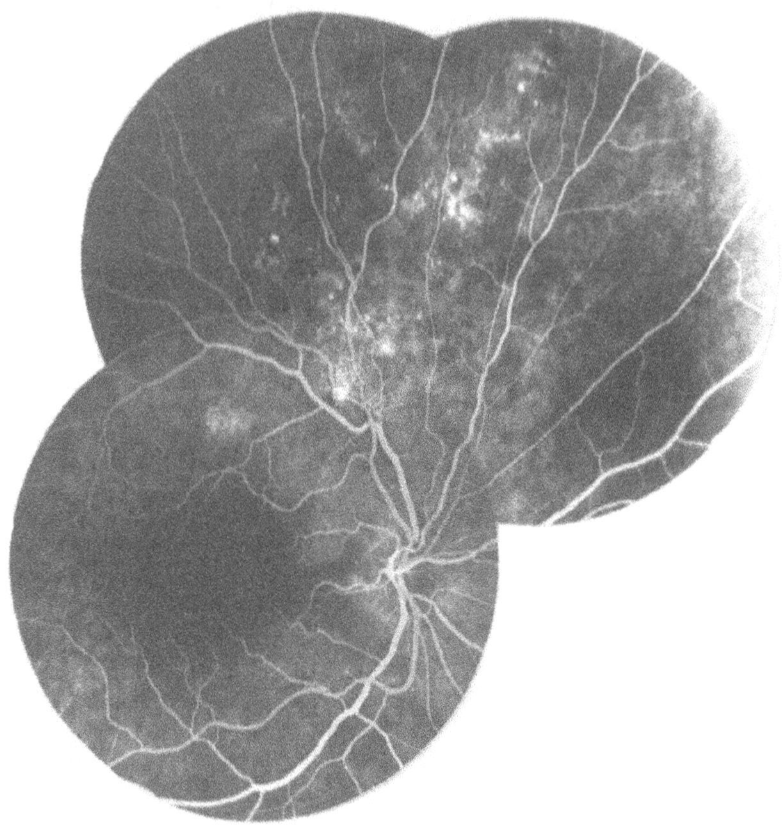

Fig. 1. Superotemporal **BRVO** with an arterial macroaneurysm associated with two collateral macroaneurysms.

perfusion was considered severe when at least five disk areas of capillary non-perfusion were detectable. Collateral vessels were defined as few or several on the basis of standard angiographic frames.

Each angiogram was evaluated in a masked fashion by two authors (MBP, SS); agreement between the two authors was achieved in 95% of cases, and uncertain cases were defined by a third author (SDP). Statistical analysis was performed using the χ^2 test.

Results

Table 1 summarizes general and ophthalmologic characteristics of the considered population. Out of a total of 133 patients, 22 (16.5%) developed macroaneurysms (Group A); the remaining 111 patients, with no evidence of

Table 1. Summary of general and ophthalmologic characteristics of the considered population

	Group A	Group B
Patients	22 (16.5%)	111 (83.5%)
Age, years (mean SD)	65.3 ± 10.1	66.4 ± 9.6
Diabetes, cases	3 (13.6%)	17 (15.3%)
Hypertension, cases	14 (63.6%)	69 (62.1%)
Severe capillary non-perfusion, cases	17 (77.3%)	85 (76.6%)
Amount of venous collaterals, cases		
Few	17 (77.3%)	49 (44.1%)
Several	5 (22.7%)	62 (55.9%)

Group A: BRVO with macroaneurysms. Group B: BRVO without macroaneurysms.

macroaneurysms, constituted the control group (Group B). The mean age of patients in group A was 65.3 ± 10.1 (SD), with 63 females (56.8%) and 48 males (43.2%). The mean age of patients in group B was 66.4 ± 9.6, with 14 females (36.3%) and 8 males (63.7%).

Three patients of group A (13.3%) and 17 of group B (15.3%) were affected by diabetes mellitus, whereas 14 patients of group A (63.6%) and 69 of group B (62.1%) suffered from hypertension (Table 1). The total number of detected macroaneurysms was 42; nine (21.4%) were large, 14 (33.3%) were of medium-size and 19 (45.2%) were small. Three lesions had an arterial origin, 22 were capillary and 17 were from collateral vessels; no lesion originated from venous vessels (Table 2). Fourteen patients had only one lesion, three patients had two lesions, and five patients had three or more lesions. Four patients had a combination of two or more macroaneurysm types. In 18 cases (81.8%) the lesions were located outside the macular region, and in 4 cases (18.2%) in the macular region. The lesions were associated with sorrounding intraretinal haemorrhage in seven cases (31.8%), while in only two cases (9%) sorrounding lipid exudation was noted, with involvement of the fovea absent in all cases.

The mean time for the detection of macroaneurysms was 19.2 months (range: 0–49). In two cases spontaneous involution of the lesions noticed, after 13 and 25 months respectively. Additional lesions developed in two cases, after 16 and 21 months respectively. Five patients of Group A (22.7%)

Table 2. Summary of size and type of macroaneurysms

Type	Small	Medium	Large	Total lesion per type
Capillary	12	5	5	22
Collaterals	7	7	3	17
Arterial	0	2	1	3
Venous	0	0	0	0
Total lesions per size	19	14	9	42

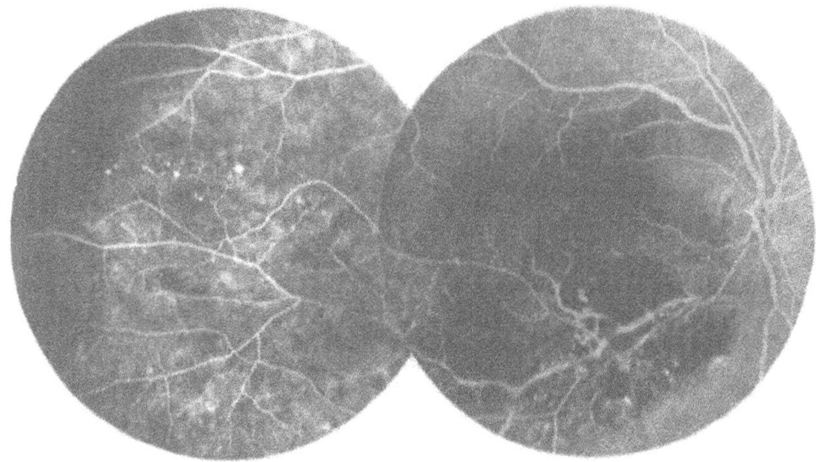

Fig. 2. Inferotemporal BRVO showing two peripheral capillary macroaneurysms.

and 26 of Group B (23.4%) developed retinal and/or optic disc neovascularizations, and underwent scattered photocoagulation. In 17 out of 22 patients (77.3%) of Group A, there was a severe capillary non-perfusion, compared with 85 out of 111 patients (76.6%) of Group B. Statistical analysis showed no significant difference. On the contrary, when the amount of retinal venous collaterals was considered, 17 patients (77.3%) in Group A showed few collaterals as against 49 patients (44.1%) in Group B. Statistical analysis revealed a significant difference ($p < 0.004$) and the relative risk of the development of macroaneurysms was 1.7 in the cases with few collaterals.

Two patients of group A developed an exudative retinal detachment involving the affected retinal quadrant and the macular region.

Discussion

Among the possible vascular changes following BRVO, macroaneurysms were present relatively frequently. The prevalence of 16.5% found in the present study appears very similar to that reported by Cousins (16.3%). However, there are hints in the clinical evidence that macroaneurysms in BRVO are more frequently encountered than in central retinal vein occlusion, in which they may be rare[2,7]. In their report Cousins and colleagues[5] came to the conclusion that macroaneurysm occurrence is associated with severe capillary non-perfusion on fluorescein angiography. Our data do not confirm this statement since comparing group A, with macroaneurysms, with group B, without macroaneurysms, the prevalence of severe capillary non-perfusion is very similar, with no statistically significant difference between them. The

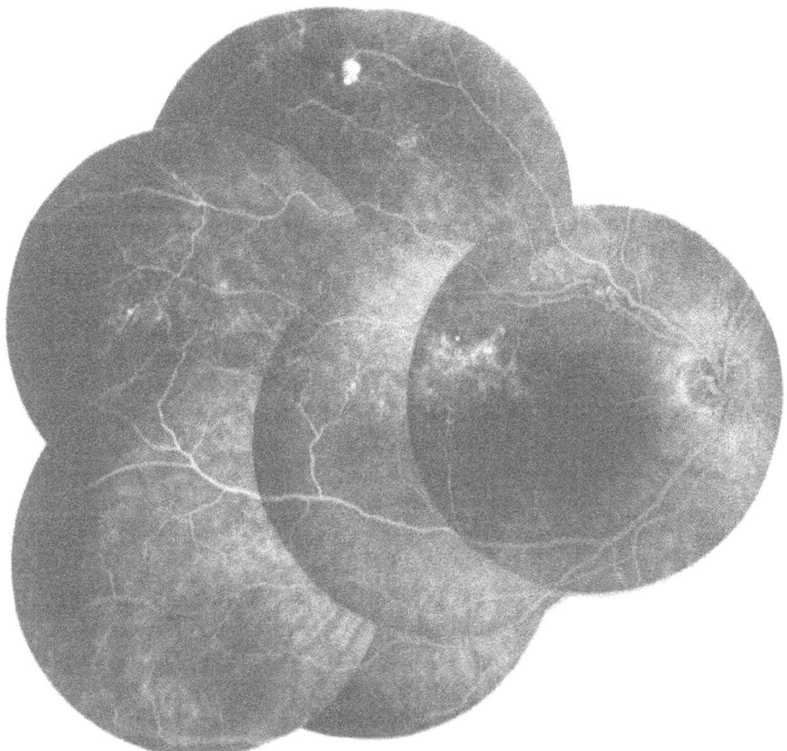

Fig. 3. Superotemporal BRVO with three capillary and two collaterals macroaneurysms.

percentage of patients affected by hypertension or diabetes mellitus is also similar in the two considered groups and corresponds to those in the study by Cousins[5].

A critical factor in the pathogenesis of macroaneurysms in BRVO seemed to be the number of retinal venous collaterals; indeed, collaterals were found more frequently in patients with macroaneurysms than in those without macroaneurysms. The consequence of the paucity of retinal venous collaterals may be a haemodynamic overload with possible dilation of some vascular segments and development of macroaneurysms. Thus, the insufficient number of retinal venous collaterals may be considered the most important contributory factor in the development of macroaneurysms secondary to BRVO. The paucity of retinal venous collaterals also affects the development of exudative retinal detachment secondary to BRVO[7], as was noted in two patients of Group A.

A further consideration is the relative rarity of sorrounding intraretinal haemorrhage and lipid exudation found in our study, combined with a frequent peripheral location of macroaneurysms. This feature explains the low risk of impairment of the central visual function.

References

1. Magargal, L.E., Augsburger, J.J., Hyman, D., Townsend, R. Venous macroaneurysms following branch retinal vein obstruction. Ann Ophthalmol. 1980; 12: 685–687.
2. Schulman, J., Jampol, L.M., Goldberg, M.F. Large capillary aneurysms secondary to retinal vein obstruction. Br J Ophthalmol. 1981; 65: 36–41.
3. Sandborn, G.E., Magargal, L.E. Venous macroaneurysms associated with branch retinal vein obstruction. Ann Ophthalmol. 1984; 16: 464–466.
4. Takeda, M., Kimura, S. Large capillary aneurysms secondary to branch vein occlusion. Jpn J Ophthalmol. 1982; 36: 315–316.
5. Cousins, S.W., Flynn, H.W., Clarkson, J.G. Macroaneurysms associated with retinal branch vein occlusion. Am J Ophthalmol. 1990; 109: 567–570.
6. Branch Vein Occlusion Study Group. Argon laser photocoagulation for macular edema in branch vein occlusion. Am J Ophthalmol. 1984; 98: 271–282.
7. Battaglia Parodi, M., Bondel, E., Ravalico, G. Macroaneurysms in central retinal vein occlusion. Ophthalmologica. 1995; 209: 248–250.
8. Battaglia Parodi, M., Isola, V. Branch retinal vein occlusion and exudative retinal detachment: pathogenetical aspects. Ophthalmolgica. 1994; 208: 29–31.

Eye Clinic
University of Trieste
Italy

74. Decrease of PKC activity by a peptide fraction from porcine factor VIII in endothelial cells CPA-47

L. PAZZAGLI, C. CECCHI, M. BERTINI and G. BATTISTA GERVASI

(Florence and Pisa, Italy)

Purpose

A peptide fraction of low molecular weight (Vueffe) prepared from porcine Factor VIII by enzymatic hydrolysis with trypsin, reduces bleeding time in laboratory animals without interfering either with platelets or blood coagulation[1]. For its molecular weight and pharmacological properties this fraction is completely different from other larger peptide fractions also derived from Factor VIII[2]. Remarkable properties of Vueffe are the low doses at which it is active, the long duration of action and the resistance to oral administration. The effect of Vueffe appears to be promising for controlling blood effusions in important areas such as the eye[3,4].

The aim of the present study was to investigate a relationship among the anti-haemorrhagic properties of Vueffe and PKC activity.

Protein kinase C (PKC), discovered in 1977 by Inoue *et al.*[5], transfers the γ-phosphate of ATP to the seryl or threonyl residues of various protein substrates[6,7]. In vascular cells, protein kinase C has been shown to modulate growth rate, DNA synthesis, hormone and growth factor receptor turn-over[8], smooth muscle contraction[9] and cAMP responses to different hormones[10]. The activation of PKC is also a common pathway by which mediators increase transendothelial permeability during tissue inflammation and in the development of diabetic vascular complications[11].

Methods

Cultured CPA-47 endothelial cells (3.6×10^7 cells per experimental point) were allowed to reach confluence in regular growth medium (MEM with 10% calf serum). All endothelial cells were subjected to an equal number of passages (range 44–50). Cells were treated with 1 μM phorbol 12-myristate 13-acetate (PMA, a PKC activator commonly used to detect its activity) and with different Vueffe concentrations (25–400 ng/ml) for 1 h. PKC was partially purified from cultured cell according to Lee *et al.*[12]. Briefly, cultured dishes were washed extensively with 20 mM Tris–HCl, 2 mM EDTA, 0.5 mM EGTA, 0.33 M sucrose, pH 7.5 (buffer A). Cells were scraped and lysed with a glass Dounce homogenizer. After centrifugation

G. Coscas and F. Cardillo Piccolino (eds.), Retinal Pigment Epithelium and Macular Diseases, pp. 427–430.
© 1998 Kluwer Academic Publishers.

at 2500 *g*, the supernatant was ultracentrifuged at 100 000 *g* for 30 min. The resulting supernatant was collected as the cytosolic fraction. The pellet were resuspended with buffer B (buffer A without sucrose) with 1% Nonidet and homogenized again. The soluble fraction obtained after centrifugation at 100 000 *g* for 30 min was retained as the membranous fraction. Both cytosolic and membranous fractions were applied to DEAE-columns. The PKC activity was measured on the eluted fractions by its ability to transfer ^{32}P from [γ-^{32}P]ATP in to the selective PKC peptide, comprising residues 4–14 of myelin basic protein (MBP$_{4-14}$), in presence of Ca^{2+}, phosphatidylserine and diacylglycerol at 37°C. PKC activities were calculated by subtracting the non specific kinase activity from the cpm obtained in presence of Ca^{2+} and lipids.

Protein determination was performed according to the Bicinchoninic Acid Protein Assay Kit (Sigma).

Results and conclusions

Administration of Vueffe to endothelial cultured cells, stimulated by PMA, decreases significantly the activity of PKC (Table 1). Taking as 100% protein kinase activity values obtained in the presence of PMA, different Vueffe concentrations caused an enzymatic activity decrease to $67 \pm 16.6\%$ (Vueffe = 25 ng/ml) and to $58 \pm 24.7\%$ (Vueffe = 200 ng/ml) (Fig. 1). No significant change was observed in the cytosolic fractions.

The anti-haemorrhagic properties of Vueffe are probably related to a decrease in endothelial permeability mediated by PKC. This is consistent also with the demonstration that Vueffe decreases capillary permeability for serum protein[13].

Further studies are in progress in order to investigate the action mechanism of this peptide fraction from porcine factor VIII.

Table 1. PKC activities (mol/min/mg) measured in membranous fractions from cultured endothelial cells exposed to 1M PMA and to different Vueffe concentrations. The five different experiments were performed in duplicate.

PMA	1.717	3.019	2.837	4.710	2.321
VF 25 ng/ml	–*	–*	2.118	3.751	1.125
VF 50 ng/ml	0.491	1.514	1.086	–*	1.023
VF 200 ng/ml	–*	1.048	0.588	3.231	–*
VF 400 ng/ml	–*	0.652	–*	–*	

*Values not determined at these concentrations.

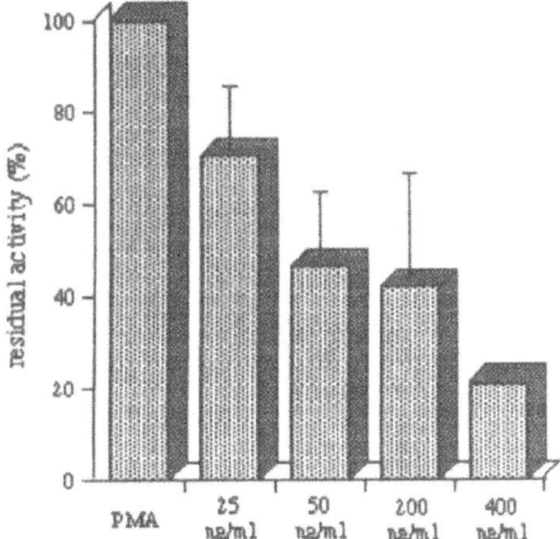

Fig. 1. Effect of different concentrations of Vueffe on PKC activities. Values are means ± SD of five independent experiments and are expressed as residual activity (%).

References

1. Gervasi, G.B., Bartoli, C., Carpita, G., Baldacci, M. Decrease of bleeding time by a peptide fraction from bovine factor VIII in laboratory animals. Arzneim-Forsch/Drug Res. 1988; 38: 1268–1270.
2. Weiss., H.J., Phillips, L.L., Rosner, W. Separation of sub-units of antihemophilic factor (AHF) by agarose gel chromatography. Thromb Diath Haemorrh. 1972; 27: 212–219.
3. Valli, A., Bellone, A., Protti, R., Bolla, N. Colour Doppler imaging to evaluate the action of a drug in ocular pathology. Ophthalmologica. 1995; 209: 117–122.
4. Cardillo Piccolino, F., Ghiglione, D., Ceppa, P. Villaggio, B., Carli, F., Allegri, P., Bertagno, R., Zingirian, M. Fundus angiography with fluorescein-labelled peptide fraction from bovine factor VIII: correlation with histologic findings. Eur J Ophthalmol. 1992; 2: 135–143.
5. Inoue, M., Kishimoto, A., Takai, Y., Nishizumka, Y. Studies on a cyclic nucleotide-independent protein kinase and its proenzyme in mammalian tissues. II. Proenzyme and its activation by calcium dependent protease from rat brain. J Biol Chem. 1977; 252: 7610–7616.
6. Newton, A.C. Protein kinase C: structure, function and regulation. J Biol Chem. 1995; 270: 28495–28498.
7. Jaken, S. Protein kinase C isoenzymes and substrates. Curr Opinion Cell Biol. 1996; 8: 168–173.
8. Hachiya, H.L., Takayama, S., White, M.F., King, G.L. Regulation of insulin receptor internalization in vascular endothelial cells by insulin and phorbol ester. J Biol Chem. 1987; 262: 6417–6424.
9. Jiang, M.J., Morgan, K.G. Intracellular calcium levels in phorbol ester-induced contractions of vascular muscle. Am J Physiol. 1987; 253: H1365–H1371.
10. Limas, C.J., Limas, C. Phorbol ester- and diacylglycerol-mediated desensitization of cardiac β-adrenergic receptors. Circ Res. 1985; 57: 443–449.
11. Lynch, J.J., Ferro, T.J., Blumenstock, F.A., Brockenauer, A.M., Malik, A.B. Increased endothelial albumin permeability mediated by protein kinase C activation. J Clin Invest. 1990; 85: 1991–1998.

12. Lee, T.S., MacGregor, L.C., Fluharty, S.J., King, G.L. Differential regulation of protein kinase C and (Na,K)-adenosine triphosphatase activities by elevated glucose levels in retinal capillary endothelial cells. J. Clin. Invest. 1989; 83: 90–94.
13. Witte, S. Surface phenomena of coagulation factors "in vivo", observed by fluorescence intravital microscopy. Ann NY Acad Sci. 1983; 416: 426–440.

Department of Biochemical Sciences
University of Florence
Italy

75. Clinical, angiographic and histopathological results after surgical removal of subfoveal choroidal new vessels

A. SCHEIDER, E.M. MESSMER, T. GRASBON, J.P. HOOPS
and A. KAMPIK
(Munich, Germany)

Introduction

Multiple papers have reported differences in outcome of choroidal neovascularization (CNV) due to age-related macular degeneration (ARMD) compared to other causes, but few have compared intra- and postoperative outcome of different CNV types in ARMD. Several papers have also described histopathological features of these membranes and their correlation with angiography, but scant information exists of intraoperative findings in correlation to both histopathology and angiography. Furthermore, it has been mentioned that surgically extracted membranes are larger than expected from the preoperative angiography. Unpublished data from Berger and colleagues reported a postoperative RPE-defect that was 145% larger than the original CNV. However, no information was given about the extracted CNV type or a possible intraoperative trauma.

The purpose of this pilot study was to find out whether more information can be obtained about intraoperative risks and the clinical course after surgical excision of subfoveal CNV in correlation to the angiographic and clinical subtype and whether a comparison of the pre- and intraoperative CNV size might give us additional information about the true size of CNV.

Methods

All eyes were examined in a regular fashion with preoperative fluorescein and, if necessary, indocyanine green (ICG) angiography. CNV was classified according to the MPS standard. The surgical procedure consisted of an extended core vitrectomy and separation of the posterior hyaloid membrane if necessary. This was followed by a temporal retinotomy, mobilization and extraction of the CNV or haemorrhage. According to the intraoperative course, the eye was subsequently filled with air, gas or silicone oil. If possible, the CNV was extracted from the eye and forewarded for routine histological

G. Coscas and F. Cardillo Piccolino (eds.), Retinal Pigment Epithelium and Macular Diseases, pp. 431–433.
© *1998 Kluwer Academic Publishers.*

sectioning and staining. A histological classification was independently suggested by two trained examiners according to the proposal of Gass (subpigmentepithelial CNV = type 1 and subretinal CNV = type 2). In case of disagreement, the best fitting classification was elaborated after discussion with a third examiner. For pre- and intraoperative CNV size comparison, optimal images of the CNV and the optic disc from each angiography and operation video were digitized and their area was calculated after marking with the mouse. Intraoperative CNV area was estimated after mobilization of the CNV in the subretinal space.

Results

Between October 1995 and May 1996, 41 eyes of 39 patients (74.4 ± 11.8 years) with subfoveal CNV or haemorrhage underwent surgery. Forty eyes had the typical signs of ARMD; three had been treated with laser before surgery. One eye had the typical signs of presumed ocular histoplasmosis syndrome. Twenty-four eyes had a subfoveal CNV with no or only few accompanying blood or exudate, 13 eyes had a subfoveal haemorrhage and four eyes suffered from a massive subretinal haemorrhage extending up to the mid-periphery. Extraction through a small retinotomy was possible in 22 of 23 eyes with CNV and in 11 of 12 eyes with subfoveal haemorrhage. A larger retinotomy, extending to or above the vascular arcade was necessary in one eye with CNV, in one eye with subfoveal haemorrhage and in all four eyes with massive haemorrhage. Laser coagulation was thought to be necessary in none of the CNV eyes, in one eye with subfoveal haemorrhage and in two of four eyes with massive haemorrhage (in the other two, rebleeding prevented an exact apposition of the retinotomy rim with the RPE). So far, 27 eyes have been followed for more than 4 weeks. Visual acuity changed from 0.01 ± 0.0027 to 0.02 ± 0.0014 in the 17 eyes with CNV only, from 0.006 ± 0.0035 to 0.0125 ± 0.0017 in the eight eyes with subfoveal haemorrhage and from 0.003 ± 0.0022 to 0.006 ± 0.007 in two eyes with massive haemorrhage. It was interesting to note that even the extraction of old scars led to unexpected satisfied patients who noted a significant decrease of their metamorphopsia.

A correlation of angiography and intraoperative CNV size could be done in 10 eyes. Two examiners found independently an intraoperative increase of 5% and 9%. Intraoperative complications were the following: choroidal haemorrhage after CNV extraction occurred in seven eyes (3/24 CNV, 2/13 subfoveal haemorrhage and 2/4 massive haemorrhage). All three eyes in the CNV group were subfoveal recurrences after parafoveal laser treatment. Central iatrogenic retinal tears during the preparation or extraction process occurred in three eyes, two after parafoveal laser, one with firm CNV adherence to retina. Peripheral retinal tears occured in nine eyes (21.9%). All were detected at the end of the operation and treated. No secondary retinal detachment was detected. A correlation of intraoperative complications, central retinal tears and intraoperative choroidal bleeding with the clinical CNV type demonstrates that recurrences after parafoveal laser have the highest incidence for both.

Clinicopathological correlation of 11 CNV demonstrated that four CNV with angiographically well defined borders were classified as type 2 membranes, three CNV, that had both classic and occult components could be confirmed as being mixed types whereas type 1 membranes were either ill defined or had some classic components.

Conclusion

This pilot study demonstrates that acceptable short-term results are possible after the surgical extraction of subfoveal CNV in ARMD. However, since we operated only on eyes with comparatively advanced disease and a visual acuity of mostly below 20/200, a comparison with the results of other current treatment modalities is difficult. Our comparative analysis demonstrated that CNV are larger than angiographically expected. However, for smaller CNV that are the usual indication for laser treatment, this difference should probably not necessitate a change of the suggested treatment technique. Although the numbers of CNV for clinicohistopathological comparison are small and will be subject to reappraisal in the future, correlation of angiography, intraoperative findings and histopathology indicate that well defined membranes in ARMD are type 2 membranes and comparatively easy to remove surgically whereas mixed types or ill defined membranes, being type 1 membranes, have a higher risk of intraoperative bleeding and significant loss of RPE and choriocapillaris possibly due to their firmer interlacing with RPE and Bruch's membrane. A single small intraoperative bleed that was usually observed after the extraction of well defined type 2 CNV could indicate that such membranes usually have only one feeder vessel.

Our study so far indicates that different histopathological membrane types seem to have a different intraoperative outcome. It was therefore reassuring that these types can be differentiated by fluorescein angiography that allows for a better patient selection. Although there is still an ongoing debate about its usefulness, surgery seems suitable for eyes with well defined subfoveal CNV or subfoveal haemorrhage.

Augenklinik der Ludwig-Maximilians-Universität
80336 München
Germany

76. Subfoveal choroidal neovascularization in punctate inner choroidopathy: surgical management and pathological findings

T.W. OLSEN, A. CAPONE Jr, P. STERNBERG Jr,
H.E. GROSSNIKLAUS, D.F. MARTIN and T.M. AABERG Sr

(Atlanta, Georgia)

Background

Punctate inner choroidopathy[1], multifocal choroiditis[2], and multifocal choroiditis associated with progressive subretinal fibrosis[3] may all appear quite similar clinically. Patients affected with these conditions, which may represent either variants of single disorder or a spectrum of disease, have a similar profile: they are commonly young myopic females with multiple focal areas of inflammation at the level of the choroid/Bruchs' membrane/retinal pigment epithelium complex. The aetiology and incidence of these conditions is unknown. Visual outcome in punctate inner choroidopathy is generally good, barring the development of subfoveal choroidal neovascularization (CNV)[1].

Conventional management options in the treatment of subretinal CNV include observation, photocoagulation, and the administration of local or systemic steroids. Uncontrolled case series published to date suggest that macular surgery may be a viable therapeutic option in patients with CNV due to ocular histoplasmosis[4-6]. Choroidal neovascularization in punctate inner choroidopathy is similar to that in ocular histoplasmosis in that the neovascular membranes grow in the subretinal space anterior to the retinal pigment epithelium.

We propose that surgical intervention may offer the best opportunity for visual recovery in cases of punctate inner choroidopathy complicated by subfoveal choroidal neovascularization. Herein we review the records of six eyes of five patients with punctate inner choroidiopathy who underwent submacular surgery for subfoveal choroidal neovascularization. Surgical specimens were examined using light and transmission electron microscopy. The histopathology and ultrastructure of the excised subretinal tissue are described, and a classification system is proposed which characterizes the development of choroidal neovascularization with associated subretinal fibrosis.

G. Coscas and F. Cardillo Piccolino (eds.), Retinal Pigment Epithelium and Macular Diseases, pp. 435–437.
© 1998 Kluwer Academic Publishers.

Results

Five young myopic female patients ranging from 20 to 48 years of age presented with fundus lesions consisted with the diagnosis of punctate inner choroidopathy. Four cases were bilateral, one was unilateral, none had evidence of anterior chamber inflammation, and only one had rare posterior vitreous cells. Six eyes of these five patients underwent subretinal surgery for the excision of subfoveal choroidal neovascular membranes.

While standardized visual acuity testing was not performed, visual improvement from preoperative levels using best corrected Snellen visual acuity was noted in all six eyes. Preoperative visual acuities ranged from 20/70 to 20/300. Best postoperative vision ranged from 20/20 (two cases) to 20/200. Follow-up range from 8 to 36 months (median 14 months). Recurrences were common and occurred in four of six eyes. Half of the six recurrences required additional procedures. Three were managed surgically, two with laser photocoagulation, and one with observation. 'Bridging' of separate foci of choroidal neovascularization resulted in a stellate or dumbbell-shaped areas of subretinal fibrosis in four of six eyes.

Histopathological evaluation of the excised choroidal neovascular complexes was performed in all cases. Findings included endothelial line vascular channels, fibrocytes, retinal pigment epithelial cells, collagen fibrils and lymphocytes.

Conclusion

Subfoveal choroidal neovascularization in punctate inner choroidopathy may be managed effectively with submacular surgery. Recurrences are common and may result in substantial visual loss. Based on our experience with the above cases and other patients with punctate inner choroidopathy who have developed extrafoveal or juxtafoveal choroidal neovascularization, we suggest that five stages may occur in the evolution of bridging neovascularization associated with this condition. Stage 1 is the initial, presumably inflammatory reaction that occurs at the level of the choriocapillaris or possibly retinal pigment epithelium and results in a focal injury to Bruchs' membrane. In Stage 2, the early neovascular phase, neovascular buds growth for the injured area of Bruchs' membrane within the subretinal space. Stage 3 represents the 'bridging phase' where two or more separate neovascular foci coalesce to form a single, larger choroidal neovascular complex. Reactive pigment epithelial hyperplasia occurs at the borders, engulfing the neovascular membranes. Fibrocytes invade the core of the complex, laying the groundwork or Stage 4, the contractile phase. Contraction of the coalesced of neovascular complexes causes the stelloid or dumbbell-shaped areas of subretinal fibrosis seen clinically. Stage 5 is the cicatricial phase seen clinically as a fibrotic plaque with the destruction of the overlying photoreceptors. Small neovascular buds may involute, or the distance between neovascular buds may be too great for the bridging phase to occur. The time frame of the stages is variable, but typically occurs over several weeks.

References

1. Watzke, R.C., Packer, A.J., Folk, J.C. et al Punctate inner choroidopathy. Am J Ophthalmol. 1984; 98: 572–584.
2. Morgan, C.M., Schatz, H. Recurrent multifocal choroiditis. Ophthalmology. 1986; 93: 1138–1147.
3. Cantrill, H.L., Folk, J.C. Multifocal choroiditis associated with progressive subretinal fibrosis. Am J Ophthalmol. 1986; 101: 170–180.
4. Thomas, M.A., Kaplan, H.J. Surgical removal of subfoveal neovascularization in the presumed ocular histoplasmosis syndrome. Am J Ophthalmol. 1991; 111: 1–7.
5. Thomas, M.A., Grand, M.G., Williams, D.F. et al. Surgical management of subfoveal choroidal neovascularization. Ophthalmology. 1992; 99: 952–968.
6. Berger, A.S., Kaplan, H.J. Clinical experience with the surgical removal of subfoveal neovascular membranes. Short-term postoperative results. Ophthalmology. 1992; 99: 969–976.

77. Vitrectomy in Coats' disease

F. MIRANTI, M. MENGA and L. BAUCHIERO

(Ivrea, Italy)

Introduction

Coats' disease is a retinophathy characterized by the presence of retinovascular alterations, more frequently located in the temporal region, with massive macular exudation. The initial lesion affects the vascular wall, first arterioles, then capillaries and veins, causing the disappearance of endothelial cells and perycities, the gradual thinning of basal membrane with dilatation of vessel wall, and alteration of the blood–retinal barrier with plasma transudation[1–5].

The disease may be divided into two forms, the juvenile and the adult, with similar clinical manifestations. It is primarily monolateral and it affects males with a frequency three times that of females. The ophthalmoscopic findings are characterized by the presence of yellowish retinal and subretinal exudation and by vascular abnormalities variously associated as teleangectasis, deformation of the vessels wall, which assume the shape of micro and macroaneurysms, arteirovenous shunts, intraretinal new vessels, microvascular alterations with extensive capillary diffusion and non-perfusive capillaropathy. Vascular alterations are more frequently located in the retinal temporal region with presence of macular exudation. Macular exudates may be associated with vascular anomalies located solely in peripheral areas. Spontaneous evolution is usually progressive with possible retinal detachment secondary to massive subretinal exudation and vitreal traction. Uveitis, cataract, rubeosis or neovascular glaucoma with bulbar atrophy may develop. In some cases spontaneous remissions with obliteration of the vessels and resorption of exudation occur[6–8].

Medical therapy with antibiotics and corticosteroids, as recommended in the past, is unsatisfactory. The most effective treatment is laser photocoagulation of the vascular alterations causing massive exudation, possibly associated with cryosurgery of the more peripheral lesions which are not accessible to laser treatment.Vitreoretinal and episcleral surgery allow treatment of cases which present vitreoretinal fibrosis and tractional retinal detachment[8–13].

Case report

A 27-year-old male Caucasian with a one-month history serious loss of central vision, associated with metamorphopsia came to our observation.

G. Coscas and F. Cardillo Piccolino (eds.), Retinal Pigment Epithelium and Macular Diseases, pp. 439–445.
© 1998 Kluwer Academic Publishers.

The fundus examination revealed a marked retinal exudation with hyaloid fibrosis and distortion of the vessels of the perimacular circle, perifoveal microaneurysms (Fig. 1); in the superior temporal periphery an area of tele-angectasis with shunts, macroaneurysms and retinal oedema.

Fluoroangiography revealed posterior pole oedema due to leakage of the microanurysms and the vessels of the perifoveal circle, which appeared to be stretched and dilated by the epiretinal membrane (Fig. 2), and the presence of ischaemia and leakage of the vessels in the superior temporal periphery (Fig. 3). Visual acuity was 1/20.The 30° visual field revealed a reduced central retinal sensitivity of the foveal threshold.

The left eye had a normal fundus and presented 20/20 visual acuity. First we performed scatter photocoagulation of the peripheral ischaemic areas and of the vascular anomalies; the patient was further submitted to a pars plana vitrectomy. After the removal of the central and peripheral vitreous, we peeled the epimacular membrane, combined with an extensive and accurate removal of the posterior hyaloid as far as the equator, in order to prevent possible post-surgery retraction. Episcleral cryopexis was accomplished at the extreme retinal periphery to complete the treatment of the vascular alterations respon-sible for exudation. We did not perform silicone oil or gas tamponade, and no episcleral indentation was involved. At the end of the operation we pre-ferred not to remove the subretinal exudates. A few days later we performed a focal photocoagulation of the microaneurysms present in the perifoveal area

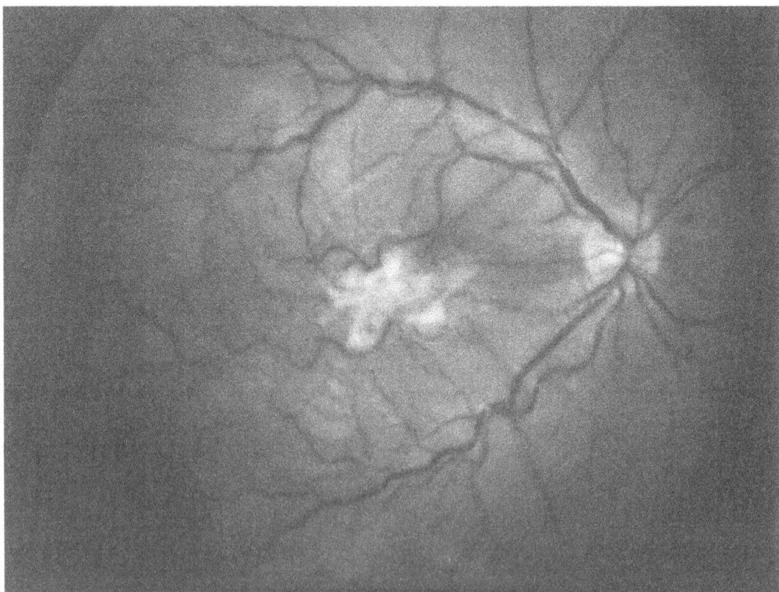

Fig. 1. Macular involvment in Coats' disease.

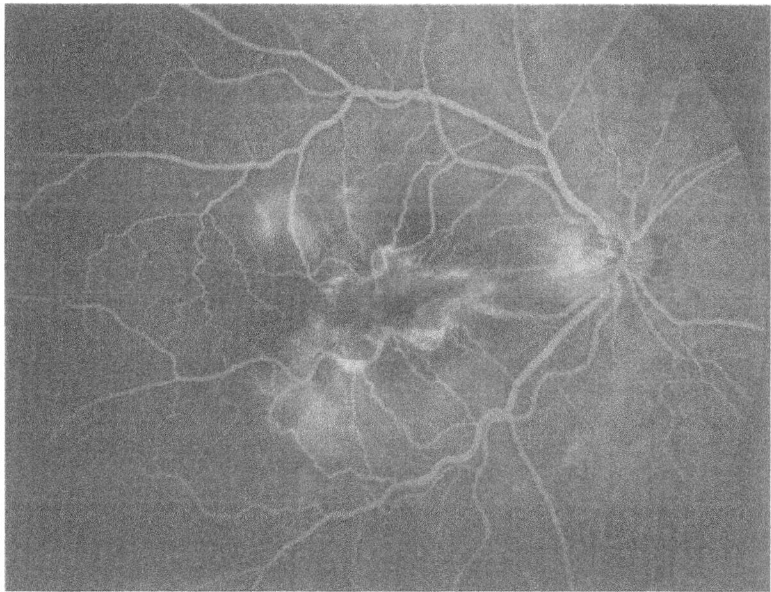

Fig. 2. Fluoroangiographic appearance of the posterior pole.

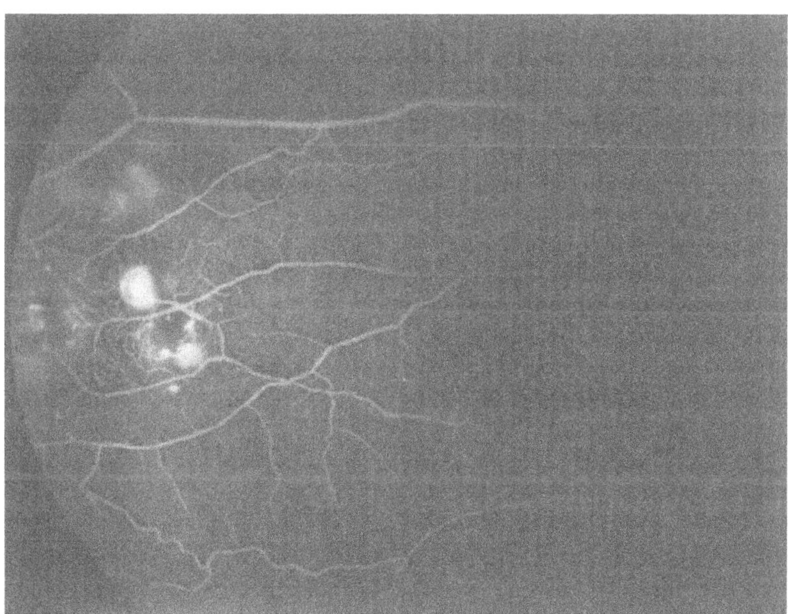

Fig. 3. Fluoroangiographic appearance of the temporal periphery.

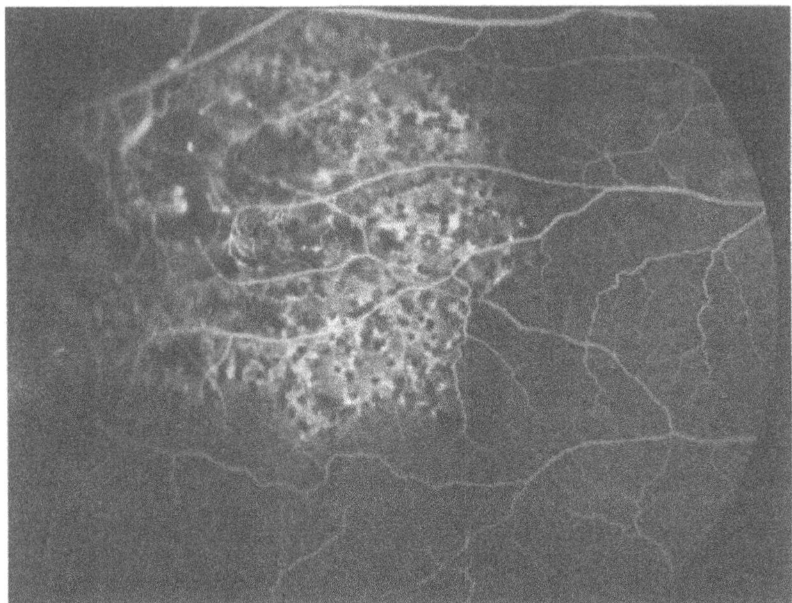

Fig. 4. Fluoroangiographic evidence of laser treatment of the temporal periphery.

to facilitate the resorption of exudates and to prevent a possible relapse of retinal oedema. Postoperatively we obtained a substantial reduction of metamorphopsia and a progressive gradual improvement of visual acuity which reached 16/20 three months later with an enhancement of the central 30° visual field (Humphrey 30/2 test).

A follow up fluoroangiographic examination performed 1 month later showed vascular abnormalities not completely involved by laser or cryoscar (Fig. 4); further laser photocoagulation was performed (Fig. 5); six months after surgery subretinal exudation was completely resolved. Finally, two years after the operation visual acuity was 20/20, the 30° visual field showed a normal sensitivity; the patient did not complain of metamorphopsia, the macular region showed no biomicroscopic or fluoroangiographic signs of retraction or oedema, whereas the foveal reflex has reappeared (Fig. 6, 7).

Conclusion

The peculiarity of the case reported was the severe macular disruption caused by the epiretinal membrane, a strong adhesion between the fibrotic hyaloid and the retina, and the need to delaminate the points of adhesion using membrane spatula and scissors. No serious surgical complication occurred

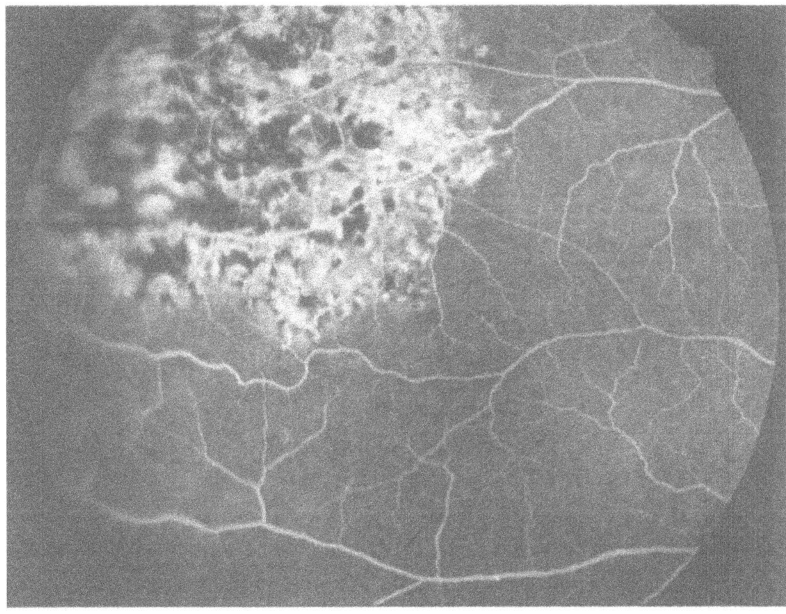

Fig. 5. Fluoroangiographic appearance after second laser retreatment of the temporal periphery.

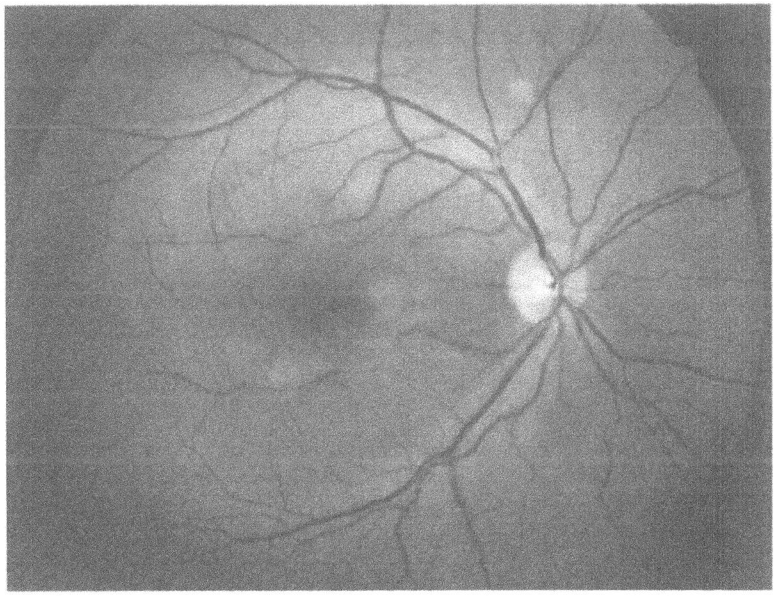

Fig. 6. Retinography 2 years after surgery.

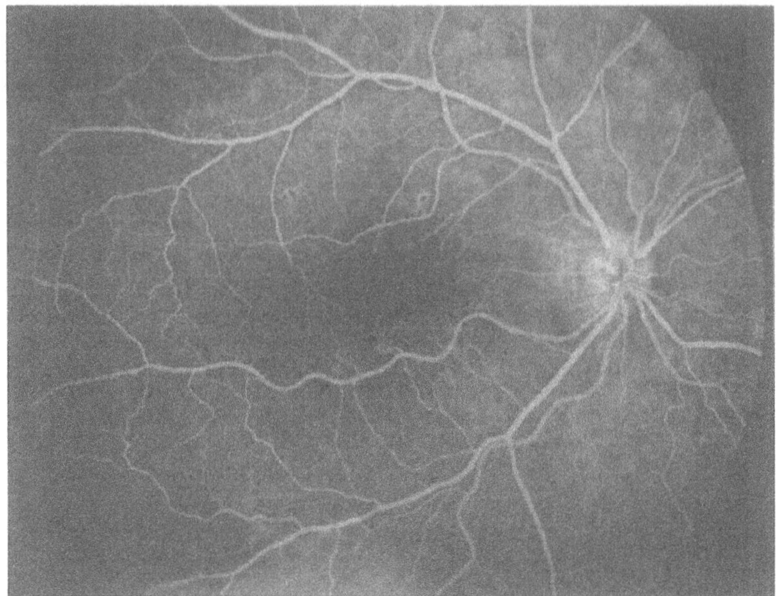

Fig. 7. Fluoroangiographic appearance 2 years after surgery.

except for the slight haemorrage of a perimacular capillary; however, a particularly strong retinovitreal adhesion may be responsible for such complications.The refinement of surgical instruments and surgical techniques has extended the indications of vitrectomy and has improved the prognosis in the macular disorders which cannot be treated by medical or physical therapy alone. The case reported has undoubtedly benefited from surgery thus solving the anatomical alterations and complete functional recovery.

References

1. Coats, G. Forms of retinal disease with massive exudation. Ophthal Hosp Rep. 1908; 17: 440–525.
2. Gass, J.D., Blodi, B.A. Idiopathic juxtafoveolar retinal telangiectasis. Update of classification and follow-up study. Ophthalmology. 1993; 100: 1536–1546.
3. Haut, J., Monin, C., Daghfous, F., Les maladies propres des vaisseaux retiniens. Encycl Med Chir (Paris France) Ophtalmologie. 21240 E20 p. 8.
4. Kubota, T., Kurihara, K., Ishibashi, T., Inomata, H. Proliferative vitreoretinopathy in Coats disease. Clinicohistopatological case report. Ophthalmologica. 1995; 209: 44–46.
5. Tripathi, R., Ashton, N. Electron microscopical study of Coats disease. Br J Ophthalmol. 1971; 55: 289–301.
6. Senft, S.H., Hidayat, A.A., Cavender, J.C. Atypical presentation of Coats disease. Retina. 1994; 14: 36–38.
7. Taillanter-Francoz, N., Bonnet, J., Baserer, J. Formes mineures du sindrome de Leber-Coats (Observations cliniques). Bull Soc Ophthalmol Fr. 1981; 81: 487–489.

8. Tarkkanen, A., Laatikainen, L. Coats' disease: clinical, angiographic, histopatological findings and clinical management. Br J Ophthalmol. 1983; 67: 766–776.

9. Berzas, C., Richard, G. Therapie der ablatio retinae bei morbus Coats. Fortschr Ophthalmol. 1991; 88: 598–602.

10. Han, D.P., Pulido, J.S., Mieler, W.F., Johnson, M.W. Vitrectomy for proliferative diabetic retinopathy with severe equatorial fibrovascular proliferation. Am J Ophthalmology. 1995; 119: 563–570.

11. Haut, J., Van Effenterre, G., Marre, J.M., Dureuil, J., Moulin, F., Traitement par photocoagulation au laser à l'argon de la maladie de Coats. Bull Soc Ophtalmol Fr. 1979; 79: 463–465.

12. Spitznas, M., Joussen, F., Wessing, A. Treatment of Coats' disease with photocoagulation. Graefes Arch Klin Exp Ophthalmol. 1976; 199: 31–37.

13. Schmidt, Erfurth, U., Lucke, K. Vitreoretinal surgery in advanced Coats disease. Ger J Ophthalmol. 1995; 4: 32–36.

City Hospital of Ivrea (Italy)
Department of Ophthalmology
Piazza Credenza, 2
10015-Ivrea (TO)
Italy

78. Automated perimetry variations found on epiretinal macular membranes

D. VILAPLANA, M. HORAS, R.P. CASAROLI and J. BARRAQUER

(Barcelona, Spain)

Introduction

Automated perimetry is a method which has largely proved its utility in the diagnosis and follow-up of certain ophthalmic pathologies[1-3], as well as its functional repercussions[4-6]. We carried out a randomized prospective study to assess the variations in the retinal sensitivity with automated perimetry in two groups of population affected by a macular epiretinal membrane. We performed a vitrectomy with a membrane peeling in one group, while we kept the other group under observation.

Materials, methods and patients

Twenty-nine eyes from 29 patients suffering from an epiretinal macular membrane were chosen. A vitrectomy with peeling was performed on 15 of them, selecting 14 for control.

For this study we chose those patients showing a degree I or II according to Gass classification, the visual acuity of whom was ≤0.4 for far vision (any crystalline sclerosis must be minor). Patients with corneal opacities, retinal vasculophaties such as diabetes, venous obstructions or vasculitis were excluded from the survey as these can alter visual field indexes. Other exclusion criteria were vitreous opacities and lack of cooperation in answers to automated perimetry.

We studied 14 variables (sex, age, refraction, time of evolution, etiology, cardiovascular history, lipoprotein abnormalities, smoking habits, severity of retinal distortion, vitreous changes, angiography, control date, visual field indexes and vitreous changes in the contralateral eye) to obtain two groups of population as homogeneous as possible.

We carried out a central visual field study prior to surgery in the group of operated patients, and one on the day of the first visit for patients of the control group; this was repeated 2 months later in the two groups.

Central visual field evaluation was performed using the macula program M1 of the Octopus 500 EZ perimeter which tests 37 points in the central 10° area and 22 peripheral points to a 24° eccentricity. Patients with percentages of false positive or false negative answers higher than 20%, short-term fluctua-

G. Coscas and F. Cardillo Piccolino (eds.), Retinal Pigment Epithelium and Macular Diseases, pp. 447–452.
© *1998 Kluwer Academic Publishers.*

tion higher than 2.2, or lack of cooperation judged by the perimetrist, were primarily excluded.

A vitrectomy to remove epiretinal membrane was performed by removing the central vitreous gel first for further withdrawing of peripheral vitreous. After completing as wide a vitrectomy as possible, we proceeded with the peeling of the macular membrane with the aid of a dissection instrument and a forceps. Whenever we found a retinal detachment in the inmediate post-operatory course, this was solved by means of cryocoagulation and SF6.

To analyse the statistical data, we used the system SPSS Windows 6.01. To evaluate the study homogeneity among the fourteen variables we employed the U Mann-Whitney, Chi-square and Kruskal-Wallis tests. To asses changes in visual acuity before and after the survey we used the Wilcoxon test, which was also used to study the visual field indexes at the beginning and at the end of the survey. We used the Mann-Whitney U test to analyse the variations in the visual indexes as well as the evolution of visual acuity, comparing it between operated and non-operated patients, as well as the evolution degree of the epiretinal membrane and its influence on these parameters.

Results

We studied 29 eyes from 29 patients: eight women and 21 men, aged 15–80 years old. Eighteen cases were idiopathic, two post-traumatic and nine post-retinal detachment surgery. We observed an improved mean sensitivity when comparing pre- and post-surgery values (mean 20.07 and 22.67 dB respectively; $p = 0.0131$). This improvement was also observed in the mean defect, with a pre-surgery mean of 8 and post-surgery mean of 5.4 ($p = 0.0084$). No significant change was observed in the loss of variance ($p = 0.9773$) and in the corrected loss of variance ($p = 0.8888$) after surgery.

We noticed significant improvements after 2 months in the control group, both in the mean sensitivity (23.71 and 25.00, respectively; $p = 0.0099$), and in the mean defect (3.79 and 2.57, respectively $p = 0.0068$).

No significant differences were observed when comparing the improvements in visual field indexes in the operated group and the control group. The mean improvement in mean sensitivity in the operated group was 2.60, while in the control group it was 1.29 ($p = 0.2777$). The same happened with the mean defect, where there was an improvement of 2.60 in the operated group compared with 1.21 ($p = 0.2600$) in the-non operated group. The mean of the differences in the loss of variance of the operated group was 0.47, while in the non-operated group it was 2.86 ($p = 0.3922$). The mean of the corrected loss of variances was 0.20 in the operated group and 1.93 ($p = 0.5672$) in the non-operated group.

When comparing visual field indexes with the global population studied (operated and control groups), there were significant differences between groups. Table 1 shows a mean sensitivity of 23.29 in grade I, and 20.47 in

Table 1. Mean sensitivity.

Decibels	Grade I	Grade II
16	–	1
17	–	1
18	–	3
19	1	2
20	1	1
21	–	–
22	3	3
23	3	1
24	2	2
25	1	1
26	2	–
27	1	–
Total	14	15
Mean	23.29	20.27
SD	2.27	2.85

Wilcoxon $p = 0.0121$

The mean sensitivity in decibels is better in grade I than in grade II according to Gass classification.

Table 2. Mean defect.

Decibels	Grade I	Grade II
1	1	–
2	1	–
3	4	2
4	2	2
5	3	1
6	–	2
7	2	–
8	1	2
9	–	1
10	–	1
11	–	3
12	–	–
13	–	–
14	–	1
Total	14	15
Mean	4.29	7.53
SD	2.02	3.42

Wilcoxon $p = 0.0088$

The mean defect in decibels is lower in grade I than in grade II according to Gass classification.

grade II ($p = 0.0121$). Table 2 shows a mean defect of 4.29 for grade I, and 7.53 for grade II ($p = 0.0088$), while Table 3 shows a mean loss of variance in grade I of 8.5, while for grade II it is 19.80 ($p = 0.0117$). Table 4 shows that variations in corrected loss of variance are 5.21 for grade I and 16.53 for grade II ($p = 0.0052$). There was no significant correlation between visual field indexes and a greater or lower visual acuity.

Discussion

Since Machemer[7] in 1978 first described the peeling of epiretinal membranes, many authors[8–12] have treated this pathology.

Despite post-surgery vision improvements, which we have been able to verify in our group of population, we had no knowledge of any work evaluating the alterations in retinal sensitivity caused by this pathology with the aid of automated perimetry, and which could justify the fact that anatomical results which were surprisingly good were accompanied by bad functional results.

Table 3. Loss of variance.

Decibels	Grade I	Grade II
3	1	–
4	1	–
5	3	1
6	1	1
7	4	1
8	–	1
9	–	1
10	1	–
11	–	1
13	3	2
14	–	1
15	–	1
17	1	1
20	–	1
23	1	–
27	–	1
55	–	1
77	–	1
Total	14	15
Mean	8.50	19.80
SD	5.60	20.05

Wilcoxon $p = 0.0117$

The loss of variance in decibels is lower in grade I than in grade II according to Gass classification.

Table 4. Corrected loss of variance.

Decibels	Grade I		Grade II
2	2	1	
3	3	–	
4	5	1	
6	1	3	
7	1	2	
9	–	2	
10	1	–	
11	–	1	
12	–	1	
17	1	1	
25	–	1	
52	–	1	
75	–	1	
Total	14		15
Mean	5.21		16.53
SD	4.00		20.35
Wilcoxon $p = 0.0052$			

The corrected loss variance in decibels is lower in grade I than in grade II according to Gass classification.

We observed that greater degrees of the macular disease, were associated with a greater deterioration of retinal sensitivity, as we noticed when comparing the mean sensitivity and the mean defect in grade I or in grade II. The relative scotomas generated by such pathology are localized and deeper as the epiretinal membrane evolved. We evaluated this fact through a significant increase observed in the values of the loss of variance and the corrected loss of variance, and that these persist even after surgery.

An important finding has been that the increased sensitivity appearing 2 months after surgery is not really such an increase, but is due to some learning effects, if compared to that of the control group. This leads us to think that the alterations produced are, to a certain extent irreversible, or show a very slow recovery.

Automated perimetry was useful in revealing the alterations produced in the retinal sensitivity, but these do not correlate with any higher or lower post-surgery degree of vision.

This method shows that the retinal damage is not exclusively constrained to the macular region but affects the whole area of the posterior segment.

Conclusions

The more the macula is damaged, the more the retinal sensitivity becomes altered. Alterations in retinal sensitivity produced by epiretinal membranes are either irreversible or they show a very slow recovery. Post-surgery improvement in visual field indexes in this pathology is due to learning effects. Automated perimetry contributes to document functional alterations in these patients.

References

1. Flammer, J., Drance, S.M., Zulauf, M. Differential light threshold. Short- and long-term fluctuation in patients with glaucoma, normal controls, and patients with suspected glaucoma. Arch Ophthalmol. 1984; 102: 704–706.
2. Flammer, J. The concept of visual field indices. Graefe's Arch Clin Exp Ophthalmol. 1986; 224: 389–392.
3. Gramer, E., Althaus, G., Leydhecker, W. Localization and depth of glaucomatous visual field defects in relation to the size of the neuroretinal rim area of the disc in low-lesion glaucoma, glaucoma simplex and pigmentary glaucoma; clinical study with the Octopus 201 perimeter and the optic nerve head analyzer. Klin Mbl Augenheilk. 1986; 189: 190–199.
4. Vilaplana, D., Barraquer, J., Massana, J., Lucas, R., Moreno, V. Temporal branch vein occlusion: laser photocoagulation and its visual field effects. Lasers Light Ophthalmol. 1992; 4: 201–207.
5. Duch Mestres, F., Vilaplana, D., Rutllan Civit, J., Torres, F., Barraquer, J. Static perimetry evaluation of argon green and dye red laser treatment for choroidal neovascular membranes. Lasers Light Ophthalmol. 1993; 6: 27–32.
6. Vilaplana, D., Moreno, V., Barraquer, J. Temporal branch vein occlusion: diode laser photocoagulation. Lasers Light Ophthalmol. 1995; 7: 37–43.
7. Machemer, R. Die chirurgische entferhung von epiretinalen makula membranen. Klin Monatsbl Augenheilkd. 1978; 173: 36–42.
8. Michels, R.G. Vitrectomy for macular pucker. Ophthalmology. 1984; 91: 1384–1388.
9. von Gunten, S., Pournaras, C.J., de Gottrau, Ph., Brazitikos, P. Facteurs prognostiques du traitement chirurgical des membranes épirétiniennes. Klin Monatsbl Augenheilikd. 1994; 204: 309–312.
10. Rice, T.A., De Bustros, S., Michels, R.G., Thompson, J.T., Debanne, S.M., Rowland, D.Y. Prognostic factors in vitrectomy for epiretinal membranes of the macula. Ophthalmology. 1986; 93: 602–610.
11. Grewing, R., Mester, U. Results of surgery for epiretinal membranes and their recurrences. Br J Ophthalmol. 1996; 80: 323–326.
12. Bryselbout, E., Turut, P. Les membranes épirétiniennes idiopathiques et secondaires. J Fr Ophtalmol. 1991; 14: 265–285.

Laforja 88
08021 Barcelona
Spain

79. Relaxing retinotomies: visual results and macular findings

Ch. KOUTSANDREA, M. APOSTOLOPOULOS, D. CHATJOULIS,
E. PARIKAKIS and G.P. THEODOSSIADIS

(Athens, Greece)

Background

Relaxing retinotomies are sometimes necessary in the treatment of complicated cases of retinal detachment. Our purpose was to study the poor visual outcome in eyes treated with vitrectomy and relaxing retinotomy, in association with the postoperative macular findings.

Materials and methods

Thirty-seven successfully treated eyes from a series of 54 cases, treated with vitrectomy and relaxing retinotomy for severe proliferative vitreoretinopathy (PRV), were evaluated retrospectively. Twenty-one of the 37 eyes (56.7%) suffered from retinal detachment with advanced PVR, 14 of the 37 eyes (37.8%) from retinal detachment due to trauma, while the remaining two patients (5.4%) had tractional retinal detachment due to proliferative diabetic retinopathy.

In this study we defined as relaxing retinotomy the circumferentially extended retinotomy equal to or more than 90°. Cases with postoperative band keratopathy or macular detachment were excluded from the study. In all our cases we performed lensectomy, when the eye was phakic, vitrectomy, complete membrane removal, flattening of the retina with perfluorocarbon (PFCL), and direct PFCL/silicone oil exchange.

The preoperative and postoperative examination included measurement of the visual acuity, biomicroscopic and indirect ophthalmoscopy, colour photographs and fluorescein angiography. The 37 cases were divided into three groups according to the retinotomy size: Group A (90–179° 17/37 eyes), Group B (180–269°, 11/37 eyes), Group C (270–360°, 9/37 eyes). The statistical analysis was made by the χ^2 test for linear trends. The follow-up period ranged from 18 to 54 months.

Results

The visual results of our cases were rather poor. Visual acuity of 5/200 or better was obtained in 11 (29.7%) cases, counting fingers in 15 (40.5%) and

G. Coscas and F. Cardillo Piccolino (eds.), Retinal Pigment Epithelium and Macular Diseases, pp. 453–454.
© *1998 Kluwer Academic Publishers.*

hand movements to light perception in 11 (29.7%) of the cases. The most common macular lesions were retinal pigmentary abnormalities in 67.5% of the eyes (25/37) and macular eterotopia in 43.2% of the eyes (16/37). In five eyes (13.5%) macular pucker was observed, two eyes had a scar at the macular area (5.4%) and one a macular hole (2.7%). The correlation between the retinotomy size and the functional results, as well as between the macular findings and the functional results was not statistically significant. No statistically significant difference was also found between the retinotomy size and the macular findings, although there was a trend for macular eterotopia in eyes of group C (the group of large retinotomy size).

Conclusions

The functional results in the cases studied were rather poor. Visual acuity of $\geq 5/200$ was found in 29.7% of the cases. The poor visual outcome could be attributed to macular lesions observed postoperatively, such as retinal pigmentary abnormalities and macular eterotopia. Macular pucker, scar formation and macular hole were also found. There was no statistically significant difference between functional results and retinotomy size, between functional results and macular findings, and between macular findings and relaxing retinotomy size (although eterotopia was found in a greater percentage in the large retinotomy size group).

Athens University
Department of Ophthalmology
Greece

Author Index

G. Coscas and F. Cardillo Piccolino (eds.), Retinal Pigment Epithelium and Macular Diseases, pp. 455–457.
© 1998 Kluwer Academic Publishers.

Documenta Ophthalmologica Proceedings Series

1. J. François (eds.): *Symposium on Light-Coagulation*. Argon Laser and Xenon Arc (Ghent, Belgium, 1972). 1973   ISBN 90-6193-141-X

2. J.T. Pearlman (ed.): *10th ISCERG Symposium* (Los Angeles, Calif., USA, 1972). 1973   ISBN 90-6193-142-8

3. H.E. Henkes (ed.): *Photography, Electro-Ophthalmology and Echo-Ophthalmology in Ophthalmic Practice*. 1973   ISBN 90-6193-143-6

4. E. Dodt & J.T. Pearlman (eds.): *11th ISCERG Symposium* (Bad Nauheim, Germany, 1973). 1974   ISBN 90-6193-144-4

5. W.J. Holmes (ed.): *Public Health Ophthalmology*. Papers Presented at the Conference on the Prevention of Impaired Vision and Blindness (Paris, France, 1974). 1975   ISBN 90-6193-145-2

6. A. Th. M. van Balen (ed.): *First International Symposium on Artificial Lensimplantation* (Utrecht, The Netherlands, 1974). 1975   ISBN 90-6193-146-0

7. A.F. Deutman (ed.): [Symposium on] *New Developments in Ophthalmology*. (Nijmegen, The Netherlands, 1975) 1976   ISBN 90-6193-147-9

8. O. Hockwin (ed.): *Progress of Lens Biochemistry Research*. In Honour of Prof. Dr. med. J. Nordmann. 1976   ISBN 90-6193-148-7

9. J.J. de Laey (ed.): *International Symposium on Fluorescein Angiography* (Ghent, Belgium, 1976). 1976   ISBN 90-6193-149-5

10. R. Alfieri & P. Solé (eds.): *12th ISCERG Symposium* (Clermont-Ferrand, France, 1974). 1976   ISBN 90-6193-150-9

11. E. Auerbach (ed.): *Experimental and Clinical Amblyopia. 13th ISCERG Symposium* (Kibbutz Ginossar, Israel, 1975). 1977   ISBN 90-6193-151-7

12. E.L. Greve (ed.): *Symposium on Medical Therapy in Glaucoma* (Amsterdam, The Netherlands, 1976) 1977   ISBN 90-6193-152-5

13. T. Lawwill (ed.): *ERG, VER and Psychophysics. 14th ISCERG Symposium* (Louisville, USA, 1976). 1977   ISBN 90-6193-153-3

14. E.L. Greve (ed.): *2nd International Visual Field Symposium* (Tübingen, Germany, 1976). 1977   ISBN 90-6391-154-1

15. J. François & A. De Rouck (eds.), J.T. Pearlman and J. Kelsey (co-eds.): *Electrodiagnosis, Toxic Agents and Vision. 15th ISCEV Symposium* (Ghent, Belgium, 1977). 1978   ISBN 90-6193-155-X

16. H.-J Merté (ed.): *Genesis of Glaucoma*. Contributions of the Wessely Symposium in Munich (October 1974) with final Considerations by H. Goldmann. 1978   ISBN 90-6193-156-8

17. A.F. Deutmann & J.R.M. Cruysberg (eds.): *5th International Congress on Neurogenetics and Neuro-Ophthalmology* (Nijmegen, The Netherlands, 1977). 1978   ISBN 90-6193-159-2

18. O. Hockwin & W.B. Rathbun (eds.): *Progress in Anterior Eye Segment. Research and Practice*. In Honour of Prof. J.E. Harris. 1979   ISBN 90-6193-158-4

19. E.L. Greve (ed.): *3rd International Visual Field Symposium* (Tokyo, Japan, 1978). 1979   ISBN 90-6193-160-6

Documenta Ophthalmologica Proceedings Series

20. J. François, S.I. Brown & M. Itoi (eds.): *Proceedings of the Symposium of the International Society for Corneal Research* (Kyoto, Japan, 1978). 1979
ISBN 90-6193-157-6

21. J. François, E. Maumenee & I. Esente (eds.): *First International Congress on Cataract Surgery* (Florence, Italy, 1978). 1979　　ISBN 90-6193-162-2

22. E.L. Greve (ed.): *Glaucoma Symposium.* Diagnosis and Therapy (Amsterdam, The Netherlands, 1979). 1980　　ISBN 90-6193-164-9

23. E. Schmöger & J.H. Kelsey (eds.): *Visual Electrodiagnosis in Systemic Diseases.* Proceedings of the 17th ISCEV Symposium (Erfurt, GDR, 1979) 1980
ISBN 90-6193-163-0

24. A. Hamburg (ed.): *Symposium on Uveal Melanomas.* On the Occasion of the Snellen Medal Presentation to Dr W.A. Manschot (Utrecht, The Netherlands, 1979). 1980
ISBN 90-6193-722-1

25. H. Zauberman (ed.): *Proceedings of the Conference on Subretinal Space* (Jerusalem, Israel, 1979). 1981　　ISBN 90-6193-721-3

26. E.L. Greve & G. Verriest (eds.): *4th International Visual Field Symposium* (Bristol, UK, 1980). 1981　　ISBN 90-6193-165-7

27. H. Spekreijse & P.A. Apkarian: *Visual Pathways: Electrophysiology and Pathology.* 18th ISCEV Symposium (Amsterdam, The Netherlands, 1980). 1981
ISBN 90-6193-723-X

28. H.C. Fledelius, P.H. Alsbirk & E. Goldschmidt (eds.): *3rd International Conference on Myopia* (Copenhagen, Denmark, 1980). 1981　　ISBN 90-6193-725-6

29. J.M. Thijssen & A.M. Verbeek (eds.): *Ultrasonography in Ophthalmology.* Proceedings of the 8th SIDUO Congress (Nijmegen, The Netherlands). 1981 ISBN 90-6193-724-8

30. L. Maffei (ed.): *Pathophysiology of the Visual System.* Proceedings of a Workshop (Pisa, Italy 1980). 1981　　ISBN 90-6193-726-4

31. G. Niemeyer & Ch. Huber (eds.): *Techniques in Clinical Electrophysiology of Vision.* 19th ISCEV Symposium (Horgen-Zürich, Switzerland, 1981). 1982
ISBN 90-6193-727-7

32. A.Th.M. van Balen & W.A. Houtman (eds.): *Strabismus Symposium* (Amsterdam, The Netherlands, 1981). 1982　　ISBN 90-6193-728-0

33. G. Verriest (ed.): *Colour Vision Deficiencies VI.* Proceedings of the 6th Symposium of the International Research Group on Colour Vision Deficiencies (Berlin- Steglitz, Germany, 1981). 1982　　ISBN 90-6193-729-9

34. A. Roucoux & M. Crommelinck (eds.): *Physiological and Pathological Aspects of Eye Movements.* Proceedings of a Workshop (Pont d'Oye Castle, Habay- la-Neuve, Belgium, 1982). 1982　　ISBN 90-6193-730-2

35. E.L. Greve & A. Heijl (eds.): *5th International Visual Field Symposium* (Sacramento, Calif., USA, 1982). 1983　　ISBN 90-6193-731-0

36. R. Birngruber & V.-P. Gabel (eds.): *Laser Treatment and Photocoagulation of the Eye.* Proceedings of an International Symposium (Munich, Germany, 1982). 1984
ISBN 90-6193-732-9

Documenta Ophthalmologica Proceedings Series

37. H.E.J.W. Kolder (ed.): *Slow Potentials and Microprocessor Applications.* 20th ISCEV Symposium (Iowa City, USA, 1982). 1983 ISBN 90-6193-733-7
38. J.S. Hillman & M.M. Le May (eds.): *Ophthalmic Ultrasonography.* Proceedings of the 9th SIDUO Congress (Leeds, UK, 1982). 1984 ISBN 90-6193-734-5
39. G. Verriest (ed.): *Colour Vision Deficiencies VII.* Proceedings of the 7th Symposium of the International Research Group on Colour Vision Deficiencies (Geneva, Switzerland, 1983). 1984 ISBN 90-6193-735-3
40. J.R. Heckenlively (ed.), G.H.M. van Lith & T.Lawwill (ass. eds): *Pattern Electroretinogram, Circulatory Disturbances of the Visual System and Pattern-Evoked Responses.* 21st ISCEV Symposium (Budapest, Hungary, 1983). 1984

ISBN 90-6193-503-2
41. E.C. Campos (ed.): *Sensory Evaluation of Strabismus and Amblyopia in a Natural Environment.* In Honour of Prof. Bruno Bagolini. 1984 ISBN 90-6193-508-3
42. A. Heijl & E.L. Greve (eds.): *6th International Visual Field Symposium* (Santa Margherita Ligure, Italy, 1984). 1985 ISBN 90-6193-524-5
43. E.L. Greve, W. Leydhecker & C. Raitta (eds.): *2nd European Glaucoma Symposium* (Hyvinkää, Finland, 1984). 1985 ISBN 90-6193-526-1
44. P.C. Maudgal & L. Missotten (eds.): *Herpetic Eye Diseases.* Proceedings of an International Symposium (Leuven, Belgium, 1984). 1985 ISBN 90-6193-527-X
45. B. Jay (ed.): *Detection and Measurement of Visual Impairment in Pre-Verbal Children.* Proceedings of a Workshop (London, UK, 1985). 1986 ISBN 0-89838-789-2
46. G. Verriest (ed.): *Colour Vision Deficiencies VIII.* Proceedings of the 8th Symposium of the International Research Group on Colour Vision Deficiencies (Avignon, France, 1985). 1987 ISBN 0-89838-801-5
47. P.L. Emiliani (ed.): *Development of Electronic Aids for the Visually Impaired.* Proceedings of a Workshop on the Rehabilitation of the Visually Impaired (Florence, Italy, 1984). 1986 ISBN 0-89838-805-8
48. K.C. Ossoinig (ed.): *Ophthalmic Echography.* Proceedings of the 10th SIDUO Congress (St. Petersburg Beach, Florida, USA, 1984). 1987 ISBN 0-89838-873-2
49. E.L. Greve & A. Heijl (eds.): *7th International Visual Field Symposium* (Amsterdam, The Netherlands, 1986). 1987 ISBN 0-89838-882-1
50. D. BenEzra, S.J. Ryan, B.M. Glaser & R.P. Murphy (eds.): *Ocular Circulation and Neovascularization.* Proceedings of the First International Symposium (Jeruzalem, Israel, 1986). 1987 ISBN 0-89838-892-9
51. J.M. Thijssen, J.S. Hillman, P.E. Gallenga & G. Cennamo (eds.): *Ultrasonography in Ophthalmology 11.* Proceedings of the 11th SIDUO Congress (Capri, Italy, 1986). 1988 ISBN 0-89838-378-1
52. B. Drum & G. Verriest (eds.): *Colour Vision Deficiencies IX.* Proceedings of the 9th Symposium of the International Research Group on Colour Vision Deficiencies (Annapolis, Md., USA, 1987). 1989 ISBN 0-89838-403-6
53. R. Sampaolesi (ed.): *Ultrasonography in Ophthalmology 12.* Proceedings of the 12th SIDUO Congress (Iguazú Falls, Argentina, 1988). 1990 ISBN 0-7923-0765-8

GPSR Compliance
The European Union's (EU) General Product Safety Regulation (GPSR) is a set
of rules that requires consumer products to be safe and our obligations to
ensure this.

If you have any concerns about our products, you can contact us on

ProductSafety@springernature.com

In case Publisher is established outside the EU, the EU authorized
representative is:

Springer Nature Customer Service Center GmbH
Europaplatz 3
69115 Heidelberg, Germany